DIETARY FATS, PROSTANOIDS AND ARTERIAL THROMBOSIS

DEVELOPMENTS IN HEMATOLOGY AND IMMUNOLOGY

VOLUME 4

1. Lijnen HR, Collen D and Verstraete M, eds: Synthetic Substrates in Clinical Blood Coagulation Assays. 1980. ISBN 90-247-2409-0
2. Smit Sibinga C.Th., Das PC Forfar JO, eds: Paediatrics and Blood Transfusion. 1982. ISBN 90-247-2619-0
3. Fabris N: Immunology and Ageing. 1982. ISBN 90-247-2640-9

series ISBN 90-247-2432-5

DIETARY FATS, PROSTANOIDS AND ARTERIAL THROMBOSIS

GERARD HORNSTRA, M.D.
University of Limburg
Department of Biochemistry
P.O. Box 616
6200 MD Maastricht
The Netherlands

with an introductory chapter by
A. BLEAKLEY CHANDLER, M.D.
Department of Pathology
Medical College of Georgia
Augusta, GA 30912
USA

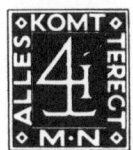

1982
MARTINUS NIJHOFF PUBLISHERS
THE HAGUE / BOSTON / LONDON

Distributors:

for the United States and Canada

Kluwer Boston, Inc.
190 Old Derby Street
Hingham, MA 02043
USA

for all other countries

Kluwer Academic Publishers Group
Distribution Center
P.O. Box 322
3300 AH Dordrecht
The Netherlands

Library of Congress Cataloging in Publication Data   CIP

Hornstra, Gerard.
   Dietary fats, prostanoids and arterial
thrombosis.

   (Developments in hematology and immunology ;
v. 4)
   Bibliography: p.
   1. Thrombosis--Nutritional aspects. 2. Pro-
staglandins--Physiological effect. 3. Thromboxanes
--Physiological effect. 4. Acids, Fatty--Metabolism,
I. Title. II. Series. [DNLM: 1. Dietary fats--
Metabolism. 2. Dietary fats--Adverse effects.
3. Fatty acids--Metabolism. 4. Thrombosis--
Etiology. W1 DE997VZK v. 4 / WG 540 H816d]
RC694.3.H67   616.1'35   82-6396

ISBN-13:978-94-009-7578-1   AACR2

ISBN-13:978-94-009-7578-1   e-ISBN-13:978-94-009-7576-7
DOI: 10.1007/978-94-009-7576-7

CONTENTS

PREFACE

Knowledge of mechanisms involved in the pathogenesis of occlusive arterial diseases is fundamental for the design of prevention and treatment. A series of studies based on in vitro investigations, the experimental animal and the human being have slowly increased our understanding of cardiovascular diseases and unveiled their secrets to us. Over the last 60 years it has been generally assumed that dietary fats and lipids and the occurrence of atherosclerosis are closely related. Yet, even if epidemiological studies clearly indicate the existence of an association between the amount of composition of dietary lipids and morbidity and mortality of cardiovascular disease, our basic knowledge on cause and effect is still hidden in a cloud of uncertainty.

The present book discusses the relation between dietary lipids and arterial thrombosis, which latter process has been observed in the coronary arteries in up to 90% of subjects with acute myocardial infaction. In this volume Dr. Hornstra, who has occupied himself with thrombosis research with never-failing enthusiasm, great skill and critical approach for the last fifteen years, tries to establish possible links between lipid metabolism and thrombosis. His literature studies are comprehensive and his investigations are impressive in that they give a new dimension and a new methodology to research of lipids and thrombosis.

His presentation is fascinating and answers some questions, raises many more and ranges from brilliant analysis to provocative statement. His approach to the subject will make this book a source of inspiration to the scientist, the clinician and the epidemiologist.

ARNE NORDØY
Professor Dr. Med.
University of Tromsö
Institute of Clinical Medicine
Tromsö
Norway

ACKNOWLEDGEMENTS

This book could only be written owing to the indispensable cooperation of a great many collegues. Some of them were of essential value in this respect: Edward Haddeman and Jan Don who, over the years, have performed a great deal of the experiments described, and Cor Gardien who was involved in most of the artwork. Mary Peters and Mariet Molenaar typed, and re-typed, the manuscript; I am very grateful to them for their constant help. The valuable contribution of Puck Muller in many of the coagulation studies is also greatly acknowledged.

I also want to thank many colleagues who sent me reprints of their most recent work. They enabled me to discuss te various aspects of arterial thrombosis in relation to the latest findings and in doing so they contributed significantly to the topicality of this volume. I sincerely hope that they – and others – will let me know their criticism and keep me informed about their progress in future research.

It is true that the energy and time invested in this book might also have been spent in quite a different way. For this reason I would like to thank my family and friends for their respecting my choice.

Maastricht, March 1982   Gerard Hornstra

1. ARTERIAL THROMBOSIS, PLATELETS AND ATHEROGENESIS

As much as arterial thrombosis is recognized as a major factor in cardiovascular disease, its true contribution to arterial disease and ischemia is often masked. In this chapter, the pathology of arterial thrombosis and the interrelatonships of the thrombotic process and atherogenesis will be considered. Thrombotic ischemia may result either from acute obstruction of arteries by thromboemboli and rapidly forming mural thrombi or from a long-term effect whereby thrombi contribute to the growth and progression of atherosclerotic lesions.

The incorporation of thrombi into atherosclerotic plaques is a clear-cut mechanism of plague growth that has not been given substantial recognition as a factor in atherogenesis, in part because of the paradoxical nature of the process that causes thrombi to lose their identity as they are transformed to plaques. The frequency and, consequently, the morbidity and mortality of arterial thrombosis, has not been subject to accurate assessment for the very reason that thrombi intimately contribute to plaque formation and the progression of atherosclerosis.

The major subject of this volume deals with the relation between dietary fats and arterial thrombosis. Dietary and plasma lipids may affect thromboatherogenesis by altering the thrombogenic properties of blood as well as by contributing to the fat content of thrombi. Thrombosis may be looked upon as a reparative process when thrombi seal injured sites on a vessel wall. Platelets form part of the thrombus that initially covers intimal defects. They may also have a more permanent effect on vascular repair. In vitro experiments have recently demonstrated that a hormonal growth factor contained in the platelet stimulates smooth muscle and other connective tissue cells to replicate. As with many reparative processes, the endresult of vascular repair may incur a net pathologic deficit. For example, mural thrombi that are organized by smooth muscle cells may be converted into sclerotic intimal plaques. The relative importance, however, of the platelet-derived growth factor in the proliferative phase of atherogenesis remains to be determined.

* By A. Bleakley Chandler, M.D.

1.1. PATHOLOGY OF ARTERIAL THROMBOSIS

The formation of thrombi in arteries can usually be related to their development on localized lesions of the arterial wall, notably atherosclerotic lesions. Haemodynamic factors and thrombogenic properties of blood may modify the reaction, but an underlying lesion of the arterial wall seems essential. Obstructive thrombi may produce ischemia in any arterial bed that lacks sufficient collateral circulation. The ischemic consequences of thrombi and thromboemboli in the coronary circulation illustrate many general features of thrombotic ischemia, while exhibiting some effects peculiar to the heart. In this organ, thrombotic ischemia, in effect, may generate additional thrombi over myocardial infarcts and, at times, may precipitate lethal cardiac arrhythmias. The potential significance of microembolic phenomena in producing transient ischemic injury in the heart, as is known to occur in the cerebral and retinal circulation, is the subject of much interest and investigation.

1.1.1. *Pathogenesis of arterial thrombosis*

Thrombi form in arteries from flowing blood. Repeated observations in the experimental animal, and more recently in man [91], have shown that platelets quickly separate from the axial stream of the flowing blood and accumulate at a site of vascular injury to build a thrombic mass. The platelets first adhere to the injured vessel and then cohere to each other to form aggregates. Even though the platelet and vascular wall are sources of thromboplastin, the initial response of platelets is independent of fibrin coagulation. Fibrin appears subsequent to platelet adhesion and aggregation to stabilize the thrombus. In Chapter three, a detailed analysis of basic mechanisms and regulators of thrombogenesis involving platelets, the vessel wall and the coagulation system is presented.

In arteries, mixed thrombi usually develop in situ over an underlying intimal lesion. The basic structure of mixed thrombi, which are composed of platelet-fibrin units bordered by leucocytes and variable numbers of entrapped red blood cells, is similar at any site of formation. In general, the site of formation and local conditions of blood flow influence structure. Thrombi that form in fast-moving pulsatile arterial blood are apt to contain more platelets and fewer entrapped red cells and to be more compact than thrombi that have formed in slower currents of veins [129].

By far the most frequent arterial lesions associated with thrombi are those of atherosclerotic origin. Benson in 1926 [43] noted that coronary thrombi customarily develop in narrowed and sclerotic arteries in which the luminal or plaque surface is physically disrupted. Disruption of the plaque surface, variously described as intimal tears or ulcerations, plaque fissures, or plaque ruptures, is associated with a significant number of arterial thrombi [43, 136, 142, 153, 320, 484, 724]. Despite the early awareness of ulcerative plaques, little is still known of their pathogenesis. Intramural or plaque haemorrhage, a suction Venturi effect through an area of stenosis, and failure of endothelium to regenerate have been cited as factors in the genesis and perpetuation of these lesions [133]. Whatever the cause, rupture or ulceration of an atherosclerotic plaque clearly exposes to the lumen thrombogenic elements within the arterial wall. Exposed connective tissue fibers promote platelet adhesion and aggregation, while both collagen and tissue thromboplastin activate the coagulation system to generate thrombin.

In reviewing these aspects of the pathogenesis of arterial thrombosis, it should be recognized that the association between plaque rupture and thrombosis, although impressive, is not universal. Arterial thrombi may develop over minor intimal breaks of largely fibrous plaques in the absence of underlying haemorrhage or rupture of a necrotic atheroma [247, 384, 439]. Hemodynamic factors, too, may interact with acute arterial injury to promote thrombosis. The separation of platelets from blood and their deposition at sites of injury is enhanced in zones of slowed or turbulent flow, and the removal of thrombogenic substances generated in the blood or released from an injured vessel wall may be retarded. The shearing effect of flow and the associated turbulence around stenoses may lead to endothelial injury as well as augment contact of the cellular elements of the blood with the arterial wall [589]. Thus, while a single precipitating event in a vessel wall may initiate thrombosis, the extent of the reaction may depend upon hemodynamic factors and the thrombogenic potential of blood. It should be emphasized that thrombi are not static structures. They are constantly changing by resolution, by organization or by further growth.

Once formed, a mural thrombus may provide a nidus for its own subsequent growth. Many thrombi have layers of differing age, which suggests that they were formed episodically over a period of time. Though recurrent thrombosis is commonly observed [142, 163, 724], the mechanisms governing this form of growth remain unexplained. It has been proposed that the older thrombus may absorb and accumulate on its surface thrombogenic substances form the blood until a critical level initiates another episode of thrombosis [129].

1.1.2. *Thrombotic ischemia in arterial disease*

The pathologic effects of thrombi are related to obstruction of blood flow, ischemia and, at times, to further alteration of the arterial wall by repair of the thrombotic-vascular lesion. Thrombi that form on atherosclerotic plaques may lead to acute obstruction of the lumen and consequent ischemia. Once formed, a mural thrombus often persists to become incorporated into the arterial wall, thereby contributing to the growth of the plaque and perpetuation of the ischemia. Not all thrombi produce obvious acute ischemia, especially small non-occlusive mural thrombi, which nevertheless may in time contribute to stenosis of the lumen and progression of ischemia by becoming part of the arterial wall.

In situ thrombi may form rapidly or they may build up slowly to obstruct an artery, often in episodes, whereas obstruction is usually sudden and complete in the case of embolic phenomena. Thrombosis and thromboembolism of the coronary circulation are emphasized below as important examples of thrombotic ischemia.

1.1.3. *Thrombosis in the coronary circulation*

The frequency and role of occlusive coronary thrombi in myocardial infarction have been the subject of sporadic and vigorous debate. A number of investigators have reported a relatively low frequency of occlusive thrombi and some have concluded that the thrombi are younger than the associated infarcts [134]. As a result, it has been argued that coronary arterial thrombosis is a consequence rather than a cause of acute infarction. One step toward clarification of this issue has been the recognition that only one form of acute myocardial infarction is usually associated with coronary thrombosis. Thrombotic occlusion is frequently found in regional transmural infarction, but is infrequent in subendocardial infarction [134, 171, 261, 557].

The pathologists who hold that coronary thrombi caue infarcts point out that the thrombi are consistently located at a proximal position in the artery supplying the infarcted myocardium and that the thrombi, in most cases, are found to arise at specific sites of rupture or ulceration of atherosclerotic plaques [134, 171, 344, 694]. The striking and consistent spatial relationships between occlusive thrombi and myocardial infarcts in conjunction with the high frequency of thrombi in transmural infarction provide strong evidence that prior thrombosis is critical to the development of transmural myocardial infarcts.

A recent clinical study utilizing coronary angiography has shown that occlusive coronary thrombosis is frequently present within four hours after the onset of the manifestations of transmural myocardial infarction [187]. Other clinical studies have shown the effects of therapeutic removal of occlusive thrombi. The lysis of coronary thrombi in acute infarction by administration of streptokinase under selective coronary angiography, followed by improvement in cardiac status, has lent additional weight to the concept that thrombi cause infarcts [690].

Further evidence of the causal role of coronary thrombosis in myocardial infarction has been obtained by means of tagging fibrinogen with radioisotopes. The incorporation of ^{125}I-fibrinogen into coronary arterial thrombi after the onset of typical ischemic chest pain and electrocardiographic changes of recent anteroseptal infarction was first interpreted by Erhardt and coworkers [231] as evidence that thrombosis occurs after infarction. However, after additional studies their views were modified to suggest that part of the occlusive thrombus may form by propagation after the onset of necrosis [232]. At about the same time, Fulton [274, 275] showed by means of more detailed correlative morphologic appraisals that the central occlusive portion of a thrombus subtending an infarct is characteristically radionegative, which would indicate formation of the thrombus before administration of radiofibrinogen and antecedent to infarction.

The infrequent association of coronary thrombosis with subendocardial multifocal infarcts raises several questions. In some instances, small thrombi responsible for correspondingly small infarcts may escape detection. As Friedberg and Horn

[261] and more recently Ridolfi and Hutchings [694] suggested, many of these patchy subendocardial lesions may result from anomalies of perfusion from causes other than acute thrombosis. Lastly, one should take into account the possibility that some small necrotic foci may result from causes other than ischemia and therefore should be excluded from the category of infarcts.

Not all occlusive coronary thrombi, of course, are associated with myocardial infarction. If the collateral circulation is adequate, an infarct may not develop following an acute thrombotic occlusion [74, 724]. At times, acute thrombi are present in patients who die suddenly *before* an infarct has had time to develop. This phenomenon may occur in coronary embolism [848] or in cases of severe coronary atherosclerosis with acute coronary thrombosis. The immediate fatal event in these cases is probably a cardiac arrhythmia [698]. It should be emphasized that coronary thrombosis is by no means found in all cases of sudden cardiac death occurring in the presence of advanced coronary sclerosis [734]. Coronary thrombosis occurs in about one-third of the cases in patients dying within 10 min to 2 h of the onset of the fatal illness and in even fewer cases in those patients who die instantaneously [5, 33, 264, 323, 775]. Clearly, explanations in addition to coronary thrombosis must be sought for precipitating causes of lethal arrhythmias in sudden cardiac death.

1.1.4. *Arterial thromboembolism and microembolism*

Thromboemboli may arise from in situ thrombi on the valvular endocardium, the mural endocardium, usually in association with infarcts, cardiomyopathies or auricular arrhythmias and from ulcerated plaques or aneurysms of the aorta and great vessels. Alternatively, they may form de novo entirely in the bloodstream. Large emboli arising from thrombi in the left side of the heart frequently produce clinical manifestations by obstruction of the circulation in the cerebral, mesenteric, renal, splenic, and lower limb arteries. Indeed, acute arterial thromboembolism is not an uncommon presentation of an hitherto unrecognized or silent myocardial infarction. Mural aortic thrombosis often gives rise to renal artery thromboembolism, which may be important in the genesis of some instances of renal disease and hypertension [569]. Similarly, aortic emboli of either thrombotic or atheromatous material may contribute to ischemia in some cases of chronic mesenteric or peripheral vascular insufficiency.

While the pathological basis for and effects of, large thromboemboli are well known, microembolic disease is assuming a greater degree of clinical and pathological importance, largely as a result of the landmark observations of Russell in 1961 [707] on retinal artery microembolism and the subsequent study of Gunning and his colleagues in 1964 on retinal and cerebral ischemia [320]. Microthromboemboli, like their larger counterparts, may be derived from mural thrombi of arteries and the left side of the heart, particularly from bland and infected valvular thrombotic vegetations. Microemboli may be platelet-fibrin thrombi or composed largely of aggregated platelets.

Although many platelet microthrombi and emboli originate in the blood-vascular interface, it is important to recognize that embolic microthrombi may also form within the circulation without any apparent contact with the arterial wall. For example, in both the rat [609] and the pig [436] infused platelet aggregants and releasing agents such as adenosine diphosphate result in the production of transient intravascular microthrombi of aggregated platelets. In the pig, intracoronary artery infusions of adenosine diphosphate are associated with transient platelet aggregation in the myocardial microcirculation and a high frequency of lethal arrhythmias, which may be induced by ischemia of the conduction system, possibly in conjunction with the release of platelet constituents and metabolites [436]. The dense granules of platelets have been shown to contain serotonin and adenosine diphosphate, while constituents of the alpha-granules include fibrinogen and a number of lysosomal enzymes [378, 444]. Thromboxane A_2, an unstable metabolite of prostaglandin endoperoxides that promotes platelet aggregation and is a powerful vasoconstricter, may be formed and released with other constituents [771]. These released products may enhance ischemia and promote the development of lethal cardiac arrhythmias through vasoconstriction and platelet aggregation [368, 771, 799].

The role of platelet microthrombi and microemboli in the pathogenesis of some cases of sudden cardiac death has been the subject of increasing interest. Jørgensen, Haerem and their associates have observed platelet microthrombi and emboli in the coronary vasculature in a number of cases of sudden cardiac death, occurring instantaneously or within a few minutes of the onset of the fatal illness [321, 322, 438]. Haerem [325] suggested that such emboli could play a causal role in the pathogenesis of sudden coronary death, particularly in diseased hearts in which the myocardial substrate subjected to ischemia is more vulnerable to the development of arrhythmia. Coronary microemboli may arise from thrombi in the coronary arteries, the heart and the ascending aorta, or, alternatively, may form within the circulation itself. At least some intramyocardial microthrombi may have arisen by embolization from mural thrombi in the more proximal segments of the coronary arteries [228, 270, 323]. Similar observations in the experimental animal have associated ischemic myocardial injury with platelet and platelet-fibrin microemboli from proximal mural thrombi [257, 572, 578].

Apart from the potential role of platelet microemboli in the genesis of some cases of sudden cardiac death, there appears to be little doubt that microthromboemboli are important in the pathogenesis of transient monocular blindness and cerebral ischemia [320, 707]. Rapidly accumulating knowledge of the function of platelets in thrombosis and of the significance of the thrombotic process in atherogenesis, along with the concomitant development of platelet-inhibitory drugs, has prompted a number of clinical intervention trials with platelet-active agents [92]. Many of the drugs employed appear to be effective in preventing thrombotic phenomena [290].

1.2. THROMBOSIS AND ATHEROGENESIS

Over a hundred years ago in his 'Manual of Pathological Anatomy', the pathologist Carl von Rokitansky [697] first postulated what has become widely known as the thrombogenic hypothesis of atherosclerosis. Rokitansky proposed that the disease is the result of an excessive intimal deposition of blood components, including fibrin. He maintained that localized thickening, atheromatous change, and calcification of the arterial wall are due to the repeated deposition of blood elements and their subsequent metamorphosis and degeneration on the lining membrane of the vascular wall. This hypothesis was not generally accepted at the time. The main objection was that the lesion of atherosclerosis is in the intima not on the surface and, therefore, could not be due to a surface deposit [498]. This seemingly important objection turned out to be unfounded when it was shown that endothelium can grow over a thrombus and incorporate it into the intima [131]. Thrombi participate in atherogenesis primarily by contributing to the growth of plaques on which they form and, at times, by initiating atherosclerotic lesions on a previously normal arterial wall [135, 263, 570, 872]. Atherosclerosis, of course, may arise by other means, but the various causes are not mutually exclusive (350). These causative factors may act alone or in combination in the development of lesions. Arterial thrombosis is only one factor that must be assessed in atherogenesis.

1.2.1. *Organization and metamorphosis of thrombi*

As a mural thrombus is organized and covered by endothelium, it may be converted into a lesion that is typically atherosclerotic [202]. Occlusive thrombi and thromboemboli can also be converted into intimal plaques by first shrinking and retracting to an eccentric parietal position to create a single channel between the thrombus and opposing vessel wall. Duguid [202] emphasized that as a thrombus is transformed to an atherosclerotic plaque it loses its identity, so that eventually the lesion's thrombotic origin is obscured.

The arterial wall reacts to a thrombus by organizing or converting it to living tissue. Organization takes place by an ingrowth of connective tissue while adjacent endothelium grows over the thrombus to reestablish continuity of the vascular lining [202]. Small mural thrombi are organized by an avascular process [161, 203, 353], whereas larger thrombi tend to become vascularized by an ingrowth of capillary sprouts from the newly formed overlying endothelium [161, 288, 575]. The connective tissue, which is fibromuscular in character is derived from modified smooth muscle cells capable of synthesizing collagen [348, 349, 573, 575]. In vitro, arterial smooth muscle cells synthesize types I and III collagen [483]. These cells, which often exist in the intima of arteries, may also be derived from endothelium by metaplasia [7, 130, 131, 349]. Endothelium is now known to be capable of synthesizing in vitro both basement membrane, type IV, and pericellular type V collagen [420, 510].

In relation to the Benditt's monoclonal genetic mutation theory of plaque origin [41, 42, 650, 651], it is of interest to note that the cells organizing a thrombus tend to become monoclonal as measured by sex-linked enzyme markers [652]. The monoclonal theory suggests that atherosclerotic plaques arise by the proliferation of a single clone of cells. The monoclonality of the majority of fibrous plaques has been cited as evidence that thrombi cannot play a role in atherogenesis [41, 42] on the basis that the cells organizing a thrombus would be polyclonal. Pearson and his associates [652] provided objective evidence in their study that monoclonal characteristics similar to those in fibrous plaques develop in arterial thrombi as they become organized.

Atherosclerotic plaques vary in composition from those that are sclerotic and largely fibromuscular to those that contain much lipid and are atheromatous. Many transitional forms of fibrofatty plaques exist between these extremes. Thrombi also vary considerably in composition, but all thrombic elements – fibrin, cellular elements and plasma – influence plaque development. Fresh arterial thrombi characteristically contain numerous platelets. A thrombus, however, may change in composition after it has formed. Experimental studies have shown that mural platelet-fibrin thrombi are apt to undergo fibrinous transformation [437, 873], whereas occlusive thrombi tend to retain their platelets even when shrunken to a mural position before incorporation into the arterial wall [338]. The recently described growth factor derived from platelets may stimulate smooth muscle cells to proliferate and make collagen [700]. Fibrin in thrombi also seems to stimulate the production of collagen actively [347, 514, 575], perhaps by serving as a scaffold.

Crawford and Levene [161] observed that the sequestered remnants of an incompletely organized thrombus may undergo regressive changes to grummous fatty material. Both cellular elements and plasma lipids may contribute to the fat content of thrombi. Among the cellular elements in thrombi, platelets are a major source of lipid [128, 338]. They are especially rich in cholesterol, which seems to be present in platelets in proportion to plasma levels [740]. Foam cells characteristic of those in atherosclerotic plaques can be derived from macrophages that have phagocytized lipid-rich platelets [128]. Although cholesterol in platelets is not esterified as much as it is in plasma and in plaques [762], it has been shown by experiments in the rabbit that macrophages [173] and foam cells [672] can esterify ingested cholesterol. Macrophages may also interact with platelets to accumulate and esterify cholesterol of plasma lipoproteins [255]. Plasma lipids may be entrapped in a forming thrombus and continue to be absorbed as it is organized [735, 843, 870]. Weigensberg and coworkers [793, 842, 843] have shown that mural aortic thrombi in the normolipemic rabbit absorb and retain substantial amounts of radiolabelled plasma cholesterol while evolving into fibrofatty plaques, particularly during the first eight weeks of organization.

The rate of each reaction engaged in metamorphosis of a thrombus could influence the type of lesion that develops. Variations in the rate of endothelialization and organization relative to that of thrombolysis could significantly influence the amount of thrombus incorporated into the arterial wall [170]. Endothelial regeneration in man is fairly slow, taking up to eight days to cover such small areas as an arterial needle puncture wound [162]. Since the rate of endothelialization seems relatively constant, the size of the thrombus could materially affect the outcome. It is likely that mural microthrombi are rapidly incorporated and quickly lose their identity. Conversely, a large thrombus would be organized more slowly and is more likely to retain thrombic remnants in its center for a long time [161]. How rapidly an occlusive thrombus can retract to an eccentric parietal position is not known. However, experimental occlusive coronary thrombi can retract by one week after formation and become converted to eccentric plaques by six weeks [665]. Experimental pulmonary thromboemboli can undergo metamorphosis to typical atherosclerotic plaques in as short a period as three weeks [338].

1.2.2. *Progressive thrombosis and atherosclerosis*

Thrombosis is not simply an isolated event in the course of atherosclerosis but is intimately involved in the continued development of the lesions. The stratified appearance of many plaques suggests that they were formed by repeated deposits of thrombi [142, 202, 514]. Clark and his colleagues [142] and others [163, 202, 575] have emphasized that recurrent thrombosis is an important factor in the pathogenesis of progressive atherosclerotic stenosis of coronary arteries. Deeper layers of thrombus are organized and converted into plaque as fresh uppermost layers are deposited. This form of episodic, and often silent, plaque growth may extend over months or years [163].

1.2.3. *Significance of thrombosis in plaque development*

Since the evidence of the thrombotic origin of an atherosclerotic plaque is obscured as a result of metamorphosis of the thrombus, it is difficult to ascertain the true contribution of thrombosis to plaque development. For this reason, any estimate of the incidence of incorporated thrombi in plaques would seem likely to be an underestimate. A recent survey of published data indicates that incorporated thrombi can be frequently identified in established atherosclerotic plaques [135].

Thrombotic components are most often identified within fibrous and fibrofatty plaques. By means of immunofluorescent techniques Woolf and Carstairs [871] compared aortic fatty streaks, small lipid plaques and fibrolipid lesions. Two-thirds of the fibrolipid plaques, a figure equaling 45% of all types of plaques examined, contained specific fluorescence for fibrin/fibrinogen antigen. Fluorescence in a banded, often laminated, pattern suggested it was thrombotic fibrin rather than fibrin/fibrinogen derived from infiltration or hemorrhage. Platelet antigen was also detected in the same areas in about one-half of these plaques. In the fatty streaks and small lipid plaques, a diffuse pattern of fluorescence specific for fibrin/fibrinogen antigen, but not platelet antigen, was thought to represent fibrinogen that had infiltrated along with plasma from the lumen. Little information is available on the age when thrombi begin to contribute to plaque growth. However, in one study microthrombi were found to be incorporated in plaques of coronary arteries only after the age of 25 years [132]. Although thrombosis does not appear to be a factor in the pathogenesis of superficial fatty streaks, the possibility that fatty streaks provide a base for thrombus formation and subsequent growth of the lesions should not be excluded [350, 869].

1.2.4. *Onset of plaques by thrombi*

There is limited evidence that thrombosis is a factor in the inception of atherosclerotic lesions. Occasional small mural thrombi, either uncovered or in varying stages of incorporation, have been observed on apparently healthy vessel walls [131, 203, 350, 579, 535, 490], but undetected and preexistent submicroscopic changes could be present in a seemingly normal artery [579]. Interpretation of possible early thrombotic lesions may be further complicated by the reaction of the intima to the overlying thrombus. Jørgensen and his coworkers [440] correlated the presence of aortic microthrombi with focal intimal edema and suggested that the edematous lesions resulted from injury to the to the vascular lining by the thrombi. Regardless of their mode of origin, small thrombotic-vascular lesions could represent an incipient stage of atherosclerosis. Unequivocal and strong support for the concept that thrombi can initiate plaque formation on a normal vessel wall is recognized in thromboembolism. In man [31] and in the experimental animal [131, 338], plaques can be derived from thromboemboli that have lodged in previously normal arteries.

Though still incomplete and limited by the exclusion of thrombi that have completely lost their identity in the conversion process, these observations on the frequency of intimal thrombotic lesions nevertheless provide substantial evidence that thrombosis is an important factor in the long-term development of arterial plaques. Antithrombotic measures might reasonably be directed toward reduction of the long-term effects of thrombosis and associated plaque growth as well as toward the prevention of acute thrombotic ischemia.

1.2.5. *Regression of atherosclerosis in relation to thrombosis*

Lately, much interest has arisen in the possibility that the progression of atherosclerosis may be arrested and regression of the lesions induced. Experimental evidence indicates that severe restriction of dietary lipids can be effective [863]. In addition, reports have appeared that show arrest or regression of the disease in man by use of partial ileal bypass surgery [105], and by cholestrol-lowering diets and drugs [32].

The study of experimental thrombotic atherosclerosis provides a useful method for following regression of lesions without manipulation of dietary or blood lipids [338, 265]. Studies of thrombotic atherosclerosis in normolipemic animals clearly illustrate that the lesions can undergo spontaneous regression. Both in situ and embolic thrombi will shrink while undergoing metamorphosis to a plaque and continue to reduce in size after conversion has occurred. This process of plaque formation and subsequent regression at a specific site on a previously normal arterial wall can be accurately followed in experimental studies of the fate of thrombi in coronary [665] or other arteries [131, 265, 338].

In natural disease factors may exist that increase the rate of production of thrombi or impede and prevent their resolution so that, in effect, the thrombi accumulate and produce advanced atherosclerosis [338]. The question might thus be raised whether some therapeutic approaches to the induction of arrest or regression of atherosclerosis may be mediated through an antithrombotic pathway.

1.3. THE PLATELET-DERIVED GROWTH FACTOR AND ATHEROGENESIS

1.3.1. *The concept*

A prominent feature of atherosclerotic plaques is the smooth muscle or myointimal cell [286]. Growth of myointimal cells may involve the thrombotic process or other atherogenic stimuli. These cells take part in early plaque development and are present in fatty streaks. They may continue to proliferate, produce collagen and progressively enlarge an atherosclerotic plaque. In addition, like macrophages, they may accumulate lipid as part of plaque development [61, 285, 286].

Recently, a series of studies by Ross and his associates and subsequently by other investigators has led to the concept that a growth factor released by platelets and interacting with the arterial wall may stimulate intimal smooth muscle cells to proliferate and synthesize collagen [112, 700, 701, 708, 864]. The evidence in support of this concept is largely derived from in vitro studies and, in part, from indirect studies in the experimental animal under conditions of thrombocytopenia or platelet inhibition.

The platelet-derived growth factor was initially discovered following the observation that monkey arterial smooth muscle cells cultured in a medium containing serum derived from platelet-free plasma remain quiescent. In contrast, cells cultured in a medium containing serum derived either from clotted whole blood or from platelet-free plasma with an added extract of platelets are stimulated to proliferate in a burst of growth for several days before becoming stationary [700]. A parallel series of studies by these and other workers has shown that the factor also stimulates other connective tissue cells to replicate in vitro [11, 461, 708].

Subsequently, it was demonstrated that this mitogenic factor is a basic polypeptide hormone of 13 000–16 000 daltons [12] located in the alpha granules of the platelet [444, 445]. Whether the platelet is simply a carrier of the hormone, which is produced elsewhere, perhaps in the pituitary [305, 306, 705], is not presently known. In contrast to other polypeptide hormones, the predominant delivery system appears to be the platelet rather than plasma [445]. The factor is carried through the circulation in the platelets' alpha granules in a cryptic state. Upon release of platelet constituents at sites of vascular injury or in extravascular sites, the hormone may initiate replication of connective tissue cells and the reparative process. Kaplan and his coworkers [445] commented on how remarkably specific the delivery system is for this hormone, which is potentially released only where needed at sites of injury. Unfortunately, the healing and reparative response often overreacts, or leaves in its wake the nidus on which pathologic processes begin.

The discovery and potential effects of this growth factor fit nicely into Virchow's concept of injury and repair as it applies to atherosclerosis; indeed it should be recalled that thrombosis itself is a reparative process, often being an exaggerated response to vascular injury. Nevertheless, the significance of this hormonal factor in the development of arteriosclerotic lesions remains to be determined. The future availability of a purified hormone could provide a way to verify the platelet growth factor hypothesis in vivo. In the meantime, experimental work in animals has concentrated on indirect approaches.

1.3.2. *Experimental support*

Experimental animal studies of arteriosclerosis based on injury to the arterial wall and accompanying involvement of the thrombotic process have been applied indirectly to the study of the platelet-derived growth factor in vivo. Moore and his colleagues [266, 571] have shown that the proliferative response to arterial injury and associated thrombotic phenomena are largely abolished in thrombocytopenic animals. Harker and his associates [343] found that inhibition of platelet function was also effective in preventing experimental arteriosclerosis.

In experiments by Moore and coworkers, the development of thromboatherosclerosis induced by an indwelling aortic catheter in the rabbit was greatly inhibited under conditions of severe thrombocytopenia produced by antiplatelet serum. Many of the lesions produced in animals with normal platelet levels were raised fibrofatty plaques covered by thrombi. These investigators concluded that thrombosis, not injury, was the determining factor in the development of the atherosclerotic lesions. In a related experiment, thrombocytopenia was again produced with antiplatelet serum, and a single balloon injury was used to remove endothelium from the aorta [266]. This procedure usually results in a proliferative response and the production of fibromusculoelastic lesions. The development of intimal lesions was suppressed by thrombocytopenia.

Another approach to the study of the influence of platelets on injury induced arteriosclerosis has been through the use of chemically produced endothelial denudation in conjunction with the administration of dipyridamole, a drug that inhibits platelet function [343]. Experimental homocystinemia sustained over three months in baboons causes patchy endothelial desquamation, associated platelet deposition that was reflected by increased platelet turnover, and the development of fibromusculoelastic aortic plaques with sparse intracellular lipid. Dipyridamole therapy normalized platelet consumption and prevented the development of arteriosclerotic plaques, but not the endothelial desquamation caused by the homocystinemia. The drug is a known inhibitor of platelet aggregation and release, an effect that could interfere with platelet adhesion to the arterial wall and release of the growth factor.

These workers concluded that sustained chemically induced endothelial injury results in endothelial cell loss that is followed by platelet adherence and release and the progressive development of arteriosclerotic lesions. The role of platelets in the genesis of the lesions was demonstrated by the capacity of an inhibitor of platelet function to prevent intimal smooth muscle cell proliferation and consequent lesion formation.

One other aspect of the interrelations of the platelet with the vessel wall to consider is that platelets may release lytic enzymes and vasoactive amines that injure the endothelium, make it more permeable, and thus allow such factors as the platelet-derived growth factor to have access to the subendothelial intima [400, 513]. This aspect of platelet behavior, when placed against the background of evidence that platelets also protect and nourish endothelium is paradoxial indeed, and serves to illustrate the paucity of knowledge in this area [513]. It has been suggested that atherosclerosis may be less severe in individuals with von Willebrand's disease, which is characterized by defective platelet-vessel wall interaction [90].

In a retrospective study of homozygous von Willebrand's disease in pigs it was observed by Fuster and his colleagues [276, 277] that arteriosclerotic plaques, either spontaneously occurring or induced by dietary cholesterol, were less frequent and less severe than in control animals although the diseased pigs frequently developed fatty streaks. This finding suggested on the one hand that the endothelium in these animals is more permeable to plasma proteins and on the other hand that the stimulus for proliferation is diminished in this desease even though active growth factor is contained in the platelets [239]. These investigators have initiated a long-term prospective study on spontaneous and dietary induced atherosclerosis. Interim reports indicate the same trend in that the pigs with homozygous von Willebrand's disease appear to be resistant to the development of atherosclerosis [278, 279]. A more recent report by Griggs and coworkers [309] has shown that absence of the von Willebrand factor in pigs is associated with limited resistance to dietary induced atherosclerosis but does not affect the extent of fatty streaking.

The one known clinical-pathologic study on the frequency of atherosclerosis in von Willebrand's disease does not follow these experimental observations. Silwer and his associates [751] found clinical evidence of arteriosclerotic disease in 14 of 31 patients over 40 years of age. The autopsy protocols of three other cases of patients over 40 years of age were reviewed and atherosclerosis of varying degrees of severity was noted in all cases though it was sparse and minimal in one case. It should be emphasized that in contrast to the pigs with homozygous von Willebrand's disease, the severity of the hemorrhagic disease in the human cases varied considerably. These observations in man are supported by the findings of Fuster, Griggs and their coworkers [278, 309] who have shown that carrier pigs do not appear to be resistant to the development of atherosclerosis.

1.3.3. *Comment*

At present, it is difficult to assess fully the significance of the platelet-derived growth factor in atherogenesis, for it could be argued that the experimental conditions of catheter or chemically induced injury of arteries associated with thrombocytopenia and platelet inhibition are not comparable to those that obtain in naturally occurring disease. Nevertheless, smooth muscle cells participate in atherogenesis and it is possible that the platelet growth factor may be one of several mitogens, including lipoproteins [863], that stimulate these cells to proliferate. Regardless of the ultimate significance of the platelet factor, it remains clear that thrombi organized by smooth muscle cells can contribute to atherogenesis. Hence, there is reason to anticipate that intensive investigation of this factor will continue and therapeutic intervention of thromboarterial disease by antithrombotic and platelet inhibitory measures will be increasingly evaluated.

2. BIOCHEMICAL PHYSIOLOGY OF DIETARY FATS

Dietary fats mainly consist of fatty acids esterified to glycerol. For a long time, they have been considered as a condensed source of energy but this view changed completely after the structural and metabolic functions of fatty acids had been recognized.

2.1. STRUCTURE AND NOMENCLATURE OF FATTY ACIDS

Although some naturally occurring branched-chain and even ring-chain fatty acids are known, the vast majority of fatty acids consists of an aliphatic chain of carbon atoms (–C–) with a terminal carboxyl group (–COOH). In saturated fatty acids, all available C-bonds are occupied by hydrogen atoms (–H, Fig. 2.1). In unsaturated fatty acids, not all free C-bonds are 'saturated' with H-atoms, resulting in a double bond between two adjacent C-atoms (–^{H}C = C^H–). Mono-unsaturated fatty acids contain one unsaturated bond and polyunsaturated fatty acids two or more (Fig. 2.2). Double bonds may have a *cis*- or *trans*-configuration. In the *cis*-configuration, the H-atoms immediately adjacent to the double bonds are located on the same side of the C-chain plane. In the *trans*-configuration, these H-atoms are situated on opposite sides of this plane (Fig. 2.3). Natural oils and fats contain fatty acids with

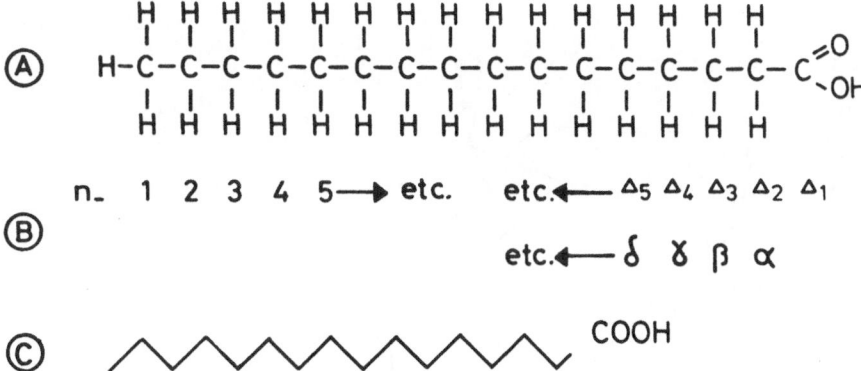

Fig. 2.1. Composition and structure of palmitic acid (16:0) A, extensive notation; B, numbering of C-atoms; C, simplified notation

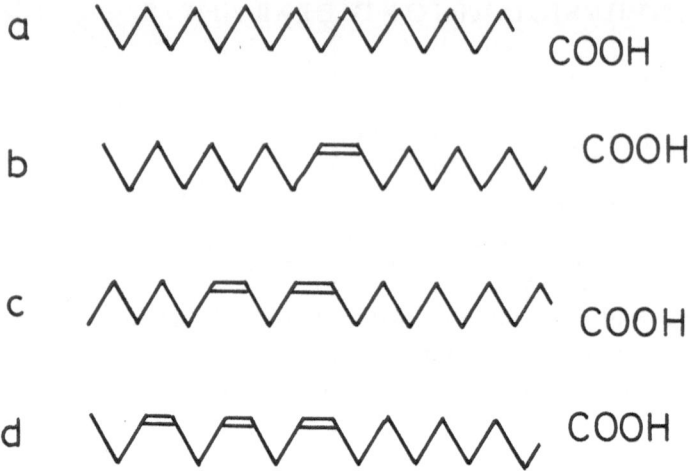

Fig. 2.2. Structure of some common fatty acids. a) stearic acid, 18:0; b) oleic acid, 18:1 (n − 9); c) linoleic acid, 18:2 (n − 6); d) α-linolenic acid, 18:3 (n − 3)

almost exclusively *cis*-isomers, However, small amounts of *trans* fatty acids are present in certain animal fats, while the oil of *Aquilegia Vulgaris* is relatively rich in columbinic acid, which has a *trans*-double bond between the 13th and the 14th C-atom (Fig. 2.4, see Chapter 6, section 2.4). Moreover, partial hydrogenation of oils results in the formation of *trans*-isomers of fatty acids in an approximate ratio of 2:1 with *cis*-isomers [209]. In natural fatty acids, two double bonds are practically always separated by one methylene group $(-C^H = C^H - CH_2 - C^H = C^H-)$. More-over, they contain almost exclusively an even number of C-atoms. Depending on the length of this C-chain, fatty acids are designated as short-chain-(≤ 6 C-atoms),

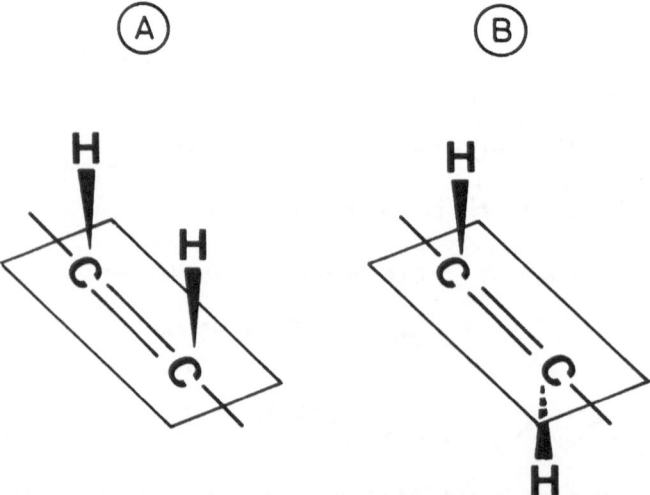

Fig. 2.3. *Cis* (A) and *trans* (B) configuration of double bonds

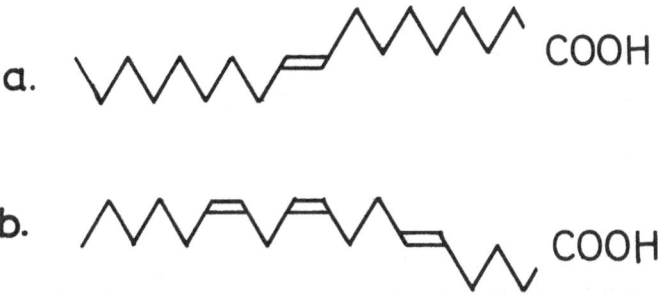

Fig. 2.4. Structure of some fatty acids containing a *trans* double bond. a) elaidic acid, 18:1 (n–9$_t$); b) columbinic acid, 18:3 (n − 6$_c$, 9$_c$, 13$_t$)

medium-chain- (8 or 10 C-atoms) or long-chain fatty acids (12 or more C-atoms).

   The systematic designation of fatty acids is rather complex and, therefore, trivial names are more frequently used. For practical purposes, we will denote fatty acids as x : y (n–z), in which x is the total number of C-atoms, y the number of double bonds and z the position of the first C-atom involved in a double bond (counted from the terminal methyl group). Figure 2.2 gives some examples of fatty acid structures and their notation. The molecular structure of the fatty acids is an important determinant of their physical properties and thereby of their structural functions. The physical properties of acids containing *trans* double bonds resemble those of saturated fatty acids more closely than those of *cis* compounds.

2.2. FATTY ACID SYNTHESIS

Depending on the special requirement of various tissues, the body needs an ever-changing variety of different fatty acids. To meet this demand, it is not completely dependent on a certain dietary fatty acid intake, because the body is able to synthesize a great variety of fatty acids itself, starting mainly from pyruvate, a product of carbohydrate metabolism. The major product of this pathway of de novo fatty acid synthesis is palmitic acid (16:0).

2.2.1. *Chain elongation*

The greater part of palmitic acid is converted into stearic acid (18:0) by chain elongation. This reaction – and the formation of longer-chain saturated fatty acids – is catalysed by an elongase enzyme system and results in the incorporation of two methylene groups from malonyl ∼CoA into the fatty acid chain just proximal to the carboxyl group:

$$R_1 - C \overset{O}{\underset{\sim}{=}} CoA + HOOC - C\overset{H_2}{\underline{}} C \overset{O}{\underset{\sim}{=}} CoA$$

$$\xrightarrow[\substack{2NADPH \\ + 2H^+}]{\substack{CO_2 \quad CoA \quad H_2O \\ \nearrow \quad \nearrow \quad \nearrow \\ \\ \searrow \\ 2NADP^+}} R_1 - C\overset{H_2}{\underline{}} C\overset{H_2}{\underline{}} C \overset{O}{\underset{\sim}{=}} CoA$$

The elongase system contains three different enzymes, which are located on the membranes of the endoplasmatic reticulum. Another fatty acid chain/elongation system is located in the mitochondria. It differs from the microsomal system in that it does not use malonyl~CoA, but acetyl~CoA. Therefore, this latter pathway can be considered as the reverse route of the catabolic process of β-oxidation (see section 2.4). Polyunsaturated fatty acids (PUFA's) are better elongated than saturated fatty acids (SAFA's), especially when the double bonds are located closely to the carboxyl groups. It is not known whether different elongase systems are required for the elongation of fatty acids of different chain lengths [779].

2.2.2. Desaturation

Starting from mainly stearic acid (18:0), the body can produce quite a number of long-chain (poly-)unsaturated fatty acids by the alternating action of a desaturase enzyme complex and the elongase described. For this purpose, various desaturases are available, which are microsomal enzyme complexes allowing the introduction of double bonds into fatty acid molecules [427]. For their activity, they require a reduced pyridine nucleotide and molecular oxygen. They act only on activated fatty acids (acyl~CoA) according to the following overall reaction

$$R_1 - C\overset{H_2}{\underline{}} C\overset{H_2}{\underline{}} R_2 \sim CoA + NAD(P)H + H^+ + O_2 \xrightarrow{}$$

$$R_1 - C\overset{H}{\underline{}} = C\overset{H}{\underline{}} - R_2 \sim CoA + NAD(P)^+ + 2H_2O$$

The various desaturases all act on a specific site of the fatty acid molecule. The Δ_9-desaturase introduces a double bond into a saturated fatty acid between the 9th and the 10th carbon atom, counted from the carboxyl group (the $\Delta_{9,10}$-position, see Fig. 2.1.B). The Δ_6-desaturase does the same between the 6th and the 7th C-atom but only in those fatty acids which have already a double bond at the $\Delta_{9,10}$-position. The Δ_5-desaturase introduces a double bond between the 5th and the 6th C-atom. It needs a substrate fatty acid already desaturated in the $\Delta_{11,12}$- and $\Delta_{8,9}$-position. Also, a Δ_4-desaturase has been described, being highly specific for substrate fatty acids with double bonds at the $\Delta_{13,14}$-, $\Delta_{10,11}$- and $\Delta_{7,8}$-positions. It introduces a double bond between the 4th and the 5th C-atom, again counted from the carboxyl group.

So far, no other desaturases have been found in mammalian tissue and the conditions mentioned above therefore imply that:
- no double bonds can be introduced between the Δ_1 and the Δ_9 psition (see Fig. 2.1)
- any further double bond is introduced between the carboxyl group and the nearest double bond present.

Consequently, starting from a (n–9) fatty acid, only another (n–9) fatty acid can be formed and from a (n–7) fatty acid only another (n–7) fatty acid. Therefore, endogenously formed polyunsaturated fatty acids can be classified as members of the (n–9)- or the (n–7)-family. Figure 2.5 shows the major steps of the biosynthesis of these families. The desaturase enzyme system is stimulated by dietary carbohydrates and SAFA's. Insulin has also been reported to have a stimulating effect, which is most probably indirect. To attain an optimum activity, the desaturase enzyme complex requires the presence of certain cytoplasmic proteins. These proteins most probably act as fatty-acid binding proteins and may regulate the supply of fatty acids (or its CoA-esters) to the enzyme. For PUFA synthesis, Δ_6-

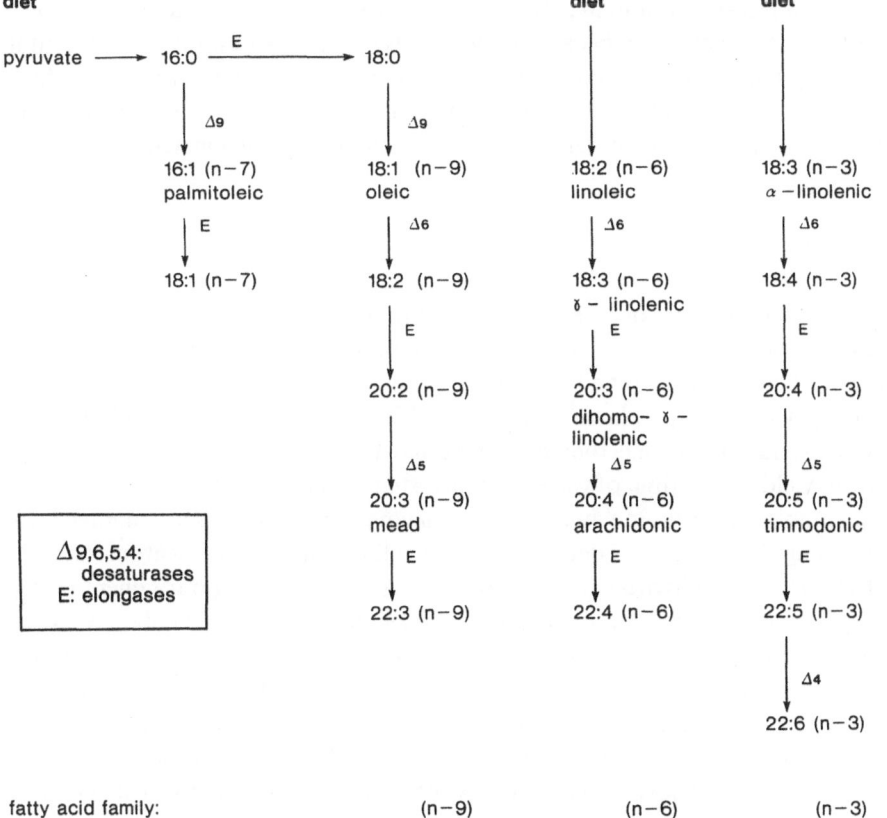

Fig. 2.5. Major biosynthetic pathways of fatty acids

desaturase activity is rate-limiting. The affinity of substrate fatty acids for this enzyme is higher, the higher the number of double bonds. Therefore, desaturation of linoleic acid (18:2(n–6)) is inhibited by α-linolenic acid (18:3(n–3)) and other long-chain PUFA's [94]. Only when these fatty acids are present in minute amounts, can oleic acid (18:1(n–9)) become desaturated and chain-elongated. This occurs in essential fatty acid deficiency (vide infra) and results in the formation of mead acid, 20:3(n–9) [374, 537].

2.3. ESSENTIAL FATTY ACIDS

Saturated fatty acids and fatty acids of the (n–9) and (n–7) families are insufficient to maintain normal life in mammals. This was shown as early as 1929 by Burr and Burr [113], who observed that rats, after being fed on a rigidly fat-free diet, developed severe deficiency symptoms and ultimately died. This deficiency could be cured only by administering small amounts of oils containing polyunsaturated fatty acids of the (n–3) and/or (n–6) series. Similar results were obtained in a wide variety of animal species and in man [1, 340, 375]. Obviously, mammals need (n–3) and/or (n–6) fatty acids and because they lack Δ_{12}- and Δ_{15}-desaturases (present in plants), they depend for these fatty acids on dietary intake. Therefore, these fatty acids are called essential fatty acids (EFA's). Figure 2.5. shows the major steps of the metabolism of 18:2(n–6), linoleic acid, and 18:3(n–3), α-linolenic acid.

2.4. FATTY ACID DEGRADATION

Fatty acid degradation occurs for the greater part by a process known as β-oxidation. This process is located in the mitochondria and only 'activated' fatty acids (esterified with CoA) can be oxidized. Activation of fatty acids requires energy and takes place in the cytoplasm. The activated fatty acids enter the mitochondria as carnitine esters after which they are converted back into CoA-esters. Fatty acid oxidation yields a multiple of the energy invested in their activation.

By a complex process, in which various enzymes and cofactors are involved, the fatty acyl (e.g. 16:0) $\sim$ CoA is dehydrogenated at the α- and β-carbon atoms (see Fig. 2.1), hydrated and dehydrogenated again, after which a 2-carbon fragment (acetyl $\sim$ CoA) is split off. The remainder of the molecule (14:0 $\sim$ CoA) enters a second degradation cycle ... etc., until the fatty acid molecule is degraded completely. The β-oxidation of unsaturated fatty acids requires some additional reactions, the nature of which still gives rise to some controversy [469]. The electrons removed in the two hydrogenation steps travel to oxygen via the respiratory chain, accompanied by oxidative phosphorylation of ADP. The acetyl $\sim$ CoA formed enters the Krebs cycle and is oxidized to CO_2 and H_2O. In this way, one molecule of palmatic acid yields 131 molecules of ATP, which represents 40% of the standard free energy of the oxidation reaction.

2.5. FATTY ACID DERIVATIVES

Fatty acids, especially the long-chain types, have strong deterging properties and are very toxic for the organism. Therefore, under normal circumstances, tissue free fatty acid levels are very low. Most fatty acids are present as triglycerides – serving as a general reserve (adipose tissue) – or as (mainly membrane-)phospholipids performing a structural function or acting as quickly mobilizable precursor substances (e.g. for prostaglandins).

2.5.1. *Triglycerides*

Triglycerides (triacyglycerols) are esters of glycerol and fatty acids. One molecule of glycerol can bind three fatty acid molecules (Fig. 2.6). These fatty acids may be similar or (partly) different. In the body, triglycerides constitute the major fatty acids depot located in the adipose tissue. When the body requires fatty acids, adipose tissue triglycerides are hydrolized by the action of a hormone-sensitive lipase. (See section 2.7.)

2.5.2. *Phospholipids*

Phospholiids have a glycerol backbone, like triglycerides, but in the 3-position it is esterified to phosphoric acid. Hydrocarbon groups are attached to the 1- and 2-positions (Fig. 2.7). At the 2-position this group is largely a (poly-)unsaturated fatty acid; at the 1-position, it usually is a saturated fatty acid. Sometimes, the hydrocarbon chain is attached to the 1-position of the glycerol moiety via an ether

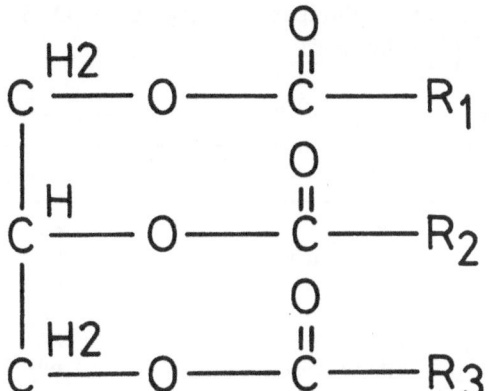

Fig. 2.6. Structure of triglyceride molecule. R_1, R_2 and R_3: fatty acid residues

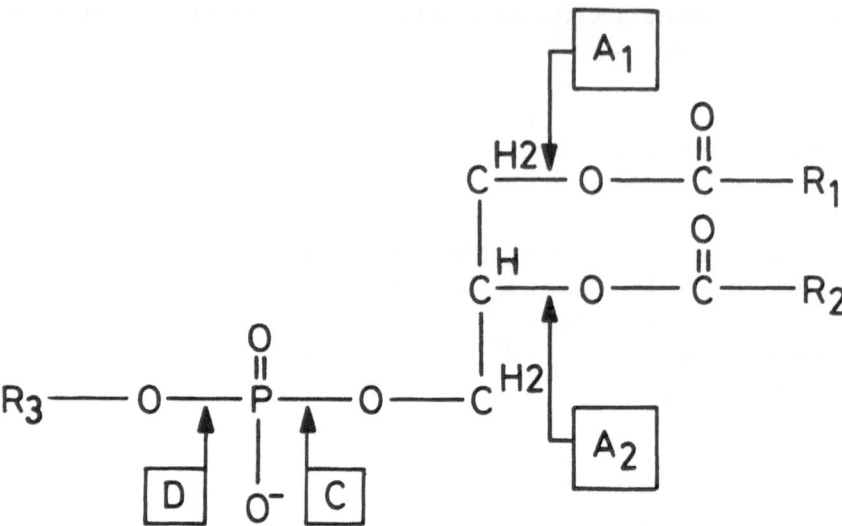

Fig. 2.7. Structure of phospholipid molecule. R_1 and R_2: fatty acid residues; R_3: alcohol group. A_1, A_2, C and D: site of action of respective phospholipases

linkage, forming an alkyl ether phosphoglyceride. Plasmalogens are alkyl ether phosphoglycerides in which the ether-linked alkyl chain contains a double bond between the Δ_1 and Δ_2 positions. The greater part of the phosphoric acid groups form diesters with the hydroxyl groups of choline, ethanolamine, serine or inositol. The major phospholipid classes and the codes used are shown in Table 2.1.

For practical purposes, sphyngomyelin (SPH) is also regarded as a phospholipid, although it does not fit our general description of such a compound. In fact, it is a sphyngolipid, a sphyngosine derivative, containing, one amide-linked (mainly saturated or mono-unsaturated) long-chain fatty acid and a phosphorylcholine group (as in PC) attached to the terminal hydroxyl group of sphyngosine.

Phospholipids (including SPH) can be hydrolyzed by special enzymes which, according to their sites of action, are called phospholipase-A_1, -A_2, -C or -D (See Fig. 2.7). Sphyngomyelinase is a C-type phospholipase.

Table 2.1. Survey of major phospholipid classes

Name	Alcohol group	Code
Phosphatidyl choline	choline	PC
Phosphatidyl ethanolamine	ethanolamine	PE
Phosphatidyl serine	serine	PS
Phosphatidyl inositol	inositol	PI
Phosphatidic acid	–	PA
Phosphatidal ethanolamine (plasmalogen)	ethanolamine	PPE

2.5.3. *Cholesterol esters*

Cholesterol is the major sterol in the human body. It serves quite a number of important functions which are not relevant here. However it is briefly mentioned because, in esterified form, it is one of the fatty acid 'carriers'. Cholesterol esters contain mainly polyunsaturated fatty acids, esterified to the 3-β-hydroxyl group of the steroid ring system. Cholesterol is the precursor of bile acids, which are important in fat absorption. It is also an important component of cell membranes and plasma lipoproteins.

2.6. FAT ABSORPTION

Vegetable or animal fats contain over 99% triglycerides. Depending on their origin, the fatty acid composition of the dietary oils and fats is highly different (Tables 4.2. and 7.1.). Since dietary triglycerides cannot be absorbed as such, they must first be hydrolyzed, which is accomplished by lipolytic enzymes produced mainly by the pancreas, but also by pharyngeal and intestinal glands. To allow these lipases optimum access to the triglycerides, the fat globules in the chyme, measuring about 100 nm in diameter, are emulsified by conjugated bile acids. These compounds lower the average diameter of the lipid globule to about 5 nm, thereby increasing the accessible surface area of the lipids 20 times. This increases the efficiency of the lipases, which split the triglyceride molecule usually into a 2-monoglyceride and two fatty acids. These substances would be able to penetrate the brush border of the intestinal epithelial cells simply by diffusion but they are hardly able to reach these cells because in view of their hydrophobic nature, they cannot pass through the thin water barrier between the glycocalix and the microvilli. Again, the conjugated bile salts have an important function here. Because of their amphiphatic nature (polar head and non-polar tail [326]), they form mixed micelles containing monoglycerides, fatty acids, cholesterol and lipid-soluble vitamins. These negatively charged micelles are able to penetrate the intervillous space. Here, the monoglycerides, fatty acids etc. diffuse out of the micelles into the intestinal mucosal cells. The conjugated bile salts can be absorbed in the ileum later and enter the enterohepatic circulation.

Inside the intestinal mucosal cells, monoglycerides and fatty acids are resynthesized into triglycerides which, together with small amounts of phospholipids and cholesterol, are 'packed' by a negatively charged β-lipoprotein to form a chylomicron with a diameter of about 2 nm. After a proteinaceous meal, another type of particle forms: the very low density lipoprotein (VLDL). This is also the principal vehicle for dietary cholesterol absorption and transportation. Chylomicra and VLDL are able to diffuse through the basolateral membrane of the villous epithelium and enter the terminal lacteals. They finally enter the circulation via the thoracic duct, which drains into the left internal jugular vein. Short- and medium-chain fatty acids are directly absorbed from the intestinal epithelium into the intestinal capillaries and when bound to plasma proteins, they are transported via the portal vein towards the liver.

2.7. PLASMATIC TRANSPORT OF FATTY ACIDS

Fatty acids are transported either as free fatty acids (vide infra) or in the form of triglycerides, phospholipids and cholesterol esters. These latter compounds are poorly soluble in their transportation medium, the blood plasma. Lipid particles, made up of physically combined lipid and protein complexes, the lipoproteins, make transportation possible. Non-esterified fatty acids are also transported with the blood, largely bound to plasma proteins and to albumin in particular.

Dietary long-chain fatty acids, esterified into triglycerides or cholesterol esters and incorporated into chylomicra and VLDL are transported to adipose tissue and to the liver. On entering the adipose tissue, the lipoprotein triglycerides are hydrolyzed by a lipoprotein lipase. The fatty acids released enter the adipocytes where they are resynthesized into and stored as triglycerides.

Chylomicra entering the liver are also attacked by a lipoprotein lipase. The fatty acids liberated – together with fatty acids synthesized de novo by the liver from carbohydrates – are resynthesized to triglycerides and incorporated into VLDLs, which are transported to the adipose tissue where their triglyceride fatty acids are transferred into the adipocytes and stored as triglycerides. The remaining low-density lipoproteins chiefly contain cholesterol esters and are of minor importance for fatty acid transportation. The same holds for high-density lipoproteins.

When needed somewhere in the body, fatty acids can be released from adipose tissue triglycerides by means of a hormone- (i.e. adrenaline, noradrenaline, ACTH, glucagon) -sensitive triglyceride lipase. The resulting diglycerides are further catabolized by a diglyceride lipase, which also degrades the resulting monoglycerides. The fatty acids released enter the bloodstream and bind physically to plasma proteins (mainly albumin) in non-esterified form. There are at least three 'classes' of fatty acid binding sites, the 'tight' one being saturated at a molar fatty acid/albumin ratio of about 2, occurring at a plasma free fatty acid concentration of about 1200 μmol/l [152]. Albumin-bound, non-esterified fatty acids are in equilibrium with unbound free fatty acids. Usually, plasma free fatty acid (FFA) concentrations indicate the sum of the protein-bound and unbound fatty acids. It should be realized that the protein-bound free fatty acids are much less 'aggressive' than the free fatty acids, the concentration of which is generally very low. However, under certain conditions (e.g. myocardial infarction), fatty acid mobilization may become so massive that the binding capacity of the plasma proteins is exceeded and the plasma FFA-level increases considerably [777]. The possible implication of this condition for platelet function and arterial thrombogenesis will be discussed in Chapter 9.

2.8. FUNCTIONS OF FATTY ACIDS

The oldest recognized function of fatty acids is to serve as a source of energy. In Western societies, about 40% of the digestible energy (energy %, en %) is supplied by dietary fats. Carbohydrates, too are an important source of energy and from this point of view should be able to replace dietary fat completely. Prolonged feeding of a fat-free diet, however, causes growth retardation, dermatitis, impaired reproduction and a great many other pathological conditions ultimately leading to death [1, 113, 375]. This syndrome could only be cured by administration of polyunsaturated fatty acids of the (n–6) and (n–3) families, which were named essential fatty acids (EFAs).

It should be noted that the EFA-activity of both fatty acid families differs considerably and is also different for the various EFA-deficiency symptoms [404]. EFA-deficiency not only occurs in animals but also in man [340, 376]. The minimum human EFA requirement has been estimated to be between 1 and 5 en% but there is still no consensus on this aspect [160].

The EFA-deficiency syndrome is a convenient starting point for discussing the possible functions of fatty acids. The increased permeability of the skin to water [35], the enhanced capillary fragility and permeability [463], the higher erythrocyte fragility [509] and the enhanced mitochondrial swelling [352] all point to an important structural and functional role in relation to biomembranes. Moreover, EFAs appeared to be the ultimate dietary precursors of prostaglandins and related compounds [50, 196]. Membrane structure and function as well as prostaglandin metabolism have important implications for the regulation of thrombus formation. Therefore, these functions will be discussed in some detail.

2.8.1. Function in biomembranes

Fatty acids may be in the fluid or in the crystalline state, depending on the fact whether the environmental temperature is above or below their melting points, respectively. In the crystalline phase, the fatty acid molecules are closely packed resulting in a rigid arrangement compared to the liquid state where the molecular arrangement is largely determined by the environment. When incorporated in phospholipids, fatty acids are important constituents of cellular membranes, which serve not only as bounderies between individual cells, but also compartmentalise several major biochemical processes within the cell.

Phospholipids, including SPH, contain a polar head-group and two non-polar tails. Due to this 'amphiphatic' character and as a result of thermodynamic forces, phospholipids, when in contact with water, form structures composed of molecular bilayers with an internal hydrophobic phase and the polar heads exposed on the surface. When these structures separate two aqueous compartments they have properties very similar to those of natural cellular membranes. Under this condition, the inter- and intramolecular interaction of hydrophobic and hydrophylic groups results in a conformation and mobility of the hydrocarbon chains which is either similar to that in the 'crystalline' or 'gel' state or adopts an intermediate 'liquid-crystalline' phase. The temperature at which the hydrocarbon core of a phospholipid bilayer changes from a rigid crystalline to a more fluid liquid-crystalline phase is called the phase transition temperature. This temperature is much lower than the melting points of the fatty acids incorporated, and is determined by their chain lengths and degree of unsaturation as well as by the nature of the phospholipid head-groups. It is now generally agreed that mammalian cellular membranes indeed consist of a phospholipid bilayer with cholesterol and (non-structural) protein molecules 'floating' in this lipid 'sea' [757]. The degree of fluidity of this lipid sea is determined by various factors, such as the physical state (crystalline or liquid-crystalline) of the phospholipid-hydrocarbon groups. Because of the less rigid arrangement of these groups above the phase transition temperature, membranes are more 'fluid' in the liquid-crystalline than in the crystalline state, thus allowing a greater mobility of certain membrane proteins serving as receptor sites. Therefore, membrane fluidity may determine, at least in part, receptor availability and efficiency and, as a result, modulate a great number of membrane-located processes. Membrane fluidity is affected by the relative proportion of the different phospholipid classes, the chain length and degree of unsaturation of their fatty acid residues and the membrane cholesterol content [182, 424, 471]. Since these latter two factors can be influenced by diet, one may expect a dietary effect on membrane fluidity and on the processes depending on it. Thus it has been shown that dietary fat-induced changes in membrane fatty acid composition influenced the cooperativity of certain allosteric membrane-bound enzymes [73]. Similar effects were observed when membrane fluidity was altered by cholesterol feeding [72]. Cholesterol incorporation in platelet plasma membranes has been shown to lower their fluidity [741], to enhance the sensitivity of the platelet to certain aggregating agents [740, 874] and to increase their production of aggregation-promoting thromboxane A_2 [791, 874].

Above the phase transition temperature, the mobility of the phospholipid-hydrocarbon groups is determined by the viscosity of their micro-environment. Therefore, membrane micro-viscosity may be regarded as being equivalent to the inverse of membrane fluidity. Membrane micro-viscosity can be determined by techniques such as nuclear magnetic resonance, electron spin resonance and fluorescence polarization, using a probe inserted into the hydrophobic core of the membrane.

2.8.2. Function as prostanoid precursors

Prostanoids are a group of metabolically related compounds of great physiological importance, implicated in such vital processes as bloodpressure regulation, haemostasis, reproduction, inflammation, etc. They are produced in almost every tissue of the body and because most of them are broken down during one single passage through the lungs or liver, they closely resemble local hormones. The prostanoids comprise two different groups of compounds, prostaglandins (PGs) and thrombo-xanes (Txs). All prostanoids contain 20 C-atoms arranged in a (bi)cyclic structure, carrying two side-chains, one of which is terminated by a carboxyl group and the other by a methyl group (Fig. 2.8). Therefore, prostanoids are cyclic fatty acids. Depending on the configuration of the cyclic part of their molecule, prostanoids are divided into various prostaglandin 'families' – indicated by the capitals A to I – and into thromboxanes. Each prostanoid family consists of a 1-, a 2- and a 3-series, depending on the number of double bonds in their two side-chains. (1, 2 or 3, see Fig. 2.8).

The striking similarity in the molecular shapes of arachidonic acid and prostag-landin E_2 led to the discovery that PGs are synthesized from essential fatty acids [50, 196]. The 1- and 2-series were shown to be derived from dihomo-γ-linolenic acid 20:3(n–6)) and arachidonic acid (20:4(n–6)), respectively, while timnodonic acid (20:5(n–3)) appeared to be the direct precursor of the 3-series PGs [789]. In animals, these long-chain polyunsaturated fatty acids are formed from linoleic acid (18:2(n–6)) or α-linolenic acid (18:3(n–3)). These two essential fatty acids can, therefore, be regarded as the ultimate dietary precursors of all PGs and their derivatives.

For the greater part, the precursor fatty acids are not available as such. Most of them have to be released from phospholipids [476, 835] by means of phospho-lipases, the exact nature of which is still a controversial point (See Chapter 3). Cholesterol esters have also been mentioned as possible fatty acid donors, especially in the adrenal cortex. Recently, attention has been drawn to the importance of tissue free fatty acids as substrates for PG-synthesis [475]. The first step in prostanoid synthesis is the enzymatic conversion of a precursor fatty acid into a prostaglandin endoperoxide, PGH [330, 626]. The enzyme involved (prostaglandin endoperoxide synthase or cyclo-oxygenase, CO) is present in virtually all tissues of the body.

The PG-endoperoxide PGH has only a short half-life because it is converted by

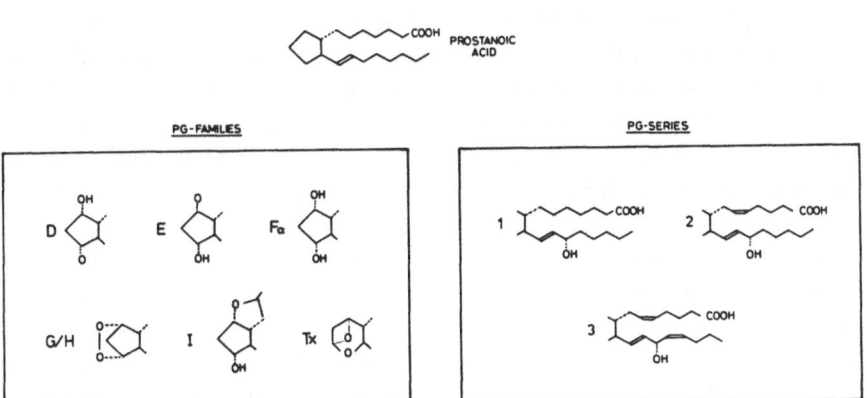

Fig. 2.8. Structural features of some prostanoid families

various, mostly membrane-bound, isomerases into other PGs [330, 626] or into thromboxanes [333]. The activities of the different isomeras are quantitatively different in the various tissues resulting in a different profile of end-products [646]. In blood platelets, the vast majority of the PG-endoperoxides are converted into thromboxanes [333]. In the vessel wall, PGs of the I-family predominate [176, 564]. Since these platelet and vascular compounds are of great importance for hemostasis and thrombosis, their formation, effects and metabolism will be discussed in more detail in Chapter 3.

The amounts of PGs formed depend on the availability of their substrate fatty acids (See Chapter 8) as well as on the efficiency of the enzyme-substrate interaction [477, 789]. Since in most tissues, the arachidonic acid content is much higher than that of dihomo-γ-linolenic acid, and because timnodonic acid is a poor substrate for the CO enzyme system [315, 598, 789], the 2-series are likely to be the most important PGs quantitatively and are, therefore, studied most extensively.

The majority of the PG-effects are mediated by changes at the intracellular level of adenosine-3'-5'-monosphate (cAMP), following PG-binding to specific receptors at the surface of the target cells [19, 301, 555, 748]. cAMP is also implicated in PG-synthesis; it has a stimulating effect in some cells and an inhibitory effect in other ones [717]. An example of a cAMP-mediated PG-effect is the antilipolytic action of PGEs observed by Steinberg and coworkers [785], which is possibly of great importance for the regulation of plasma free fatty acid levels [141].

2.8.3. Some other functions of fatty acids

Although they lie outside the scope of the present study, some other important functions of fatty acids deserve further attention. There is ample evidence that polyunsaturated fatty acids are implicated in a great many transport processes, e.g. in the removal of triglycerides and cholesterol from the liver [419, 608, 754] and in cholesterol excretion via the bile [168]. Dietary polyunsaturated fatty acids have also been shown to reduce the net synthesis of fatty acid synthetase, possibly leading to a reduction of the synthesis of saturated fatty acids [834]. These effects of polyunsaturated fatty acids may contribute to their benefical effect on athero-sclerosis [517, 806]. Apart from atherosclerosis, there are many other diseases in which (a defective?) fatty acid metabolism is involved (cancer, multiple sclerosis, cystic fibrosis, diabetes mellitus – see refs. 137, 403, 455, 553). This underscores the importance of fatty acids in maintaining normal health.

Polyunsaturated fatty acids have also been shown to be good substrates for a cytoplasmatic enzyme – with properties of a lipoxygenase – present in blood plate-lets, leukocytes and mast cells [80, 627]. The function of the resulting hydroxy acids are largely unknown but the arachidonate product of platelet lipoxygenase is known to be involved in the regulation of the Tx-synthase [335], in leukocyte chemotaxis [298, 456, 815] and in irreversible platelet aggregation [207, 208]. Recently, arachidonic acid was shown to be the precursor fatty acid of leukotrienes, a group of non-cyclized C_{20}-carboxylic acids with one or two oxygen substituents and three conjugated double bonds, produced by polymorphonuclear leukocytes [718]. It has been proposed that leukotriene A, the unstable intermediate in the formation of leukotrienes B, C, D, E and F, is the direct precursor of SRS-A, the slowreacting substance of anaphylaxis, and important mediator in asthma and other immediate hypersensitivity reactions [582, 658].

2.9. LIPID METABOLISM OF PLATELETS

Blood platelets have an active lipid metabolism. They are capable of de novo synthesis of fatty acids and phospholipids [123, 146, 147, 188, 372, 501, 512, 778] and activily exchange these substances with those from the surrounding plasma [47, 124, 431]. Although they contain only few mitochondria, fatty acid oxidation is yet an important source of energy [311]. Since platelets lack one or more components of the methyl-sterol demethylase system [184, 185], they are unable to synthesize cholesterol and although cholesterol biosynthesis in megakaryocytes has been reported, the most likely possibility of altering the platelet cholesterol content is via an exchange with the surrounding medium [740]. Platelet lipid metabolism is greatly stimulated upon platelet activation with aggregating agents [189, 190, 488, 492–495]. This strongly indicates that lipid metabolism is of primary importance in platelet function, which has been confirmed by the discovery of the functional implications of platelet fatty acid peroxidation [522]. Since this latter pathway is likely to be affected by dietary lipids, it will be discussed in detail in Chapter 3.

3. THE ROLE OF PROSTANOIDS IN ARTERIAL THROMBOREGULATION

3.1. INTRODUCTION

The formation of an arterial thrombus is triggered by the disruption of the endothelial barrier between blood and subendothelium either by the removal of endothelium or by its contraction [744, 745]. Endothelial damage sufficient to initiate a thrombotic response, can be caused by factors such as chronic hypercholesterolemia [702], chronic homocyteinemia [342], smoking [585], hypertension [227], wall shear forces [272], etc. Exposure of the subendothelium to blood results in the simultaneous occurrence of two closely interrelated processes: the response of blood platelets toward their activation and blood clotting. Platelet activation may lead to the formation of a fragile platelet thrombus via a series of frequently reviewed processes [259, 588, 846]. In brief, circulating platelets adhere to subendothelial tissue – collagen, microfibrils, basement membrane – which may become blood-exposed after vessel-trauma, rupture of an atherosclerotic plaque, etc. Adhered platelets release some of their constituents, such as adenine nucleotides, serotonin, Ca^{++} and adrenaline. Adenosine diphosphate (ADP), made available by this release reaction, causes blood platelets, to aggregate: passing platelets stick to the adhered ones, thus forming a mural platelet thrombus which, being unstable, is easily embolized. The platelet release reaction is also induced by platelet aggregation; so the formation of mural and circulating platelet thrombi is a self-propagating process.

Since vascular tissue has thromboplastic activity [601], vessel wall damage is likely to trigger extrinsic clotting. Moreover, subendothelial collagen, while interacting with one of the contact factors (Factor XII, ref. 604, 860) or with platelets [838, 839], triggers the intrinsic coagulation system, which is also initiated by platelets per se when activated by low amounts of ADP [837, 839]. Coagulation is accelerated by platelet factor 3 (PF3) a platelet-phospholipoprotein-associated clot-promoting entity which is normally inactive [237] but which becomes available upon platelet activation [430, 759]. The contribution of coagulation to the process of arterial thrombus formation has long been considered to be of secondary importance. This contribution would be confined to reinforcement of the fragile white platelet thrombus by fibrin. However, evidence is becoming available indicating that coagulation is of primary importance here, because thrombin formation appeared to be a prerequisite for the platelet aggregation response upon vessel wall damage [398, 400].

In recent years, much progress has been made in the elucidation of biochemical events following platelet activation and associated with the platelet release reaction. Moreover, the antithrombotic properties of the intact vessel wall can now be explained in biochemical terms. This knowledge resulted in the formulation of a homeostatic concept of the regulation of thrombosis in which prothrombotic Thromboxane A_2, produced by activated blood platelets, and antithrombotic prostacyclin, formed by the vascular wall, are considered to play a key role [566].

3.2. PLATELET PROSTAGLANDINS AND THROMBOXANES

Kloeze [458] was the first to show that prostaglandins are very active modulators of platelet aggregation in vitro: prostaglandin E_1 (PGE_1) had a strong inhibitory effect while PGE_2 was slightly stimulating. Of the later discovered natural prostaglandins, only PGD_2 [638, 766], and prostacyclin (PGI_2 ref. 564) were shown to be potent antiaggregants. Since Kloeze's observations, confirmed in later studies by himself and others [229, 386, 452, 460, 747], circulating prostaglandins have been regarded as possible regulators of platelet aggregation and, consequently, of thrombus formation.

In 1970, Smith and Willis demonstrated that, simultaneously with their release reaction, activated platelets produce prostaglandins, PGE_2 in particular [770]. One year later, they discovered that preincubation of the platelets with aspirin, which is known to block the platelet release reaction [632, 845], inhibited prostaglandin production by platelet [764]. These findings led them to postulate that PGE_2, produced by platelets upon their activation, mediated the release reaction of these platelets and, consequently, their involvement in aggregation and thrombus formation. However, a mediatory role of endogenously formed PGE_2 in the platelet release reaction was not in line with the finding that exogenous PGE_2 did not induce platelet release and aggregation. Therefore, a short-lived intermediate was proposed in the conversion of arachidonic acid into PGE_2. Such an intermediate was indeed isolated and characterized by various groups [330, 626, 857]. In fact, two intermediates were found which, because of their molecular configuration, were called cyclic endoperoxides and named PGG_2 (a hydroperoxide) and PGH_2. They were shown to be synthesized from arachidonic acid (AA) by an enzyme complex, prostaglandin synthase or cyclo-oxygenase (CO). The endoperoxides were able to aggregate blood platelets and their formation was blocked by aspirin and other nonsteroidal anti-inflammatory drugs as a result of CO-inactivation. Moreover, they appeared to be labile substances which are either quickly metabolized to the 'classical' PGs (E_2, D_2, $F_{2\alpha}$, etc.) or inactivated [331]. Yet the hypothesis that endogenously formed endoperoxides mediate platelet-release and aggregation [332] could not be maintained for a long time because the endoperoxide levels did not correlate with the degree in which these platelet reactions occurred. In fact, further studies suggested the existence of a highly unstable, very potent endoperoxide derivative. Using highly elegant 'trapping' techniques, Hamberg and coworkers succeeded in the isolation and characterization of such an endoperoxide metabolite [333, 794]. On theoretical and experimental grounds, the structure of this substance was proposed to contain an oxane ring and because of its very potent prothrombotic effect, it was named Thromboxane A_2 (TxA$_2$). TxA$_2$ appeared to be formed from PGH$_2$ by an isomerase-type of enzyme (Tx-synthase) and to have a very strong platelet-activating and vasoconstricting effect. It should be mentioned here that TxA$_2$ is identical to the so-called 'rabbit aorta contracting substance' (RCS), released from guinea-pig lungs during anaphylaxis [658].

3.3. VASCULAR PROSTAGLANDINS

Although arterial thrombosis is known to occur in close contact with the vascular wall, it was recognized only recently that vascular tissue is implicated not only in thrombus formation but in thromboregulation as well. Thus, in 1974 Heyns and coworkers [364] demonstrated that platelet aggregation could be inhibited by an aorta-intima extract. Their research resulted in the discovery that vascular tissue contains an ADPase activity which may play a role in thromboregulation. [365, 366, 489]. Saba and Mason [711] demonstrated that cultured endothelial cells produce a principle that inhibits platelet aggregation, serotonin release and clot retraction, thereby confirming that the vascular wall may have an active thromboregulatory function.

In 1976 Kulkarni and colleagues [468, 595] demonstrated that arachidonic acid (AA), perfused through coronary arteries, caused distinct vasodilatation which could be inhibited by pre-treatment of the vascular bed with aspirin and indomethacin. This suggested that AA is converted by blood vessels into a prostaglandin-like substance, different from TxA$_2$ or PGE$_2$, which both contract coronary arteries. The unknown substance appeared to be degraded to 6-keto-PGF$_{1\alpha}$ [674], a compound that had previously been shown to be produced by rat stomach homogenates [645]. In the same year it was demonstrated that vascular tissue indeed produces a prostaglandin with activities quite opposite to those of TxA$_2$ [564]. This vascular prostaglandin, PGI$_2$ or prostacyclin [429], appeared a very potent vasodilator and platelet aggregation inhibitor. It is derived from PGH$_2$ by a microsomal enzyme, prostacyclin synthase. Since the vessel wall contains AA as well as the cyclo-oxygenase enzyme system, PGI$_2$ can be produced from endogenous precursors [108]. Moreover exogenous AA and PGH$_2$ can be used for PGI$_2$-production [564].

3.4. PROSTANOID BIOSYNTHESIS AND METABOLISM

The first step in the biosynthesis of prostanoids (Figs. 3.1 and 3.3.) is the liberation of their precursor fatty acids – arachidonic acid, diomo-γ-linolenic acid and timnodonic acid – from membrane phospholipids. Since arachidonic acid is the most abundant of these prostanoid precursors its conversion will be described in detail here. However, it should be realized that the other precursor fatty acids can be metabolized in a similar way (see section 3.8.).

There is still discussion going on as to the mechanisms by which arachidonic acid (and any other precursor fatty acid) is released from membrane phospholipids and about the specificity of these mechanisms as far as donor-phospholipid classes and releasable fatty acids are concerned. An arachiconic-acid specific phospholipase A_2 has been mentioned as being the enzyme responsible for AA release [65, 534b]. Other investigators hold the view that a phosphatidyl-inositol (PI) specific phospholipase C (in combination with a diglyceride lipase) mediates AA-liberation upon platelet-

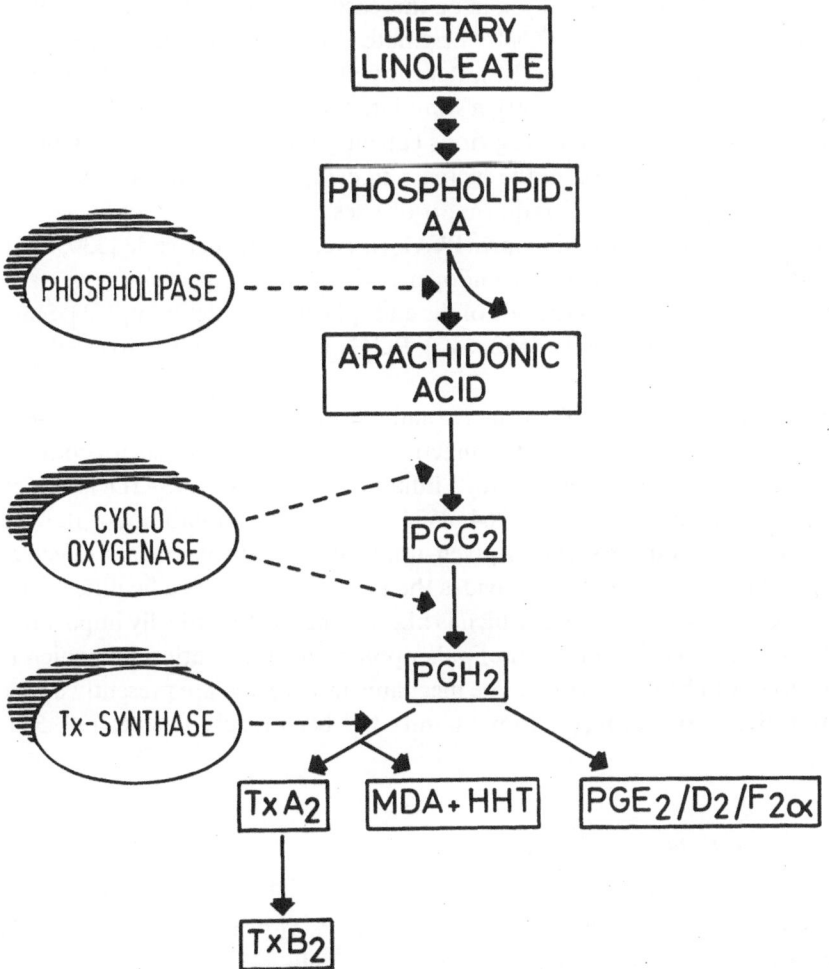

Fig. 3.1. Diagram of formation and metabolism of platelet products formed by the peroxidation of arachidonic acid by the cyclooxygenase enzyme system

triggering [40, 529, 695]. Again others stress the importance of the PI-specific phospholipase, combined with a phosphatidic acid-activated phospholipase A_2 [48, 480]. Finally, a PE specific phospholipase A_2 has been suggested to be implicated in the AA release upon platelet stimulation [99], whereas N-methylation of PE to PC is also thought to be implicated in making available PE-AA [441]. Similar controversies exist about the major AA-donor-phospholipid class: PC [65, 441], PI [40, 729], as well as PE [69, 99, 233] have been mentioned. Since platelets were demonstrated to contain phospholipase A_1 as wel [48, 765, 811] platelet activation may also lead to the liberation of fatty acids esterified to the 1-position of phospholipids.

It is generally agreed that phospholipases require Ca^{++} for their activity. One of the first effects of platelet activation (except when epinephrine is used as a platelet trigger) is platelet shape change. This phenomenon coincides with a redistribution of intra-cellular Ca^{++} stores resulting in an increase in cytoplasmatic Ca^{++} [96]. However, it is suggested that this Ca^{++} originates from a pool different from the one involved in the release reaction [95]. Recently phosphatidic acid (PA), which is formed as a result of the PI-cycle [550] in stimulated platelets [62, 98, 99, 481, 528], has been suggested to act as an endogenous calcium ionophore [48, 738]. Consequently, PA may be implicated in the increase in cytosolic calcium [48, 99, 296], thereby activating further Ca^{++}-requiring processes.

The released AA is peroxidized to form PGG_2, a cyclic hydroperoxide [330, 626]. The enzyme involved (prostaglandin endoperoxide synthase, or cyclo-oxygenase, CO) is located at the cytoplasmatic side of the endoplasmatic reticulum [773]. Since CO has also a peroxidase activity [562, 640], PGG_2 is immediately converted into PGH_2.

The CO-enzyme system is present in virtually all tissues and is a so-called self-destructive enzyme [477] because it is inactivated by the compound it produces [223]. It is inhibited by non-steroidal anti-inflammatory drugs (NSAIDs) such as aspirin and indomethacin [244, 703, 764, 857]. The degree of inhibition is not the same for the various inhibitors, while a given inhibitor is not always equally effective in all tissues [111, 525, 877]. This provides the possibility of a specific differential inhibition of CO in various tissues, which is likely to be therapeutically important.

AA, which is released from phospholipids upon platelet activation but which is not peroxidized, can be re-esterified. The mechanisms involved are presently under investigation by various groups. No unanimity has been reached as yet [99, 534, 534a, 669].

3.4.1. Platelet prostanoids

In blood platelets the vast majority of PGH_2 is converted by another microsomal enzyme Tx-synthase) into TxA_2 (Fig. 3.1.), which is very unstable and quickly hydrolizes, forming a stable but inactive derivative, TxB_2 [333, 879]. Concomitant with TxB_2 two other platelet-inactive products are formed from PGH_2 containing 17 (12-hydroxy heptadecatrienoic acid, HHT) and 3 (malondialdehyde, MDA) carbon atoms, respectively, [192, 675]. MDA is formed in equimolar amounts with TxB_2 upon platelet activation [54]. Therefore, MDA seems a suitable indicator of platelet TxA_2 formation. Inhibition of TxA_2-production by five different Tx-synthase inhibitors is linearly correlated with the inhibition of HHT formation [192]. This indicates that the Tx-synthase enzyme is also involved in the formation of HHT and that, consequently, HHT formation is a good measure for TxA_2 production. Recently, evidence has been obtained that HHT is not a decomposition product of TxA_2 [336]. Platelet endoperoxides can also be converted into the so-called classical prostaglandins (PGE_2, D_2 and $F_{2\alpha}$) but under normal conditions this only occurs to a minor degree [332, 333].

Because of the instability of TxA_2 (its half-life in a saline medium is only 30 s) its molecular configuration has not yet been confirmed. However the structure given in Fig. 3.2 is the most likely since it is the only possible one meeting the demands set by the molecular reaction sequence. TxA_2-stability is increased in plasma [768] and in albumin-containing solutions [256] which is likely to be connected with the covalent binding between TxA_2 and albumin [508]. Free fatty acids lower this TxA_2-protective effect of serum albumin [473].

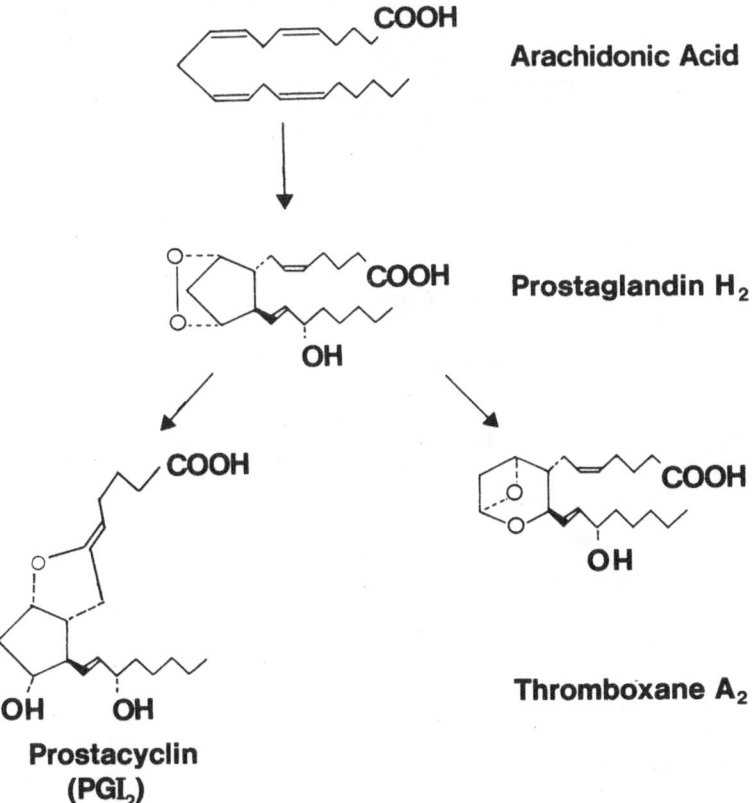

Fig. 3.2. Molecular structure of some prostanoids implicated in haemostasis and thrombosis

36

3.4.2. *Vascular prostanoids*

Although the vessel wall does produce some TxA_2 (6,416), the major vascular prostanoid is prostacyclin, PGI_2. This anti-aggregating and vasodilating compound is formed from PGH_2 [108, 313, 564] by the enzyme prostacyclin synthase (Fig. 3.3.). Vascular tissue also produces some PGE_2 [522]. Prostacyclin formation can be inhibited by inactivation of the vascular cyclo-oxygenase enzyme system [313], which initially was thought to be less sensitive towards aspirin than the platelet enzyme [34, 111]. Later experiments, however, revealed that both CO's are equally sensitive to non-steroidal anti-inflammatory drugs [115, 670] but thanks to

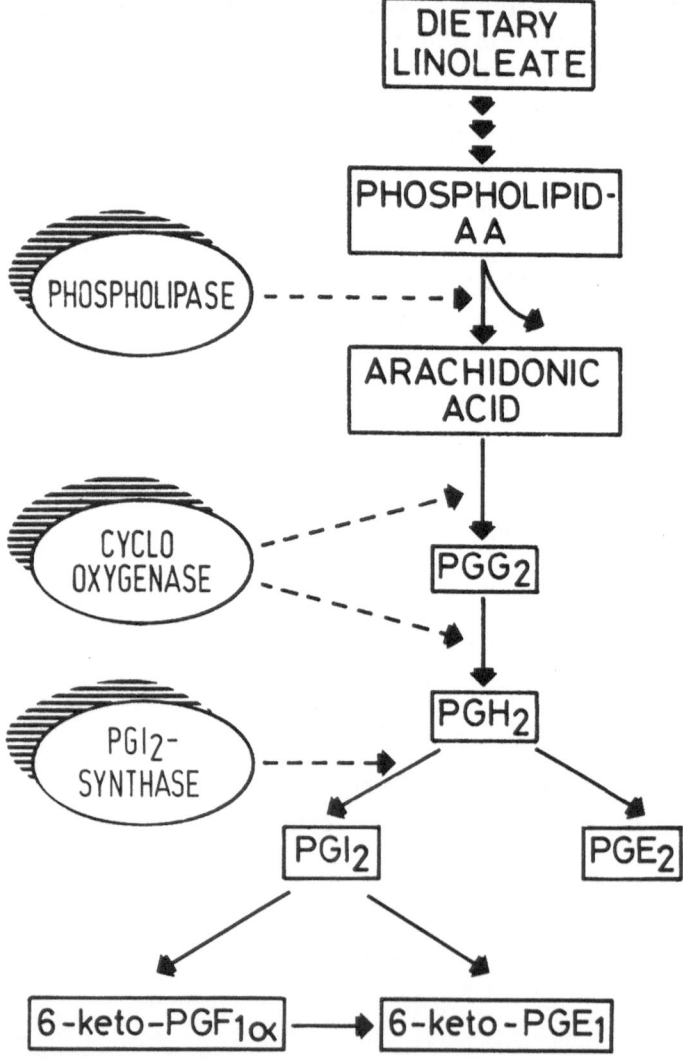

Fig. 3.3. Diagram of formation and metabolism of vascular 2-series prostanoids

endothelial protein synthesis, restoration of CO-activity takes place rather rapidly [167, 421]. Prostacyclin synthase is very sensitive to inhibition by lipid peroxides [563, 714]. The formation of PGI_2 in vivo can be influenced by various blood-borne factors such as lipoproteins [621], prostaglandins [804], β-thromboglobulin (a platelet-specific protein which is released upon platelet activation, see ref. 382), albumin-bound fatty acids [623], angiotensin [316], bradykinin [316, 380], platelet-derived growth factor [156] and other factors [505, 574, 680, 712].

Prostacyclin is a rather unstable substance and although plasma, serum and albumin have been reported to have a stabilizing effect [79, 661, 854] and prostacyclin is not inactivated in the pulmonary circulation [205, 206] its half-life in circulating blood is only 2–3 min. [139, 205, 715]. The major degradation product of PGI_2 is 6-keto-$PGF_{1\alpha}$ [429]. Recently is has been demonstrated that PGI_2 and 6-keto-$PGF_{1\alpha}$ can be enzymatically converted into 6-keto-PGE_1 [867, 868], which is a stable substance and which initially was reported to be almost as active as PGI_2 in the inhibition of platelet aggregation [20, 866]. However, later results showed the effect of 6-keto-PGE_1 to be about 1/20 of that of PGI_2 [556, 852a]. Consequently, the physiological relevance of 6-keto-PGE_1 is not clear as yet and needs further investigation.

Evidence has been presented that prostacyclin circulates in the blood, which gave rise to the concept that PGI_2 is a circulating hormone [314, 360, 565]. However, this concept has recently been contested by different research groups [70a, 140, 247a, 346, 346a, 679, 783a] and although there is still no unanimity on this point there is increasing doubt as to the validity of the view that PGI_2 would be a circulating hormone. Moreover, the importance of possible circulating PGI_2 as a constant platelet-deactivator might be doubtful because of the phenomenon of agonist-specific desensitization, which has been recognized for prostaglandin-mediated effects on platelet adenylate cyclase [154, 304, 555].

As stated before, the vessel wall generates an efficient ADPase activity [364, 366, 489]. However, the major contribution to the anti-thombotic properties of endothelium seems to be due to its production of prostacyclin [109].

3.5. INTERACTION BETWEEN PLATELET AND VASCULAR PROSTANOIDS

Since the formation of PGI_2 depends on the availability of PGH_2, an active vascular CO-enzyme system is a prerequisite for the endogenous production of prostacyclin. Consequently NSAIDs, by inhibiting CO, also inhibit vascular PGI_2-formation [313, 825]. Yet when indomethacin-treated vascular tissue, which upon incubation in buffer did not produce any PGI_2, was incubated with PRP, the vascular PGI_2-production was restored [108, 590]. On the basis of this observation it has been suggested that activated blood platelets can be a source of exogenous endoperoxides, stimulating vascular prostacyclin production and, consequently, limiting the growth of a platelet thrombus [108, 566]. Although an endoperoxide transfer from activated blood platelets to cultured endothelial cells can be demonstrated [523], there is now increasing evidence that no such transfer occurs in blood vessels under normal conditions. Thus it has been demonstrated that isolated perfused rabbit hearts showed a decrease in coronary perfusion pressure when infused with arachidonic acid, due to generation of PGI_2. However, when cyclic endoperoxides were perfused, the coronary perfusion pressure increased, suggesting that under those conditions the endothelium did not metabolize extracellular cyclic endoperoxides to PGI_2 [597]. Moreover, when isolated pulsatingly perfused rat aorta's [281] and isolated rabbit hearts [733] pre-treated with aspirin, were perfused with platelet rich plasma no prostacyclin production could be detected.

Using punched-out pieces of rat aorta, we demonstrated that under a variety of conditions, activated blood platelets do not supply the vascular wall with endoperoxides for prostacyclin formation. We also demonstrated that the results which suggested such an endoperoxide transfer [108] were artefacts, caused by a 'washout' of indomethacin from the cyclo-oxygenase enzyme system which occurs more readily in plasma than in buffer [397]. However, if platelets are prevented from using endogenously generated PGH_2 for TxA_2 synthesis, endoperoxides can escape from the platelets and can be used by the vessel wall as an exogenous substrate for PGI_2-production [596, 599, 605]. Therefore, although the 'stealing hypothesis' may be invalid as a homeostatic concept, it certainly has its value as a therapeutic concept.

3.6. FUNCTIONAL SIGNIFICANCE OF PROSTANOIDS IN HAEMOSTASIS AND THROMBOSIS

TxA_2 is an active vasoconstrictor and platelet aggregating agent, whereas prostacyclin is a potent vasodilator and inhibitor of platelet aggregation. Therefore, both substances are likely to be of regulatory importance in haemostasis and arterial thrombogenesis.

3.6.1. *TxA₂, platelet aggregation and ADP release*

As demonstrated originally by Hamberg and coworkers [333, 794] aggregation induced by collagen is preceeded by the formation of sufficient amounts of TxA_2 to mediate the release of ADP. The TxA_2 produced by and the ADP released from the collagen-activated platelets also causes other platelets to aggregate. When the platelet-TxA_2 production is inhibited by pre-treatment of the platelets with aspirin, platelet release and aggregation diminish proportionally. However, this inhibition can simply be overcome by increasing the trigger-strength [881] without reactivation of platelet TxA_2-formation [273]. Moreover, in vitro inhibition of thromboxane synthase does not necessarily result in the prevention of platelet aggregation [52]. This demonstrates that platelet aggregation and release can occur indepently from TxA_2-formation also. Consequently, TxA_2-production is not a prerequisite for these platelet reactions but potentiates them as a result of which a certain degree of platelet activation requires a low trigger strength.

Experiments performed with platelets lacking ADP in their granules revealed that TxA_2 also has a direct, ADP-independent, platelet aggregating effect [415, 453, 547], however we produced strong evidence that this direct pathway is not all that important in arterial thrombus formation. When a loop-shaped polyethylene canula is inserted into the abdominal aorta of rats, endothelial damage and flow disturbances produce the formation and growth of a fibrin-poor platelet-rich thrombus which obstructs the aortic blood flow after about 4–5 days [389] (see also Chapter 4). In an experiment in which normal rats were given sufficient amounts of

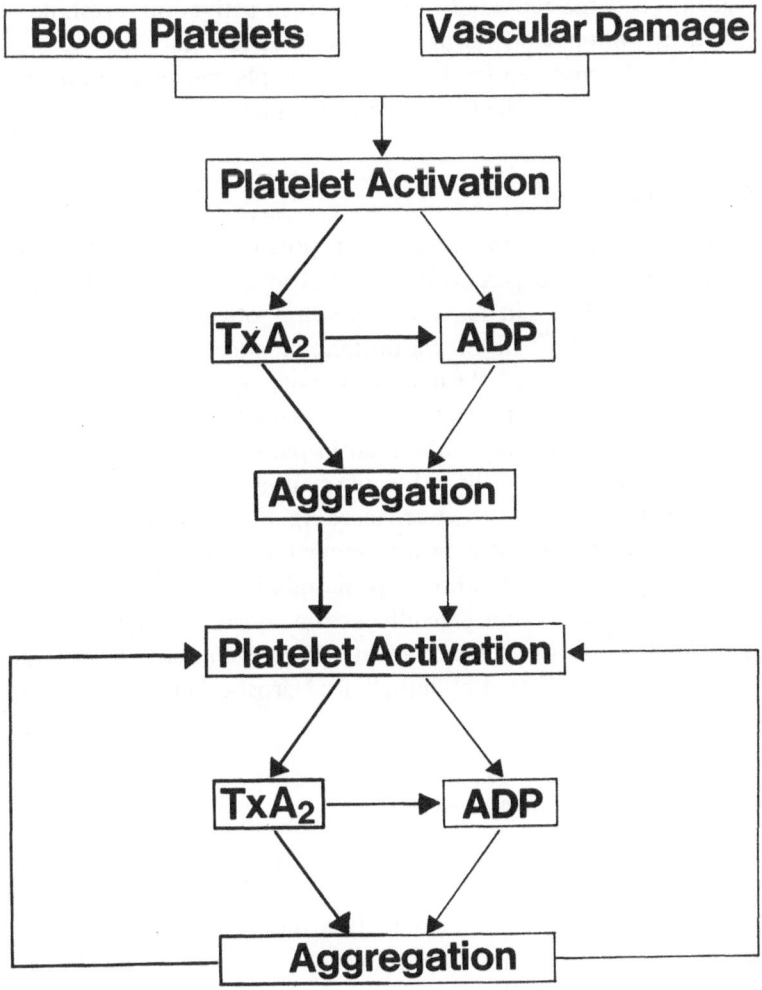

Fig. 3.4. Diagram, illustrating the role of TxA_2-formation and ADP release in platelet aggregation

aspirin to block platelet TxA_2 formation completely, this so-called obstruction time (OT) increased from 4 (no aspirin) to about 6 days. Some time ago, a special strain of rats was discovered whose platelets lack ADP in their secretion granules [673, 813]. The obstruction times of these animals appeared to be more than 26 days (see Chapter 4), although the platelets of these rats produced normal amounts of TxA_2 upon their activation [399]. This finding strongly indicates that, ultimately, the ADP release of platelets is more important for arterial thrombogenesis than their potency to produce TxA_2.

Figure 3.4 summarizes the role of TxA_2 in platelet aggregation following vascular injury. Platelets adhering to the subendothelium become activated as a result of which they release ADP and produce TxA_2 which facilitates this ADP-release. Both substances cause passing platelets to aggregate with the adhered ones. These newly aggregated platelets also become activated – provided their activation threshold is exceeded – and in turn produce and release TxA_2 and ADP, respectively, thus initiating a self-propagating and reinforcing process of platelet activation and aggregation that ultimately leads to the formation of the platelet thrombus.

3.6.2. *TxA₂ in primary haemostasis*

TxA_2 is an active vasoconstrictor and, moreover, a potent platelet aggregating agent. Since primary haemostasis depends on vasoconstriction and platelet aggregation, a functional role of TxA_2 in haemostasis seems obvious. This view is supported by the finding that the well-known prolonging effect of aspirin on the bleeding time [632, 845], coincides with the inactivation of platelet cyclo-oxygenase [244, 704, 764] as a result of which no endoperoxides and TxA_2 can be formed. Moreover, a bleeding tendency has been observed in patients with a cyclo-oxy-genase deficiency [515] and recently a thromboxane synthase deficiency has been described [545, 847] which coincides with severe bleeding. Not long ago Buchanan and coworkers [104] demonstrated that aspirin-treatment of the vessel wall leads to shortening of the bleeding time in thrombocytopenic rabbits. This strongly indi-cates that, apart from TxA_2, prostacyclin can influence haemostasis by mechanisms independent of platelet aggregation. Dejana et al. [179] even showed that the bleeding time is not necessarily affected by unbalanced prostanoid production in platelets and the vessel wall.

3.6.3. *The role of TxA₂ in arterial thrombosis*

Platelet release and aggregation are fundamental processes in arterial thrombus formation and since TxA_2 plays an important role in these processes, it is likely to be implicated in arterial thrombogenesis. Unfortunately, arterial thrombosis tendency cannot be determined in humans, so the importance of platelet TxA_2 for arterial thrombosis cannot be assessed directly. However, in various conditions known to be associated with an increased risk for myocardial infarction, the potency of activated platelets to produce TxA_2 is enhanced [428, 790, 799]. This strongly indicates that TxA_2 is of functional relevance in arterial thrombogenesis. As will be demonstrated in Chapter 6, in rats the tendency to develop arterial thrombosis is positively correlated with the TxA_2-production of activated platelets. This supports the concept that TxA_2 plays an important role in arterial thromboregulation.

3.6.4. *The thromboxane–prostaglandin balance*

The striking opposite effects of TxA_2 and PGI_2 on platelet aggregation, vascular tone and cAMP metabolism (see section 3.7.) gave rise to the concept that arterial thrombosis tendency and platelet aggregability primarily depend on the ratio between prothrombotic TxA_2 and antithrombotic PGI_2 [402, 566]. Evidence is now accumulating that this concept of balance is valid indeed. Thus, in diabetes mellitus platelet TxA_2-formation has been reported to be enhanced [327a, 428, 790] and vascular PGI_2-production to be depressed [428, 750], causing an increased TxA_2/PGI_2 ratio. Since in diabetes the tendency to develop arterial thrombosis may be enhanced (as judged from the higher risk for myocardial infarction), these findings are in agreement with the concept of balance, although it should be noted that plasma levels of TxA_2 and PGI_2 are not different from normal in diabetes [172]. In uremia the potency of stimulated platelets to produce TxA_2 is depressed, whereas vascular prostacyclin formation is increased [280, 679, 680]. Consequently, in uremia the TxA_2/PGI_2 ratio is diminished which coincides with a lower platelet aggregability.

In Chapter 6 it will be demonstrated that the tendency in rats to develop arterial thrombosis can be modified by dietary means without changing the TxA_2/PGI_2 ratio. These results in fact suggest that the prothrombotic effect of platelet TxA_2 is more important for arterial thrombus formation than the antithrombotic effect of vascular PGI_2. A similar conclusion may be drawn from the observation that in congenital CO deficiency – resulting in a profoundly reduced synthesis of both TxA_2 and PGI_2 – the haemostatic balance favours bleeding rather than thrombosis [515, 648]. Therefore, lowering platelet TxA_2-formation seems a most efficient way to decrease platelet aggregability and arterial thrombosis tendency.

3.7. PROSTANOID MECHANISMS OF ACTION

In the mechanism by which TxA_2 facilitates the ADP release of blood platelets, most probably the cytoplasmatic Ca^{++}-content is involved (Fig. 3.5). In cooperation with the Ca-binding protein calmodulin, Ca^{++} activates platelet contractile proteins, initiating an intra-platelet contractile 'wave' which forces the ADP-containing granules to empty their contents in the platelet's environment [606]. Evidence has been obtained that TxA_2 liberates Ca^{++} from intracellular stores [295, 303] and, moreover, it has been suggested that TxA_2 [292, 294], PA (see section 3.4.) and lyso-PA [296] act as endogenous Ca^{++}-ionophores and, by promoting the influx of extracellular Ca^{++}, are implicated in the increase of the cytoplasmatic Ca^{++}-concentration. Enhancement of the cytosolic Ca^{++}-content is likely to inhibit the adenylate cyclase system, resulting in a decrease in platelet cAMP [302]. Since cAMP is implicated in the sequestration of cytosolic Ca^{++} [448], this feedback mechanism keeps the cytosolic Ca^{++} content elevated and, by continuous activation of phospholipases, promotes further TxA_2 formation, platelet aggregation and ADP-release.

The platelet aggregation-inhibiting activity of prostacyclin and other anti-aggregating prostaglandins (PGE_1, PGD_2) is most probably mediated by their stimulating effect on platelet adenylate cyclase as a result of which they increase the platelet cAMP content [300, 558, 559, 696, 716, 801]. This has been shown to lower the cytoplasmatic Ca^{++}-content [448] and to inhibit the release of AA from platelet membrane phospholipids [479, 561]. Moreover, there is evidence that cAMP in-

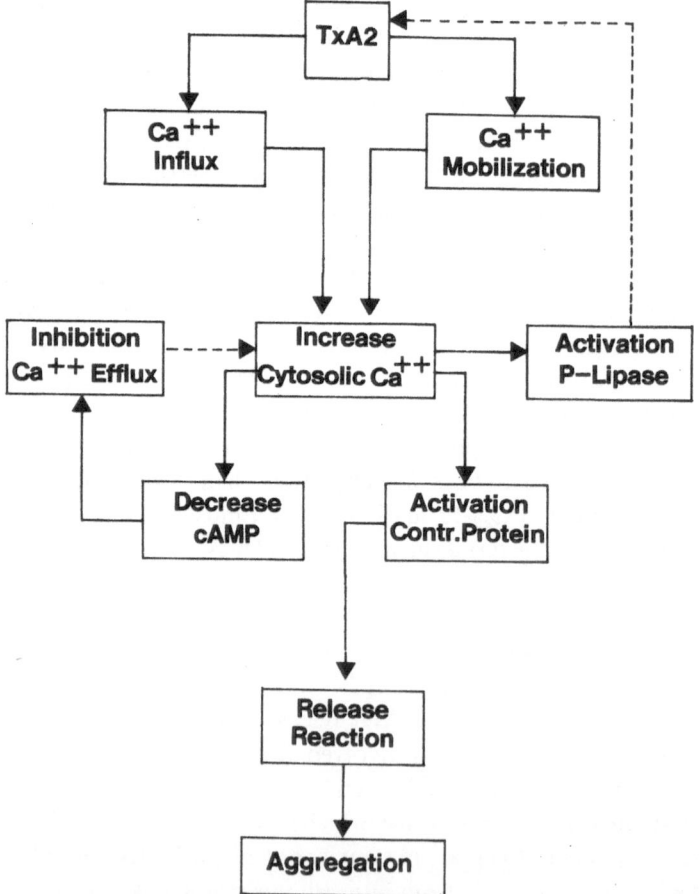

Fig. 3.5. Role of TxA_2 and Ca^{++} in the ADP-release and aggregation of activated blood platelets

hibits the oxygenation of free AA [516, 727]. Although this latter effect is still somewhat controversial [727], it is generally agreed that an increase in cAMP inhibits platelet activation, at least in part, by feedback inhibition of the generation of TxA_2, which inhibits cAMP accumulation upon adenylate cyclase stimulation [554].

The effects of thromboxane A_2 and prostaglandins on platelet function are mediated by specific receptors at the platelet surface [555, 748]. It is highly probable that the anti-aggregating prostaglandins PGD_2 and PGI_2 have different platelet receptors [506, 555, 748, 850]. The receptor for a third anti-aggregating prostaglandin (PGE_1) is probably similar to that for PGI_2 and PGE_2. These prostaglandin receptors are coupled to adenylate cyclase as a consequence of which all PG's mentioned here increase platelet cAMP [300, 558, 559, 696, 716, 801]. PGE_2 has a dual effect on platelet cAMP since it is also a strong inhibitor of cAMP via a mechanism possibly similar to that of endoperoxides and TxA_2 [76].

3.8. PROSTANOIDS OF THE 1- AND 3-SERIES

So far, only prostanoids of the 2-series have been discussed but it should be realized that the other prostanoid precursor fatty acids, dihomo-γ-linolenic acid and timnodonic acid, when present in platelets, can possibly be converted along the same pathway as arachidonic acid into TxA_1 and TxA_3, respectively. The amounts of prostaglandins formed depend on the availability of their substrate fatty acid (Chapter 8) as well as on the efficiency of the enzyme–substrate interaction [447, 789]. Platelets contain only trace amounts of dihomo-γ-linolenic acid and, consequently, TxA_1 is unlikely to be formed in significant amounts, especially because PGH_1 is a poor substrate for the Tx-synthase [192, 193, 594]. Since PGH_1 lacks a double bond at the $\Delta_{5,6}$ position, formation of PGI_1 is impossible.

In fish-eating populations arachidonic acid is partly replaced by timnodonic acid, thus creating a potential for the formation of prostanoids of the 3-series. However, as will be discussed in Chapter 7, feeding fish oil to rats does not result in the formation of significant amounts of TxA_3 and PGI_3, which is most probably due to the fact that timnodonic acid is a poor substrate for the cyclo-oxygenase enzyme system [334, 476, 789, 835].

4. EFFECT OF TYPE AND AMOUNT OF DIETARY FATS ON ARTERIAL THROMBUS FORMATION

4.1. INTRODUCTION

It is now generally accepted that the type and amount of dietary fat can affect the genesis and course of experimental atherosclerosis [307, 410, 466, 517, 807, 829, 841, 862]. Moreover, epidemiological studies clearly indicate that the type of dietary fat has a distinct influence on coronary artery disease (CAD), which is one of the clinical manifestations of atherosclerosis [363, 442, 689, 781]. Human prospective studies also showed that diets low in long chain saturated fatty acids enriched with linoleic acid are beneficial to CAD-prevention [175, 487, 552, 818]. As demonstrated in Chapter 1, there is a close relationship between arterial thrombosis and atherosclerosis, although this relationship is not exclusive [157, 158, 602, 762, 842]. However, as atherosclerosis is a multifactorial disease [84], the dietary fats may, at least in part, be effective through their influence on arterial thrombosis.

4.2. DIETARY FATS AND ARTERIAL THROMBOSIS: A LITERATURE SURVEY

When we started our investigations, the effect of dietary fatty acid compositions on arterial thrombus formation had not yet been investigated systematically. One of the reasons might have been the lack of a suitable in vivo model of arterial thrombogenesis. The body of information available at that time was mainly based on acute experiments, although 'diet' is a chronic factor, with models, the relevance of which to arterial thrombus formation is questionable. Nevertheless, a survey of the available literature in this field was thought appropriate, because earlier knowledge had to serve as a frame of reference for our own research. Another review has been published by Renaud [688]. The majority of the experiments discussed below were published before 1972. Later studies relevant to our field of interest and the work of Renaud et al [681–684] will be dealt with while discussing our own findings.

Many thrombosis models utilize the intra-arterial insertion of foreign material or are based on the application of vascular shunts or prostheses. Pearl and Friedman [649] observed that feeding dogs an unspecified hypercholesterolemic diet resulted in enhanced thrombotic complications on intra-arterial insertion of a metal wire. Evans and Irvine [234] showed that increased platelet adhesiveness is associated with a reduction of the long-term patency of Dacron ® femoropopliteal bypass grafts in men. They found that linseed and corn oil, 2×5 ml daily for one month, failed to reduce platelet adhesiveness in vitro (modified glass bead column technique [355]).

Downie et al. [200] connected a bifurcated flow chamber to arteriovenous shunts and quantified thrombotic deposits by weighing. Murphy et al. [581], using this technique in pigs, showed that the pattern and distribution of these deposits were strikingly similar to those in early atherosclerosis at comparable sites in the vascular tree. Later, it was demonstrated [407] that the structure of the deposits resembled intravascular platelet thrombi. Using the Downie technique, Mustard et al. [586] showed that enrichment of a normal stock diet with lard (final fat content 11.5%), lard (11.5%) + cholesterol (0.5%) or uncooked egg yolk (final dietary fat and cholesterol content 7.3 and 0.5%, respectively), significantly increased thrombotic deposits in pigs. There were no significantly different effects between the three dietary groups, although the deposits in the egg yolk group were three times as heavy as in the lard groups in spite of the fat content being lower. Unfortunately, this study was not continued, so it is not known whether the higher thrombogenicity of egg yolk as compared with lard is real and, if so, whether this is due to differences in fatty acid composition or to another factor.

Matheus et al. [527] used the same technique in rabbits fed a stock diet as such or supplemented with 6% coconut oil and 2% cholesterol. The enrichment significantly increased the amount of thrombotic deposits, which could be prevented by intravenous infusion of phosphatidyl serine, 30 min prior to the experiment. This antithrombotic effect of phosphatidyl serine was also observed by Mustard et al. [587] and is thought to be due to its anticoagulatory effect [583] in combination with its inhibiting action on the platelet release reaction [607]. However, when added to platelet-rich plasma (1 mg/ml), phosphatidyl serine induces mild, reversible aggregation [450].

From a physiological point of view, diet-induced thrombosis seems to be the better chronic thrombosis model. The diet normally used and originally applied by Thomas and Hartroft [803] contains 40% butter, 5% cholesterol, 2% cholic acid and 0.3% thiouracil. When fed to rats for three to four months, it produces thrombosis in about 50% of the animals, whereas myocardial infarction is observed in about 25%. As reviewed by Howard and Gresham [408], this type of diet produces hypercoagulability [544], hyperlipidemia and hyperlipoproteinemia [409]; it does not affect platelet stickiness, but increases the platelet count. The type of fat determines the thrombogenicity of the diet: butter, lard, hydrogenated coconut oil, cocoa butter, hydrogenated groundnut oil and corn oil being thrombogenic, groundnut oil being nonthrombogenic. Extrapolation of these findings to a normal dietary situation is hardly possible because the diet is highly atypical and causes widely different pathological effects.

A simpler dietary thrombosis model was devised by Ball et al. [21] who used a diet high in fat (28% lard), low in protein (8% casein) and well-balanced as to vitamins and minerals. Ad libitum feeding of a selected strain of mice [22] for about seven weeks resulted in a high incidence of organised atrial platelet-fibrin thrombi, which became lethal in 75% of the animals after thirteen weeks. Thrombosis was preceded by atrial subendothelial edema, endothelial vacuolization, thickening of basement membrane and villous projections from vascular endothelial cells [496]. Endothelial oedema completely regressed on refeeding a normal diet. Under this regimen, thrombosis did not occur although the other lesions persisted [145].

Another feature attributed to the aforementioned diet is a severe, chronic anaemia [23], which is readily reversible on refeeding a normal diet [24]. Ashburn et al. [18] showed that prevention of anaemia by intraperitoneal injections of red cells also prevented the development of atrial thrombi. It is very likely that combined local and general hypoxia (due to endothelial oedema and anaemia respectively) are the thrombogenic factors on feeding this type of diet. As low-protein diets are generally associated with anaemia [17], protein deficiency seems a prerequisite for the thrombogenic effect. The dietary fat level (6, 28 and 40%) did not clearly affect thrombosis frequency during a 12-week feeding period. Only when the experimental time was extended to 56 weeks was thrombosis incidence highest in the 40% fat group, whereas no appreciable difference was observed between the low- and medium-fat diets [144]. Using this thrombosis model, Wicks et al. [853] tested nine different dietary oils and fats for their thrombogenic effect (hydrogenated coconut oil, cod-liver oil, Wesson oil, linseed oil, olive oil, lard, corn oil, butter and cocoa butter). Although these fats had different effects on the frequency of atrial thrombosis and ventricular myocardial necrosis and calcification, little correlation existed between the fatty acid composition of the fats and their activity in producing these lesions. Maguire and Doran [511] showed that on feeding a diet high (25%) in lard and marginal (18%) in proteins, mural endocardial (atria and ventricles) thrombi develop in mice as well as in rats. In rats, this diet caused hypercholesterolemia and initially a sharp rise in triglycerides, followed by a marked decrease and the establishment of a new level at only 40% of the starting value.

From these early experiments it can be concluded that , scarce though it is, the information as to the effects of dietary fats on experimental arterial thrombosis indicates that saturated fats enhance thrombus formation, whereas unsaturated fats are not thrombogenic and may even be antithrombotic. Similar indications have been obtained in some human in vivo studies [339, 552].

4.3. NEW EXPERIMENTAL MODEL OF ARTERIAL THROMBOSIS IN RATS

Research into the effects of nutritional factors on arterial thrombus formation and its underlying processes, requires reliable, (semi-)chronic quantitative in vivo techniques to measure arterial thrombosis tendency and platelet function. Such techniques are not available for human studies. However, current developments with ultrasonic imaging of large superficial arteries [737] and scintigraphic imaging using Indium-III labelled platelets [692] are two promising noninvasive approaches for the detection of thrombi in man. Although numerous techniques to induce experimental thrombosis in animals were available when starting our project [194, 358], none of them met our specific requirements. Therefore, we devised the aorta-loop technique for investigations with rats which

- is simple and inexpensive,
- produces a high thrombosis incidence but a low mortality rate,
- allows the process of thrombus formation to be established in a simple way,
- results in a thrombus, the structure and composition of which are comparable with those of arterial thrombi in man.

This method is based on the insertion of a loop-shaped polyethylene cannula (the aorta loop) into the abdominal aorta. At places where the cannula is in permanent contact with the vessel wall, endothelial damage and flow disturbances result in the formation and growth of a thrombus, which reaches an occlusive state after about five days [389]. As the loop projects from the body and is made of translucent material, the blood flow can be checked without difficulty. If the flow is satisfactory, the colour of the blood is light-red. After the loop has become blocked, the colour rapidly changes from light-red via dark-red to blue or black.

The period between insertion and complete obstruction of the loop is called the obstruction time (OT) and is a measure of the arterial thrombosis tendency of the animal: the longer the OT, the lower the thrombosis tendency. For most experiments, it is sufficient to check the loop twice daily. To prevent the loop from being bitten, a plastic-coated cardboard collar [225] is put around the neck of the animal.

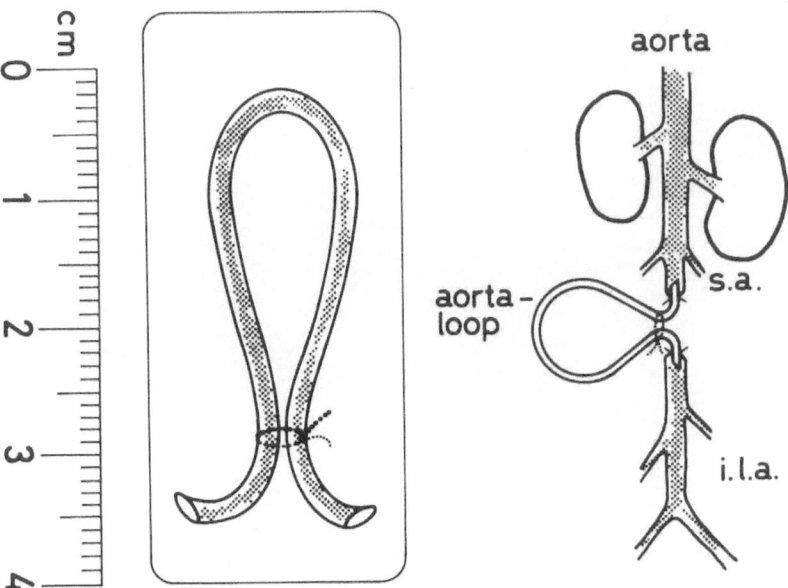

Fig. 4.1. Aorta loop and site of insertion.
s.a.: spermatic arteries.   i.l.a.: iliolumbar arteries.

When the rats are fed a normal stock diet, the obstruction tim (OT) is about five days. Once the loops have become obstructed, the animals do not die because, in the meantime, collateral vessels have developed which take over the blood supply to the hind quarters of the animal. Therefore, it remains possible to take blood samples for plasma and blood cell analyses after OT determination. Within each experimental group, the OT values show a log-normal pattern so that for a statistical evaluation of the results, logarithmic transformation of the OT is necessary.

From histological investigations it appeared that the inserted loop causes endothelial damage; the underlying tissue is denuded and platelets adhere to the affected site. Twenty-four hours after insertion of the aorta loop, large thrombi are already found at both ends of the loop. The platelets nearest to the vessel wall are swollen and have lost their internal structure. In the interstices of the platelet thrombus, numerous erythrocytes are trapped, while accumulations of polynuclear leukocytes are observed on the surface of the aggregates (Fig. 4.2). Strands of fibrin are present among the platelets. The thrombus is not homogeneos but contains several histologically different layers. The vessel wall is degenerated by the pressure of the loop and damaged by the tapered end of the loop. After two and three experimental days, the thrombi, the area of attachment to the vessel wall and the amount of fibrin have

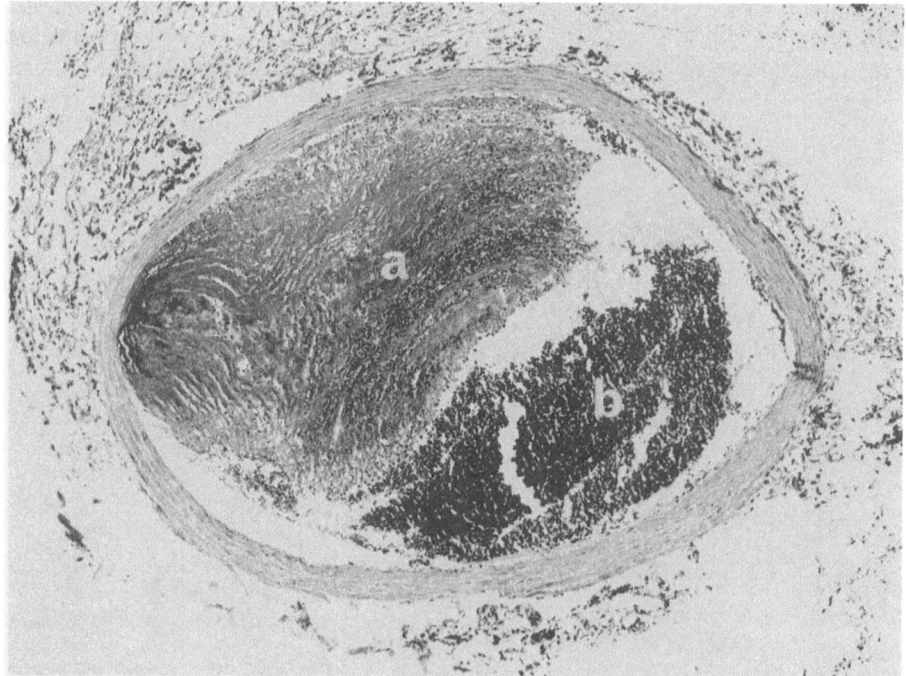

Fig. 4.2. Thrombus after three days (Masson, 55 ×)
(a) Thrombus invaded and surrounded by polynuclear and mononuclear cells.
(b) Erythrocytes.

increased. The thrombus material is invaded by polynuclear leukocytes and mononuclear cells. The trailing ends of the thrombi can be followed for a considerable
distance into the vascular lumen. After four experimental days, the vessel wall
beneath the thrombus is necrotic and in adjacent parts, the smooth muscle cells in
the media show proliferation and mitosis, while the endothelial cells of the aorta are
swollen and pyknotic. After five and six experimental days, smooth muscle cells,
fibroblasts and macrophages penetrate into the thrombus and endothelisation of
the thrombus starts. From this study it could be concluded that the structure of the
thrombi induced by the insertion of an aorta loop in rats is similar, in comparative
phases of development, to that of natural arterial thrombi in man [308] and animals
[763].

In this model, endothelial damage seems to be the initiating stimulus for thrombus formation. In rabbits it was shown, however, that endothelial damage alone

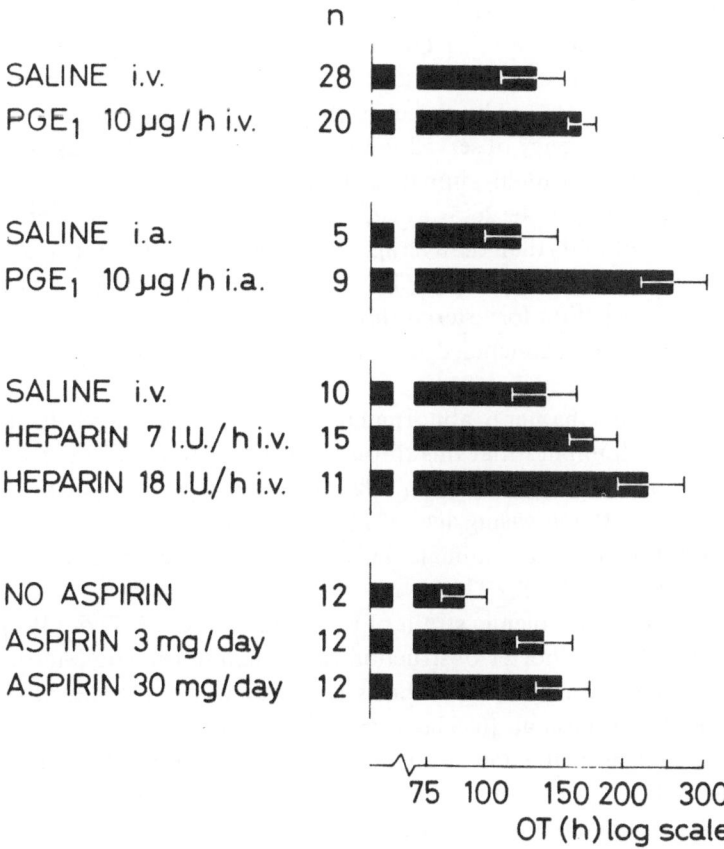

Fig. 4.3. Effect of PGE₁, heparin and aspirin on arterial thrombus formation in rats (OT±SEM).
i.v.:intravenously (jugular vein);
i.a. intra-arterially (descending aorta, just proximal of the aorta loop);
I.U. international units.

does not produce thrombosis but results in the formation of a platelet 'pseudo-endothelium' followed by layering of leukocytes, disappearance of platelets and formation of a new endothelial layer [36]. It is most probable that the turbulent flow, which will occur as a result of aorta cannulation, contributes significantly to the formation of the obstructing thrombus [784]. After loop insertion, food consumption decreases considerably. Restoration takes place rather slowly; this is not due to the cardboard collar, because in sham-operated rats having such a device, food consumption completely normalizes within three days. Haematological investigations after loop insertion showed the normal postoperative changes [221, 389].

The usefulness of the aorta loop technique was demonstrated by the observation that two platelet-function inhibiting compounds (prostaglandin E_1 and aspirin) prolonged the OT dose-dependently. The same was shown to hold for heparin (Fig. 4.3). Obstruction times were also measured in Fawn Hooded (FH) rats. This strain of rats has a hereditary defect of the platelet release reaction: their dense granules, which, in normal animals, contain ATP, ADP, Ca^{++}, seretonin, pyrophosphate and antiplasmin [378], seem to be empty, thus leading to reduced patelet nucleotide and serotonin contents [673, 813]. The defect is thought to be the underlying mechanism of the bleeding tendency observed in these animals [813], because the collagen-induced aggregation is highly impaired [673, 813]. Obstruction times measured in 15 FH rats appeared to be 26.5 days (log OT (h) = 2.80 ± 0.056) which is significantly longer ($P_2 < 0.001$) than the average OT in a group of 16 control rats (log OT (h) = 1.90 ± 0.037, OT $\sim$ 3.5 days). This clearly indicates the importance of platelet release and aggregation for arterial thrombus formation, as initited by the aorta loop. The same can be concluded from experiments with thrombocytopenic rats, performed by Reyers et al. [691].

As will be demonstrated in Chapter 6, abnormal prostanoid formation results in abnormal OT values, which implies that this thrombosis model is, at least partly, dependent on normal prostanoid metabolism. Uzunova and coworkers demonstrated that OTs decrease with increasing age [821] and also that OTs in male rats are significantly shorter than in female animals. This appeared to be connected with the effect of gonadal hormones [821, 822].

Working with a hypercholesterolemic strain of rats, Kim and coworkers [451] showed that these animals had shorter obstruction times than normocholesterolemic controls. This enhanced arterial thrombosis tendency was associated with hypercoagulability. Roncaglioni et al. [699] observed that treatment of female rats with oral contraceptives caused an enhanced tendency to thrombotic occlusion of an aorta loop. The delayed onset of a hypercoagulable state, induced by the treatment of rats with adriamycin [662], was associated with a significant reduction in the occlusion time of aorta loops [180]. Since age, sex and hypercholesterolemia are highly potent myocardial risk indicators [443, 781] and oral contraceptives have also been shown to enhance arterial thrombosis tendency [222, 518, 519] these findings support the usefulness of the aorta-loop technique.

Summarising, the aorta-loop technique provides a useful tool for measuring arterial thrombosis tendency in rats. The technique is relatively simple and inexpensive. Thrombosis frequency is 100% and the incidence of mortality is negligible. Compounds influencing platelet aggregation and blood coagulation, affect the arterial thrombosis tendency in a predictable manner. Moreover, known risk factors for atherosclerosis and thrombosis were shown to be associated with enhanced arterial thrombosis as measured by the aorta-loop technique.

4.4. RELATIONSHIP BETWEEN DIETARY FATTY ACID COMPOSITION AND ARTERIAL THROMBOSIS TENDENCY IN RATS

Three- to five-week-old Wistar rats (specific pathogen-free, SPF) were fed adequate diets, the composition of which is given in Table 4.1. The carbohydrate moiety of the diets was isocalorically replaced by various amounts of differet oils and fats, as indicated in the separate experiments. Aorta loops were inserted after feeding for 8–12 weeks. The loops were checked for obturation twice daily. Obstruction times (OT) were calculated in hours and, because of skwew distribution, transformed to their logarithmic values. Regressions were calculated using the least-squares method.

Because vegetable oils rich in poly-unsaturated fatty acids were shown to inhibit experimental atherogenesis [106, 517], experiments were started with sunflowerseed oil, which contains over 60% linoleic acid.

Table 4.1. Composition of a diet containing 50 en% fat

Ingredients	g.4184 kJ^{-1}	en%
Casein	62.0	23
Minerals ^{a}	5.4	
Vitamin mix ^{b}	1.0	
Sawdust	20.0	
Corn starch	77.1	27
Experimental fat	53.8	50
Total	219.3	100

^{a} g.4184 kJ^{-1}: KCl 0.350, MgHPO$_4$–3H$_2$O 0.956, KH$_2$PO$_4$ 0.475, KHCO$_3$ 0.719, C$_6$H$_5$Na$_3$O$_7$–2H$_2$O 0.711, CaCO$_3$ 2.014, MnHC$_6$H$_5$O$_7$ 0.0756, C$_6$H$_5$FeO$_7$–5H$_2$O 0.0439, Cu$_2$C$_6$H$_6$O$_8$ 0.0036, Zn$_3$(C$_6$H$_5$O$_7$)$_2$–2H$_2$O 0.0125, KIO$_3$ 0.00007
^{b} g.4184 kJ^{-1}: choline 0.250, vitamin E 0.020, calcium silicate 0.05, myoinositol 0.025, vitamin B$_{12}$ 0.000005, vitamin A 0.0077 niacin 0.005, pantothenic acid 0.005, riboflavin 0.0015, thiamin 0,0015, vitamin D 0.00125, vitamin K 0.000227, vitamin B$_6$ 0.0005, folic acid 0.00025, biotin 0.00005, made up to 1.00 with sucrose.

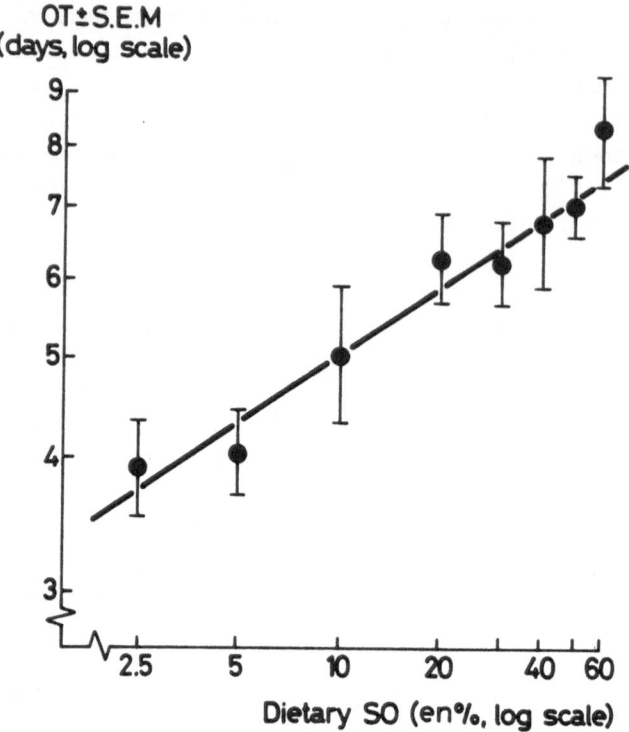

Fig. 4.4. Effect of increasing dietary sunflowerseed oil (SO) content on arterial thrombosis tendency (OT) in rats.

log OT (days) = 0.481 + 0.228 (log en% SO) r = 0.96 ; P <0.001.

Each point represents the mean OT ($\pm$ SEM) of 10–12 animals.

4.4.1. *Effect of increasing amounts of dietary sunflowerseed oil on arterial thrombus formation*

Eight groups of animals, five weeks old, were fed diets containing 2.5 to 60% of digestible energy (en%) sunflowerseed oil (SO) at the expense of carbohydrates. After twelve weeks, arterial thrombosis tendencies were measured. A significantly positive linear relationship was observed between the logarithm of the dietary SO content and the logarithm of the obstruction time (Fig. 4.4). This antithrombotic effect may be due to the increasing amount of dietary SQ or to the decreasing carbohydrate content of the diet. Therefore, in a following experiment, the dietary fat content was kept constant (60 en%) but the amounts of SO were varied by replacing it with various amounts of hydrogenated coconut oil (HCO) or butterflat (BF). In both experimental series, a positive rectilinear relationship was observed between the dietary SO content and the diet-induced thrombosis tendency (Fig. 4.5). This strongly indicates that sunflowerseed oil has an antithrombotic effect. A comparison between the fatty acid composition of sunflowerseed oil, hydrogenated coconut oil and butterfat (Table 4.2., fats No. 11–13) suggests that linoleic acid may

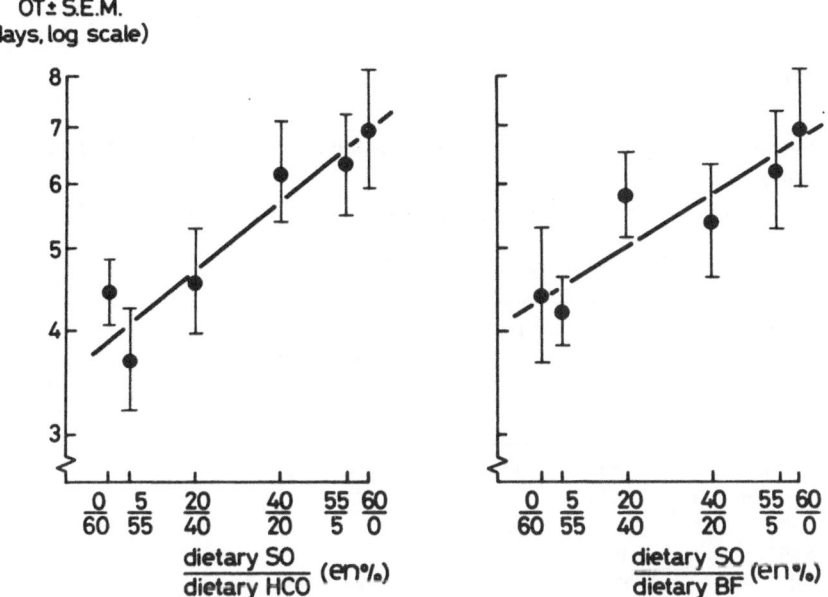

Fig. 4.5. Effect of increasing amounts of sunflowerseed oil (SO), mixed with hydrogenated coconut oil (HCO, left) or butterfat (BF, right) on arterial thrombosis tendency in rats. n = 9–11

SO/HCO : log OT (days) = 0.59 + 0.004 en% SO; r = 0.94 ; P < 0.01
SO/BF   : log OT (days) = 0.64 + 0.003 en% SO; r = 0.91 ; P < 0.02

be responsible for the antithrombotic effect of sunflowerseed oil. This suggestion is further supported by the significant positive relationship existing between the amount of dietary linoleic acid and the OT-increasig effect of the diet (Fig. 4.6.), no matter whether sunflowerseed oil is the only dietary fat or whether it is mixed with hydrogenated coconut oil or butterfat.

4.4.2. *Comparison of the effect of different fats and oils on arterial thrombus formation in rats*

Five-week-old male Wistar rats (SPF) were fed diets containing 50 en% (~ 24 w/w%) of fats with a different fatty acid composition for 9 weeks (Table 4.2, fats No. 1–11). During the last two days of the last week, the food consumption of all animals was measured and the faeces were collected to determine fat absorption. To this end, the faeces of three animals were pooled and the faecal fatty acids extracted after saponification. After weighing, the faecal fatty acids were pooled per group and quantified by gas-liquid chromatography. Fat absorption was calculated by subtracting the excreted from the ingested fat. No correction was applied for endogenous fat production. Absorption of fatty acids was calculated in the same way.

Arterial thrombus formaton was determined as described above and the optimum relationship between OT and the fatty acids absorbed was established by means of a multiple regression analysis.

4.4.2.1. *Relationship between arterial thrombosis tendency and dietary fatty acid composition*

The mean OT and log OT values of the various dietary groups are given in Table 4.3.

Table 4.2. Fatty acid composition (%) of dietary fats. Data refer to fractions $\geq 1\%$

Dietary fat			Fatty acids							
No	Name	Code	$\leq$10:0	12:0	14:0	16:0	16:1 (n-7)	17:0	18.0	18:1 (n-9)
1	Coconut oil	CO	14	44	19	10			3	7
2	Triglyceride mixture[a]	TGM		31	53	11			1	1
3	MCT-oil[a,c]	MCT	90	1		1				1
4	Whale oil[a]	WO			8	19	12	3	4	16
5	Palm oil	PO			1	44			5	39
6	Soyabean oil, hydrog.[a]	HSO				11			12	66[b]
7	Rapeseed oil	RO				3				11
8	Oliv oil	OO				11			4	71
9	Linseed oil	LO				6			6	20
10	Canbra oil	CBO				5			2	49
11	Sunflowerseed oil	SO				7			4	25
12	Coconut oil, hydrog.	HCO	14	45	18	10			13	
13	Butterfat	BF	16	4	10	20	4		12	26

Code	18:2 (n-6)	18:3 (n-3)	20:0	20:1 (n-9)	20:5 (n-3)[e]	22:1 (n-9)	22:2 (n-9)	22:6 (n-3)	24:0	24:1 (n-9)
CO	2									
TGM	2									
MCT	5									
WO	6			4	10	6[d]		4		6
PO	9									
HSO	9[b]	2[b]								
RO	13	10		7		50	2		1	
OO	11	1								
LO	13	53								
CBO	19	9		4		8				
SO	63				1					
HCO										
BF	4	1	2	1						

[a] Supplied with some glyceryl trilinoleate to prevent essential fatty acid deficiency (see Chapter 6)
[b] 58% *trans* fatty acids
[c] Medium-chain triglycerides
[d] Most probably (n-11)
[e] Plus 22:0.

Table 4.3. Arterial thrombosis tendency (OT) in rats fed diets containing 50 en% of differents fats for nine weeks

Dietary fat	No. of animals	log OT ± SEM	OT(h)
CO	12	2.13 ± 0.04	134
TGM[a]	12	1.81 ± 0.05	65
MCT[a]	12	1.89 ± 0.07	77
WO[a]	10	2.04 ± 0.08	111
PO	12	2.29 ± 0.05	195
HSO[a]	11	2.10 ± 0.04	127
RO	8	2.33 ± 0.08	214
OO	10	2.16 ± 0.04	145
LO	8	2.27 ± 0.03	186
CBO	12	2.28 ± 0.05	191
SO	12	2.24 ± 0.05	173

[a] Supplied with some glyceryl trilinoleate, to prevent essential fatty acid deficiency

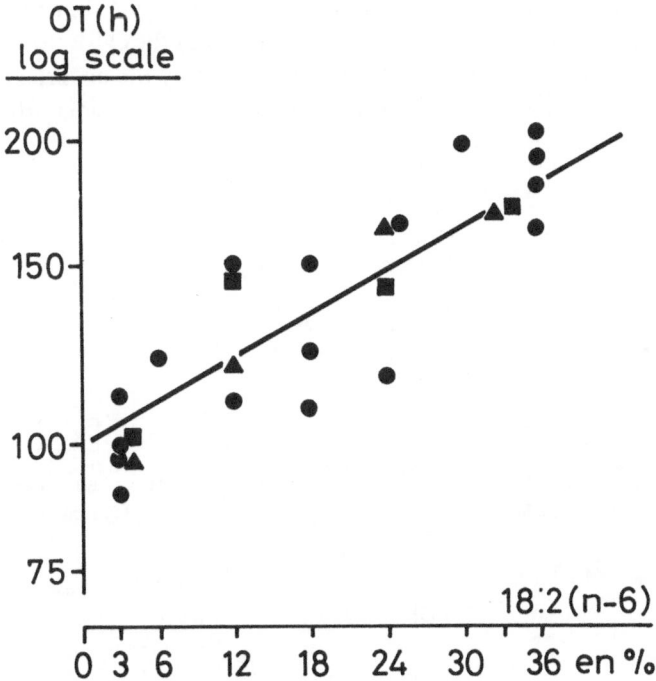

Fig. 4.6. Relationship between dietary linoleic acid content and thrombogenicity (OT). Each point represents the mean of 10–16 animals.

log OT (h) = 1.99 + 0.007 en% linoleic acid, r = 0.87 ;P <0.001

● sunflowerseed oil

▲ + hydrogenated coconut oil

■ + butterfat

56

Statistical analysis (Newman-Keuls multiple range test) showed that the dietary fats which are not connected by the same line as shown in the diagram below induce systematically different average log OT values, the confidence of this statement being at least 90%.

TGM   MCT   WO   HSO   CO   OO   SO   LO   CBO   PO   RO

Table 4.2 shows that only four fatty acids (16:0, 18:0, 18:1 and 18:2) are present in at least nine of the dietary fats. Using the rank correlation test of Spearman [776] – chosen to diminish the possibility of spurious correlations – a significant rank correlation between OT and dietary fatty acid concentration was found only for linoleic acid ($r = 0.72; P < 0.05$). However, the results given in Fig. 4.7 indicate that OT may also be related to the 16:0 content of the dietary oils. The fact that this relationship is not significant may be ascribed to the possibility that the OT is not a function of a single fatty acid and that it may also be influenced by the absorbed amount of fatty acids. As food consumption and fat absorption are considerably

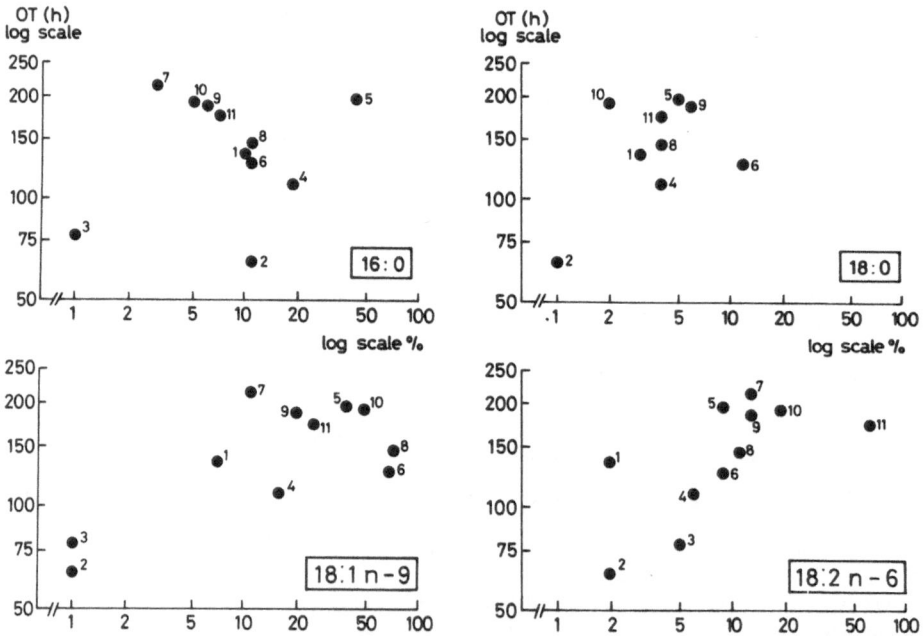

Fig. 4.7. Relationship between dietary content of some fatty acids and arterial thrombosis tendency (OT). Numbers refer to the dietary fats given in Table 4.2.

Table 4.4. Total food intake, relative fat and fatty acid absorption and absorbed amount of dietary fatty acids (Values < 20 mg.day^{-1} are not included.)

Dietary fat[a]	Food intake (g.animal^{-1} day^{-1})	Relative absorption of fat (%)	Fatty acids absorbed mg.animal^{-1}			
			$\leq$ 10:0 (100)[b]	12:0 (99)	14:0 (94)	16:0 (94)
CO	12.8	98.0	418	1339	579	286
TGM	12.4	96.1		919	1533	309
MCT	13.3	99.7	2814	31		36
WO	10.3	97.9			190	464
PO	12.7	91.8			34	1174
HSO	11.6	90.8				234
RO	10.0	91.6				79
OO	12.0	98.9				311
LO	10.8	98.6				158
CBO	12.2	97.2				155
SO	13.8	97.1				215

Dietary fat[a]	18:0 (90)	18:1[d] (97)	18:2[e] (99)	18:3[f] (99)	20:1[d] (96)	22:1[d] (87)	Rest
CO	93	224	61				
TGM	20	21	62				
MCT		36	169				
WO	94	400	202		95		935[c]
PO	138	1184	270				
HSO	258	1710	305	38			
RO		253	327	245	162	1050	57
OO	113	2051	331	20			26
LO	140	525	338	1386			
CBO	40	1425	561	266	110	222	
SO	108	827	2049				21

[a] See Table 4.2
[b] Values in brackets indicate the relative fatty acid absorption
[c] Mainly 16:1(n–7), 22:0 and 22:1(n–11)
[d] (n–9)
[e] (n–6)
[f] (n–3)

influenced by the type of dietary fatty acids [116, 117], a further investigation into their relationship with OT was done on the basis of the absorbed amounts of fatty acids (Table 4.4).

58

4.4.2.2. *Arterial thrombosis tendency as a function of the amount of absorbed fatty acids*

By means of a multiple regression analysis, we tried to describe the average log OT of a dietary group as a function of the average absorbed amount of one or more fatty acids. From ten independent variables (the different fatty acids occurring in more than one dietary fat), the multiple regression analysis computer program selects all the combinations of a given number of independent variables exceeding a pre-determined multiple correlation coefficient (R) and also selects the combination which has the highest multiple correlation coefficient. When only one independent variable is used, it appears that log OT is best described as a function of the absorbed amounts of 14:0 (R = 0.66). However, this is caused by only one dietary fat (Fig. 4.8.A; No 2, TGM), which makes the validity of this relationship very doubtful. The same holds for the results obtained by adding a second variable 8:0 + 10:0) which indeed increases the R value (0.87 significantly (P < 0.01), but this again is caused mainly by one of the dietary fats (MCT). Addition of a third (18:0) and a fourth (12:0) variable results in an R value of 0.94, which cannot be further improved significantly by including more variables.

A careful screening of the results of the multiple regression analysis used in this experiment showed [393] that, at least for up to two independent variables, the regression equation describes log OT as a function of dietary *fats* rather than as a function of constituent *fatty acids*. This is due mainly to the fairly specific fatty acid composition of the dietary fats selected for this experiment. It should also be realized that the independent variables used in this regression analysis must be considered as descriptive and not as explanatory variables for log OT.

It is striking that log OT can best be described as a function of the absorbed amount of saturated fatty acids (SAFA). This is also suggested in the literature (see section 4.2) and is further supported by the significant relationship between log OT

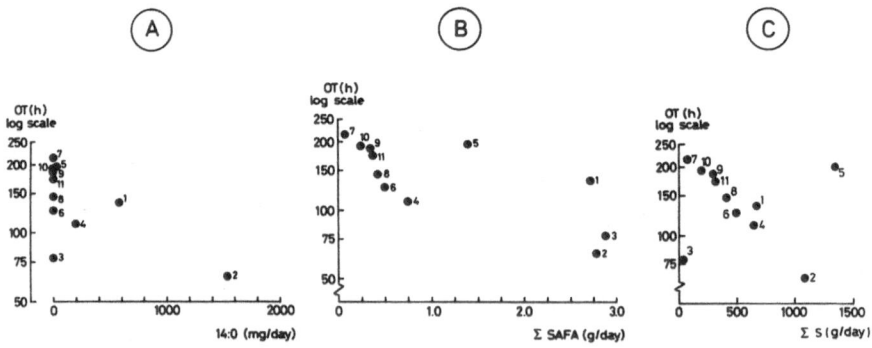

Fig. 4.8. Relationship between the amount of fatty acids absorbed and arterial thrombosis tendency (mean values per animal). Numbers refer to the dietary fats given in Table 4.2.
A : Relationship between 14:0 and OT.
B : Relationship between the total amount of saturated fatty acids (Σ SAFA) and OT.
C : Relationships between the sum of half the amount of 14:0 and the total amount of long-chain saturated fatty acids with 16 or more C-atoms (ΣS) and OT.

and the total absorbed amount of SAFA (Fig. 4.8.B; R = 0.75; P < 0.05). From Figure 4.8 it is evident that PO, CO, MCT and TGM do not fit very well: the OTs they induce seem to be too high for their SAFA-content. Three of these fats are the only ones containing 8:0, 10:0 and 12:0 (Table 4.2.), which suggests that these fatty acids are non-thrombogenic. This suggestion is consistent with the inability of 12:0 to enhance the ADP-induced platelet aggregation in vitro. In this system, 14:0 is moderately effective while 16:0 and 18:0 are highly effective [371]. Starting from these data from the literature, an attempt was made to improve the correlation between log OT and the absorbed amount of SAFA by assuming that 14:0 is only half as thrombogenic as 16:0 and 18:0. Therefore, the sum of the absorbed amount of SAFA was replaced by the sum of half the absorbed amount of 14:0 and the absorbed amount of all longer-chain saturated fatty acids ($\sum S$). When this parameter is plotted against log OT, a perfect fit is obtained, except for MCT and PO (Fig. 4.8.C).

It should be noted that almost all the fatty acids of MCT (8:0 and 10:0) are metabolised quite differently from the fatty acids with longer carbon chains. Absorption and early metabolism of 8:0 and 10:0 seem to be related more to carbohydrates, so that MCT-feeding can be considered as low fat feeding, which is known to induce a low OT (Fig. 4.4, see also ref. 387). The reason why PO is an exception is not yet known.

When log OT is plotted against $\sum S$, calculated on the basis of dietary fatty acid composition or on the basis of absorbed fatty acids, almost identical relationships are obtained. Consequently, it is sufficient to relate arterial thrombosis tendency to dietary fatty acid composition.

In sum, this experiment indicates that dietary saturated fatty acids with 14 or more carbon atoms are thrombogenic, which implies that their replacement with unsaturated fatty acids will decrease thrombogenicity.

4.4.3. *Comparison of the antithrombotic effect of oleic and linoleic acids*

To establish whether all unsaturated fatty acids are equally effective as to this 'passive' antithrombotic effect, the most common unsaturated fatty acids, oleic acid (18:1 (n–9)) and linoleic acid (18:2(n–6)) were compared as for their effects on arterial thrombosis tendency. Four groups of 12 male Wistar rats (SPF) were fed diets containing 50 en% of fat mixtures obtained by mixing hydrogenated palm oil with olive oil, safflowerseed oil and unhardened palm oil in such a way that the final mixtures contained 10 or 40% saturated acids (mainly palmitic acid) and 30 or 50% linoleic acid, the rest being oleic acid. If linoleic and oleic acid should have the same effect on arterial thrombosis tendency, the obstruction times would not be influenced by the dietary oleic/linoleic acid ratio so that, at a given saturated fat level, there would be no difference in arterial thrombus formation. This was investigated after feeding for eight weeks. The results are given in Fig. 4.9. Statistical evaluation of these results shows that, at each saturated fat level, thrombosis tendency is lower

(OT significantly longer) in the group receiving the diet highest in linoleic acid (P_2 < 0.05; analysis of variance). This finding demonstrates that linoleic acid, apart from its 'passive' antithrombotic effect when replacing long-chain saturated fatty acids, has also a specific antithrombotic effect. At comparable linoleic acid levels, the lower OT coincides with the higher saturated fatty acids, which is in agreement with the suggestion obtained from the previous experiment (section 4.4.2.).

According to the data in Table 4.2., sunflowerseed and linseed oils differ mainly in their polyunsaturated fatty acid component: in sunflowerseed oil, it is mainly linoleic acid and in linseed oil, α-linolenic acid (18:3(n-3)). Since the OTs on feeding both oils are almost similar, it is assumed that not only linoleic acid has a specific antithrombotic effect but also α-linolenic acid (see Chapter 6).

4.4.4. *Further evidence for the prothrombotic effect of dietary saturated fatty acids*

Results obtained so far, indicate that dietary long-chain saturated fatty acids promote arterial thrombosis tendency. However, if increasing amounts of hydrogenated coconut oil or butterfat are fed to rats, no shortening of the obstruction time is observed in relation to a control diet containing 5 en% sunflowerseed oil. Although this can possibly be explained by the fact that dietary carbohydrates may be equally thrombogenic as fats rich in saturated fatty acids, additional evidence is required before saturated fats can be considered prothrombotic. Some evidence was already obtained in the experiments described in sections 4.4.2 and 4.4.3. In both experimental series, the dietary carbohydrate content was kept constant. In section 4.4.2,

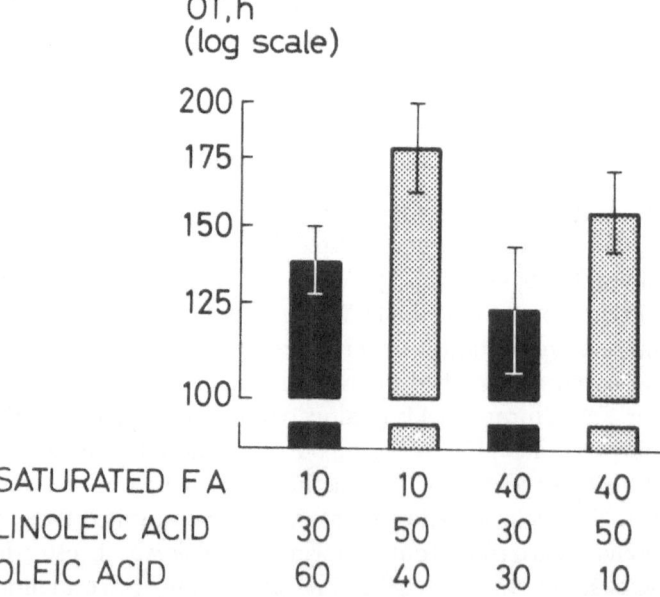

Fig. 4.9. Effect of dietary fatty acid composition (%) on thrombogenicity (OT ± SEM).

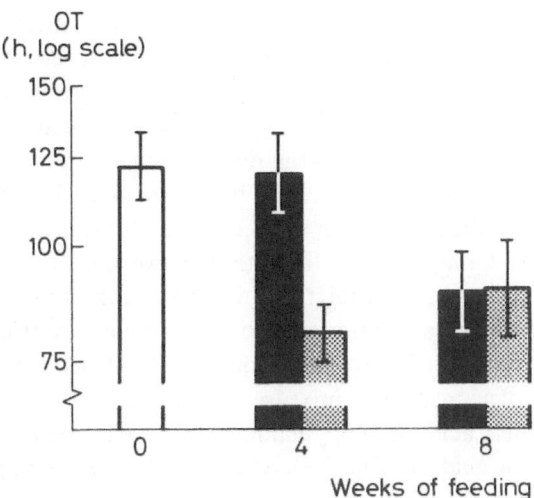

Fig. 4.10. Accelerating effect of saturated fat on the increase of thrombosis tendency in rats, following dietary changes (OT ± SEM)
□ stock diet   ■ 5 en% SO   ▨ 5 en% SO + 55 en% HCO

arterial thrombosis tendency appeared to be related to the intake of long-chain saturated fatty acids (Fig. 4.8.C.). However, this might have been due to the fact that largely fats high in long-chain saturated fatty acids contain only a small amount of antithrombotic linoleic acid. The evidence mentioned in section 4.4.3 is, therefore, more convincing: at constant dietary carbohydrate and linoleic acid contents, the arterial thrombosis tendency increases as the dietary long-chain saturated fatty acid content rises. Nevertheless, another experiment was performed in order to investigate the effect of dietary long-chain saturated fatty acids. Rats, fed a commercial stock diet, were given an experimental diet containing 5 en% sunflowerseed oil supplemented or not with 55 en% hydrogenated coconut oil. At the beginning of the feeding period (control) and four and eight weeks later, OTs were measured in part of the animals. It then appeared that after the change in diet, the OT decreased to about the same final value. However, the OT-decrease occurred more rapidly in the group receiving the HCO-supplemented diet. (Fig. 4.10). Therefore, it can be concluded that dietary fats rich in long-chain saturated fatty acids enhance arterial thrombosis tendency.

4.4.5. *Comparison of the effect of cis and trans fatty acids on arterial thrombus formation*

The organoleptic and physiochemical properties of natural oils used for the production of edible fats are improved by hydrogenation. This technological process reduces the number of double bounds and at the same time converts variable amounts of *cis* double bounds into their *trans* isomers (see Chapter 2, section 1).

These *trans* fatty acids have slightly different physical properties as compared to their *cis* isomers. Results of physiological and biochemical studies suggest that the properties of the *trans* monoenoic fatty acids are intermediate between those of saturated and *cis*-mono-unsaturated fatty acids [405, 831]. However, there are no indications that the molecular configuration around the double bonds influences the effect of unsaturated fatty acids on thrombogenesis. The hydrogenated soyabean oil used in the experiment described in section 4.4.2 contained unsaturated fatty acids about 58% of which had the *trans*-configuration. Nevertheless, this dietary group fits perfectly the curve showing the relationship between the amount of dietary saturated fatty acids absorbed and arterial thrombosis tendency (Fig. 4.8.C). In a further experiment, we compared the obstruction time in rats fed a diet containing 50 en % olive oil (80% oleic acid) or a mixture of olive oil and hydrogenated olive oil containing 40% oleic acid and 40% elaidic acid (as triglycerides; elaidic acid is the *trans* isomer of oleic acid, see Fig. 2.4). After eight weeks' feeding, the obstruction times did not differ significantly:

cis-oleic acid : $\log OT = 2.10 \pm 0.040; n = 12 ; OT = 125\,h$
$trans$-oleic acid : $\log OT = 2.02 \pm 0.058; n = 11 ; OT = 104\,h$

It is, therefore, highly likely that there is no difference between the antithrombotic effect of *cis* and *trans* unsaturated fatty acids.

4.5. SUMMARY

A model used to quantify arterial thrombosis tendency in rats showed that dietary fats rich in long-chain saturated fatty acids promote arterial thrombogenesis. Dietary linoleic acid (and most probably also α-linolenic acid) has a specific antithrombotic effect whereas mono-unsaturated fatty acids are neutral in this respect and decrease arterial thrombosis tendency only if they replace long-chain saturated fatty acids. No significant difference was observed between the antithrombotic effect of *cis* fatty acids and their *trans* isomers.

5. LOCATION OF DIETARY FAT EFFECT ON ARTERIAL THROMBUS FORMATION

5.1. INTRODUCTION

As discussed in Chapters 1 and 3, arterial thrombus formation results from platelet reactions and blood coagulation, both initiated, and possibly modulated, by the vessel wall. In order to 'locate' the dietary fat effect on arterial thrombogenesis, investigations were carried out into the effects of dietary fats on blood clotting and several thrombotic platelet functions. Most of these experiments were done with diets containing 50 or 60 en% sunflowerseed oil (SO) – an example of a linoleic acid-rich, antithrombotic vegetable oil – or hydrogenated coconut oil (HCO), which is highly saturated and has prothrombotic properties (Chapter 4). In order to prevent essential fatty acid deficiency (Chapter 6), the HCO-diet was always enriched with 5 en% SO. These experimental diets invariably induce a significant difference in arterial thrombosis tendency, as shown in Fig. 5.1.

5.2. EFFECT ON SUNFLOWERSEED OIL (SO) AND HYDROGENATED COCONUT OIL (HCO) ON BLOOD COAGULATION

In several conditions associated with thrombosis and arterial disease, coagulation and closely related platelet functions are influenced by alterations in lipids. Alimentary hyperlipemia alone may create hypercoagulability [584, 664]. A similar connection between lipids and coagulability has been noted in ischemic heart disease [63]. An increased availability and activity of procoagulant platelet phospholipids has been reported in coronary disease [615], diabetes mellitus [616], and familial hyperbetalipoproteinemia [617, 433]. Based on experimental evidence, Conner, Hoak and Warner [152] have proposed transient hypercoagulability and subsequent thrombosis may result from a sudden rise in plasma free fatty acids mobilized from adipose tissue through stress, catecholamines, or other humoral and metabolic factors.

In our studies blood for whole blood and plasma clotting time studies was obtained by a clean venepuncture of the exposed external jugular vein of ether-anaesthetised rats after overnight fasting. After some blood had drained away a syringe, prefilled or not with one part of a 3.8% (w/v) sodium citrate solution, was connected to the needle. Nine parts of blood were drawn into the syringe so slowly

64

that the vessel wall did not collapse onto the needle. After careful mixing, the anticoagulated blood was transferred into a plastic or siliconized glass tube for further processing as described for the various tests. For the measurement of activated partial thromboplastin time (APTT) and prothrombin time (PT) blood was obtained by puncturing the abdominal aorta of ether-anaesthetized animals after overnight fasting. The puncture needle was connected to a siliconized poly-vinyl tube (Portex, 4E, length 15 cm, i.d. 2 mm). Blood was collected in a calibrated plastic tube containing 1 ml 3.8% (w/v) sodium citrate. From each animal, 9 ml of blood was taken. After careful mixing and standing for at least 10 min (room temperature), PRP was prepared by centrifugation for 20 min at 190 g. The PRP was treated as described for the different tests.

5.2.1. *Whole blood clotting time*

The clotting time of native blood was measured with the rotating loop technique devised by Chandler [127]. A piece of transparent plastic tubing, length 32.5 cm, i.d. 2.3 mm; o.d. 3.9 mm, was filled with 0.5 ml of freshly drawn native blood. The tube was bent and both ends were tightly connected using a somewhat wider piece of

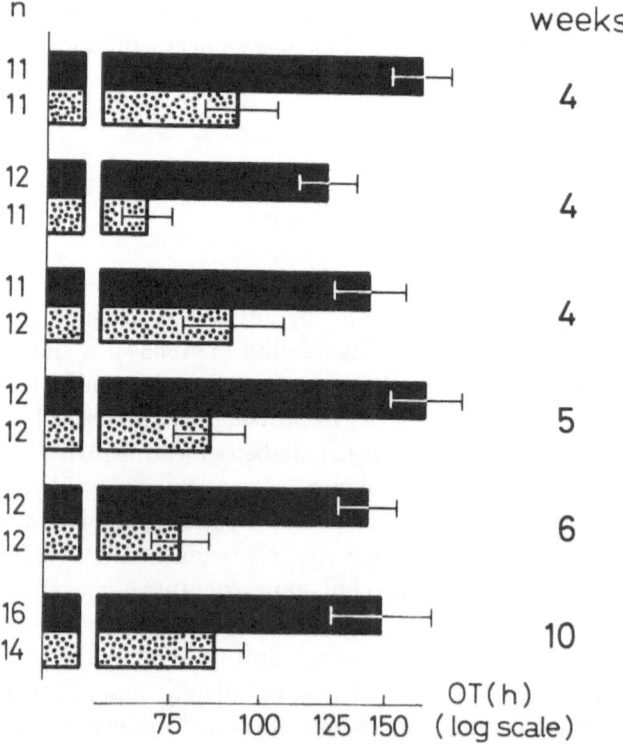

Fig. 5.1. Arterial thrombosis tendency (OT) in rats fed SO (■) and HCO (▨) diets for four to ten weeks

tubing (i.d. 3.8 mm; o.d. 5.8 mm). The loop so obtained was placed at an angle of 30° on a device rotating it at 15 rev.min^{-1}. The device is placed in a cabinet at 37° C, which is also used to prewarm the tubing. Gravity keeps the fluid blood in the lower part of the rotating loop. However, when the blood clots, it suddenly starts rotating at the same speed as the loop. The time between blood sampling and the very onset of rotation of the blood, is taken as the clotting time. This test measures blood clotting in a dynamic situation and, therefore reflects, to some extent, the in vivo situation. Clotting is preceded by visible platelet aggregation and the thrombus formed resembles a typical white-headed, red-tailed thrombus. Platelet aggregation was shown to result from thrombin formation [230]. Measurements were done after feeding for four and eight weeks. No differences were observed between the two groups (Table 5.1).

5.2.2. *Plasma recalcification clotting time (PCT)*

In 1969, Renaud published this clotting test enabling him to demonstrate a relationship between PCT and thrombosis tendency in rats as well as in man [683]. We decided to use this test to screen the intrinsic clotting system upon feeding different diets. Freshly drawn citrated blood (2.0 ml) was transferred to a siliconized glass tube and centrifuged at 130 g for 10 min. Approximately 0.3 ml of the citrated platelet-rich plasma (PRP) was collected and stored in another siliconized glass tube. The rest of the blood was centrifuged again (10 min at 4000 g) in order to obtain platelet-poor plasma (PPP). After counting its platelet content (using a Coulter Counter model FN) 50μl of the PRP was diluted with autologus PPP to a platelet concentration of about 3.10^5 μl^{-1}. This whole procedure was performed at 0° C since storage at 30° C (the temperature used by Renaud) was shown to prolong the clotting time considerably, especially in PPP. The actual clotting test was performed by transferring 0.1 ml PRP, PRP diluted with PPP or PPP, into a clear plastic tube which was placed in a waterbath (37.5° C). After a warming-up period of 30 s, 0.2 ml CaCl$_2$ (10^{-2} mol.l^{-1}) was added while a stopwatch was started. Mixing was performed by gently rotating the tube. One min later and then after every 10 s, the tube was carefully removed from the waterbath and tilted slightly to check the fluidity of the plasma. The end-point was attained when the plasma became a solid mass.

Table 5.1. Whole blood clotting time (seconds $\pm$ SEM) in Chandler's rotating loop, measured in native blood of rats fed SO or HCO-containing diets (n = 14–16)

Feeding period	Whole blood clotting time		
(weeks)	SO	HCO	P$_2$
4	138 $\pm$ 2.2	147 $\pm$ 6.5	>0.10
8	150 $\pm$ 4.8	157 $\pm$ 12.5	>0.10

The PCT measures the intrinsic clotting pathway and is greatly influenced by the number of platelets present [683]. Therefore, by comparing the clotting time of PPP with that of PRP or its dilution, an indication of the clot-promoting effect of the platelets can be obtained as well. Measurements were carried out after 15 weeks feeding. The results (Fig. 5.2) show that there is no difference between the groups. This is not in agreement with the results published by Renaud and coworkers. They clearly demonstrated that the type of dietary fat greatly influenced the PCT of PRP, which appeared to be due to a certain influence on the clot-promoting effect of the blood platelets. A striking relationship was also observed for the thrombosis tendency induced by the different dietary fats [682, 686, 687]. However, it should be noted that these researchers used an extremely hyperlipemic cholesterol and cholic acid containing diet which was shown to cause enhanced blood clotting [408, 543]. Moreover, their thrombosis model depends on endotoxin-induced activation of factor XII in the venous circulation [482] and, therefore, applies mainly to venous thrombosis for which the importance of enhanced coagulation is generally acknowledged. Recently, the same group published comparable data obtained with diets without added cholesterol and cholic acid [532]. However, when PCT measurements were carried out on the same samples at the same time and laboratory by ourselves and the Renaud group, none of us was able to discriminate between SO- and HCO-fed animals on the basis of this clotting test. It is concluded, therefore, that blood clotting, as reflected by the PCT-test, does not play a significant role in the effect of dietary fats on arterial thrombosis tendency.

5.2.3. *Activated partial thromboplastin time (APTT)*

In order to investigate the intrinsic pathway of coagulation, APTTs were measured

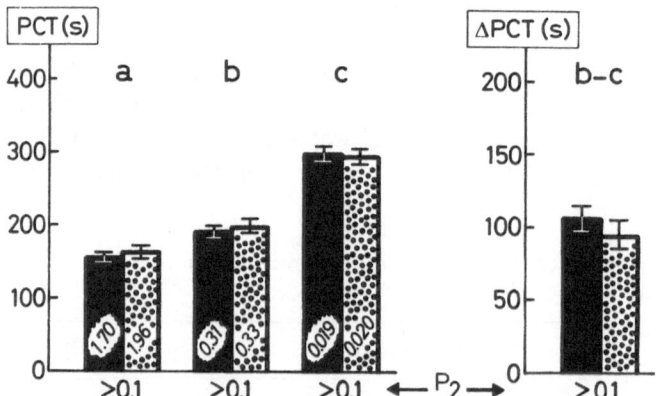

Fig. 5.2. Recalcification plasma clotting times (PCT, s ± SEM) in PRP (a), PRP diluted with autologous PPP (b) and in PPP (c) of rats fed SO (■) or HCO ▨-diets for fifteen weeks (n = 16).
(b-c) indicates clot-promoting effect of platelets. Numbers in bars × 10^6 refer to platelet concentration per μl plasma

in platelet-free plasma (PFP) after high-speed centrifugation (16.000 g for 20 min) of PPP. A standard PFP was prepared in the same way from a pool of 15 stock animals after overnight fasting. The test was performed in 0.1 ml PFP which was activated at 37° C for 2 min with 0.1 ml of Actin ® (ex Dade, B-D and Company, Rutherford, New Jersey) a liquid rabbit brain cephalin with plasma activator. Clotting was initiated with 0.1 ml CaCl$_2$ (0.033 mol.l^{-1}) and fibrin formation checked with a small metal hook. The time between CaCl$_2$ addition and the appearance of the first strand of fibrin was taken as the clotting time. Using this test system the APTT of a pool of standard PFP was 34.2 $\pm$ 0.12 s ($\bar{x}$ $\pm$ SEM, n = 4). Measurements were carried out in animals fed the SO or HCO diet for four months and also in a control group, receiving a comparable diet containing only 5 en% SO as dietary fat. The results are given in Table 5.2. from which it can be seen that intrinsic clotting is significantly lower in the HCO group as compared with both SO groups which do not differ mutually.

5.2.4. *Prothrombin time (PT)*

PT's were measured with the one-stage technique, using a rat-brain thromboplastin preparation to trigger the extrinsic clotting system. Rat-brain thromboplastin was prepared according to a procedure described by Owren and Aas [641] and modified by Muller [580a]. The preparation was diluted with Michaelis buffer [774] and gave a clotting time of 30.5 $\pm$ 0.29 sec ($\bar{x}$ $\pm$ SEM, n = 4) with undiluted standard rat PFP. PT measurements were performed in 0.1 ml PFP which was preincubated with 0.10 ml of the rat-brain thromboplastin preparation for 1 min at 37.5° C. Coagulation was triggered by adding 0.10 ml CaCl$_2$ (0.033 mol.l^{-1}) and fibrin formation was checked with a small metal hook. The time between CaCl$_2$-addition

Table 5.2. Activated partial thromboplastin times (APTT) and prothrombin times (PT), measured in platelet-free plasma of rats fed SO-(n = 14) or HCO-(n = 13) containing diets. The control group (n = 14) received a diet containing 5 en% SO.
P$_2$: significance of difference (Student's 2-samples test)

Group	APTT		PT	
	sec $\pm$ SEM	P$_2$	sec $\pm$ SEM	P$_2$
Control	41.4 $\pm$ 1.14	>0.10	31.5 $\pm$ 0.31	>0.10
SO	39.8 $\pm$ 1.08	0.009 / 0.003	32.3 $\pm$ 0.58	0.06 / 0.02
HCO	43.7 $\pm$ 0.44		30.5 $\pm$ 0.40	

and the appearance of the first strand of fibrin was taken as the clotting time. As can be seen from Table 5.2., extrinsic clotting is significantly enhanced (PT shorter) in the HCO group as compared with both SO-groups, which do not differ mutually.

5.2.5. Platelet factor 3 (PF 3)

At various stages in the coagulation cascade, activated platelets contribute to the clotting process by providing a phospholipid surface on which the activated clotting factors are concentrated and properly positioned towards each other [882]. This property of (activated) platelets is called platelet factor 3 (PF 3). It can be measured in a system in which the available phospholipid surface limits the coagulation reaction. In such a system, any additional phospholipid surface becoming available causes a reduction in clotting time. Clotting is initiated by direct activation of factor X, using a snake venom (Russell's Viper Venom, RVV). In this way, any direct influence of the intrinsic/extrinsic activation system is prevented [341]. The clotting time measured with RVV is called the Stypven Time (ST). The RVV reagent is prepared fresh daily; 0.5 mg RVV (Wellcome) is dissolved in 5 ml $CaCl_2$ (0.015 mol$:1^{-1}$) and diluted (1:20) in the same Ca^{++}-solution. This working solution is kept at room temperature.

In a first experiment, the PF3 activity, content and availability were determined in PRP, diluted with autologous PPP to a platelet concentration of about $0.3 \times 10^6.\mu l^{-1}$. PF3 activity and availability were measured by transferring 0.1 ml of the PRP + PPP dilution into a siliconised glass tube containing 0.05 ml of saline (for the measurement of PF3 activity) or a collagen suspension in saline (for measuring PF3 availability). The tubes were placed on a device at an angle of about $8.5°$ and rotated longitudinally at 30 rev.min^{-1}. After 10 min, 0.1 ml of the mixture was transferred into another siliconised glass tube and placed in a waterbath at $37.5°$ C. After 1 min, 0.1 ml of the RVV reagent was added while a stopwatch was started. After rotating the tube (mixing!), fibrin formation was checked by using an oese. The moment the

Table 5.3. Platelet count (A), platelet factor 3 activity (B), availability (C) and content (D) measured in rat platelets on feeding a diet containing SO or HCO for eight weeks (n = 16)

Parameter	Unit	SO	HCO	P_2
A. Platelet count	$\times 10^6.\mu l^{-1}$	0.30 ± 0.021	0.32 ± 0.011	>0.10
B. ST, saline	s	31.1 ± 0.83	32.9 ± 1.51	>0.10
	%	100	100	–
C. ST, collagen	s	22.9 ± 0.74	26.9 ± 1.01	<0.01
	% of saline	74 ± 1.5	82 ± 1.9	<0.01
D. ST, $3 \times$ fr/th.	s	13.9 ± 0.43	14.0 ± 0.32	>0.10
	% of saline	45 ± 1.9	43 ± 1.7	>0.10

ST = stypven time
fr/th = freezing and thawing

first fibrin strand appeared was taken as end-point. STs obtained upon saline incubation ($\sim$ PF3 activity) were taken as 100%. STs obtained after collagen addition ($\sim$ PF3 availability) were expressed in % of PF3 activity. To measure the PF3 content, the PRP + PPP dilution was frozen in a mixture of solid CO_2 and acetone ($-64°$ C) and subsequently thawn in water at $37°$ C. This procedure was repeated 3 times in order to lyse the platelets and make all their PF3 available. STs were measured and expressed as described for PF3 activity and availability. PF3 availability is better and the content higher, the lower the ST-values. The results obtained after eight weeks' feeding are shown in Table 5.3.

PF3 activity (B) and content (D) do not differ for both groups; however, PF3 availability (C) is significantly lower in the thrombogenic HCO group. This unexpected finding was confirmed in a second experiment in which PF3 availability after eight weeks' feeding was measured in citrated whole blood and followed in time after activation. One ml of freshly drawn citrated blood was divided over two siliconised glass tubes containing 0.05 ml of saline or a suspension of collagen in saline. The tubes were placed on the rotator and after 0, 4, 8, and 12 min (saline, control) or 2, 6, 10, and 14 min (collagen) STs were measured in 0.1 ml samples as described above. Due to platelet activation, PF3 becomes available causing the ST to decrease. This is shown in Fig. 5.3, sections A and B for saline and collagen-activation, respectively. Figure 5.3.C shows the time course of PF3 availability upon activation with collagen. Results are corrected for non-specific collagen-independent PF3 availability, by expressing the STs in % of the values calculated from the control (saline) series. It is evident that the HCO diet is associated with a significantly lower PF3 availability as compared with the SO diet.

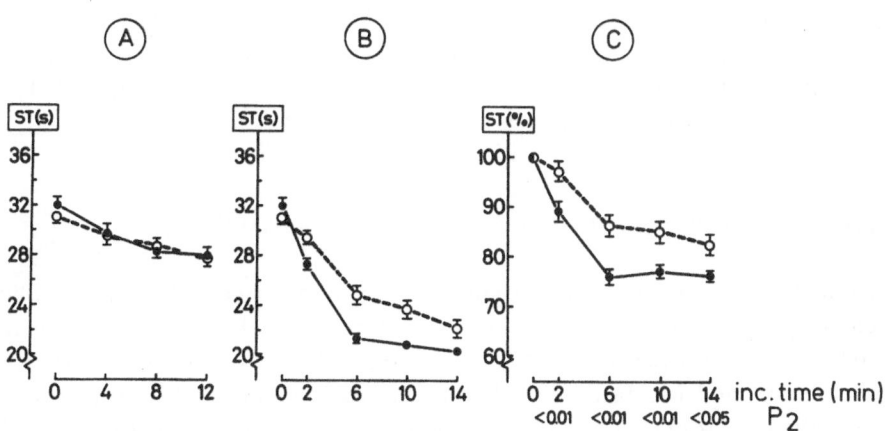

Fig. 5.3. Platelet factor 3 availability in citrated blood of rats fed SO (— ● —) or HCO (--○--) containing diets for eight weeks.

A. Course of Stypven time (ST, s ± SEM) upon incubation with saline (control series).

B. Course of ST (s ± SEM) on incubation with a collagen suspension in saline.

C. Collagen-induced PF3 availability (% ± SEM.) after correction for non-specific platelet activation as described in the text.

It has been shown that a slight degree of platelet lysis, which is inevitable when handling platelets, causes the ST to decrease considerably [430, 883]. Our results are not corrected for possible lysis so that the difference observed may be explained by the possibility that HCO platelets are more lysis-resistant than SO platelets. This has not yet been investigated. However, there is evidence to believe that HCO-platelets are less activated than SO-platelets. This will be further discussed in section 5.3.2.

From these studies it can be concluded that PF3 activity and content are not different for both groups. Since feeding the HCO-containing diet results in a *lower* PF3 availability of blood platelets upon their activation by collagen as compared to feeding the SO-diet, whereas it causes a *higher* arterial thrombosis tendency, it is unlikely that changes in PF3 are involved as a causal factor in the dietary-fat induced changes in arterial thrombosis tendency.

5.2.6. *Vessel wall induced clotting*

Blood clotting can be initiated by vessel wall damage. This clotting process is of extrinsic as well as intrinsic origin and platelets definitively contribute to it, particularly so after activation. Prostacyclin (PGI_2) was shown to inhibit vessel wall induced clotting by inhibiting platelet activation [58, 101, 398, 400].

Although initial experiments suggested that dietary fat induced differences in vessel wall induced clotting could have contributed to differences in arterial thrombosis tendency [398], later investigations did not confirm this. In fact, neither of the experiments performed showed a significant difference in vessel wall induced clotting between SO- and HCO-fed animals. Therefore, it must be concluded that the difference in arterial thrombosis tendency on feeding SO- and HCO-diets is most probably not caused by a dietary fat effect on vessel wall induced clotting. As will be discussed in Chapter 7, however, vessel wall induced clotting may be implicated in the different effects of various fish oils on arterial thrombus formation.

5.3. EFFECT OF THE DIETARY FAT TYPE ON PLATELET AGGREGABILITY

Increased platelet stickiness is perhaps most important in arterial thrombosis. The capacity of platelets to aggregate and resist the force of the blood current may be critical factors in the development of arterial thrombi. In cases of peripheral arteriosclerosis, Evans and Mustard [235] found that early failure of femoropopliteal bypass grafts by thrombotic occlusion could be directly correlated with increased platelet adhesiveness in vitro. Recently, a family with recurrent arterial thrombosis has been studied and found to have abnormal platelet function in vitro characterized by enhanced aggregability as the only apparent prothrombotic change in the blood [636].

Observations of hyperadhesive platelets in familial hyperlipoproteinemia [151,

486] and in alimentary hyperlipemia [390, 656, 689], lend further support to the concept of a pathogenetic relationship between fats and thrombotic disease. In familial hyperlipoproteinemia, hyperreactivity of platelets associated with an increased frequency of thromboembolic events is especially noted in the hypercholesterolemic type II class [486]. Hypersensitivity of platelets in type II may be mediated by abnormalities in platelet metabolism of arachidonic achid [486]; in type IIa, hypersensitive platelets have an increased cholesterol-phospholipid ratio in their membranes that may be related to the observed alterations in function [151]. These findings indicate that the dietary fat effects on arterial thrombus formation may be mediated via an effect on the platelet aggregation tendency. Before describing our own investigations in this field, the earlier literature will be reviewed.

5.3.1. *Dietary fats and platelet aggregation: a literature survey*

Most of the experiments to be described have been done in venous blood and should in fact not be included in this review on arterial thrombosis. However, several studies have been carried out in relation to arterial thrombus formation and atherosclerosis. We did therefore include them, but it is questionable whether 'venous' platelets are suitable for such a study, because there is evidence that their adenosine diphosphate sensitivity is higher than that of 'arterial' platelets [89, 884].

5.3.1.1. *Effect of a single fat dose*
By direct observation of the microcirculation in the hamster cheek pouch, Cullen and Swank [164] observed slowing of the blood flow and even complete stasis after intravenous infusion of gelatin and high-molecular-weight dextran. The same changes were observed on inducing alimentary lipemia by feeding cream via a stomach tube; this treatment was also shown to increase blood viscosity in the hamster [796]. This thrombogenic state [849] was caused by aggregation of red blood cells (rouleaux formation) and by the occurrence of platelet aggregates.

Moolten et al. [568] observed that alimentary lipemia was associated with increased platelet stickiness as measured by the glass wool braid technique [567]. They offered normal, atherosclerotic and diabetic volunteers a low-fat diet or a diet containing 36 g animal fat (cream and eggs) or maize oil. In all instances platelet-to-glass adhesion measured 2–5 h after the meal, was increased as compared with the fasting state. The effect of the animal fat diet was greatest, while the effects of the low-fat and maize oil diets hardly differed. The effects were qualitatively similar in all three groups of volunteers; only minor quantitative differences were observed.

Böhle et al. [75] performed the same kind of experiments in normal men and in patients with increased platelet aggregation (mainly atherosclerotics), who were given 50 g butterfat, olive oil, maize oil or linseed oil after overnight fasting. Platelet aggregation was determined by the PAT test of Breddin and Bauke [93] in which aggregates formed during rotation of the upper layer of sedimented citrated blood are quantified. In normal volunteers, fat-loading did not modify platelet aggregation, although it resulted in distinct hyperlipemia. In patients with increased platelet aggregation, fat-loading produced a somewhat higher degree of lipemia than in the normal volunteers. Butter and olive oil (both low in polyunsaturated fatty acids) caused a slight decrease in platelet aggregability, whereas maize oil and linseed oil, which are rich in polyunsaturated fatty acids, normalized the high aggregation values completely for a period of at least 8 h. Horlick [383] fed normal and atherosclerotic volunteers a high-fat breakfast containing 75 g of mixed animal fats (butter, eggs, cream and bacon). He measured the platelet stickiness by the glass wool braid technique of Moolten and Vroman (modified) in the fasting state and after 2, 4 and 6 h after the meal. In the normal group, no change in platelet stickiness was observed, whereas there was a significant increase in the atherosclerotic group 2 and 4 h after the meal.

Philip and Payling Wright [656] also studied the effect of alimentary lipemia on platelet function. They induced lipemia by a fatty meal consisting of bacon, fried bread, butter, eggs and double cream. Platelet stickiness in blood collected after overnight fasting and 2–2.5 h after the meal, was measured by the rotating bulb technique [875]. In this study, lipemia was associated with a significantly increased platelet stickiness as compared with that in the fasting state. Adenosine, a well-known inhibitor of platelet aggregation [83], reduced platelet retention in fasting blood strikingly. This inhibiting effect was alos present in lipemic blood, but was considerably diminished.

Gromnatskii [310], using the same technique for measuring platelet aggregation, induced lipemia in 20 normal volunteers by giving them 350–400 ml sour cream, which significantly increased the platelet stickiness. Besterman et al. [55] reported an increased platelet stickiness (Wright rotator) after a fatty breakfast (50 g) in normal as well as ischemic subjects.

Kloeze [457] induced postprandial hyperlipemia by giving fasting rats coconut oil, soyabean oil, maize oil, linseed oil, whale oil or butterfat by stomach tube in a single dose of 6 mg/cm^2 body surface/day for four days. Three h after the last load, blood was drawn by venepuncture for measuring lipemia and platelet adhesiveness in citrated blood (glass bead column technique of Hellem [354]). Although striking differences were observed in the degree of lipemia, the adhesiveness values did not differ significantly.

Lipemia can also be produced by intravenous administration of fat emulsions, a technique which is used clinically to an increasing extent. Lipofundin ®, an emulsion of cottonseed oil, when administered to rabbits (2 g oil/kg body weight), decreased the circulating platelet count significantly, but produced an inconsistent effect on platelet retention in the rotating bulb [462]. When added to blood in vitro, it invariably produced a significant increase in platelet aggregation [654]. Later investigations of Pfleiderer et al. [655], which included emulsions of a great number of fatty acids and vegetable and mineral oils, revealed that all emulsions added to citrated platelet-rich plasma or citrated blood, increased platelet stickiness. Extensive electron microscopical and biochemical studies showed that this non-specific effect of lipid emulsions is the result of a two-step process: adhesion of the fat particles to and their phagocytosis by the platelets [576]. The latter phase is associated with a considerable loss of platelet ATP [840], which might be responsible for the increase in platelet stickiness. Surface-active agents (phospholipids, albumin) are inhibitory to these processes.

Deiniger [178], connected an isolated cat heart to the arterial circulation of a donor animal, and showed that infusion of Lipofundin ® into the coronary arteries decreased the heart function due to the formation of occlusive platelet thrombi. This formation could be prevented by preincubation of the emulsion with post-heparin plasma [103]. Decreased heart function was also observed in dogs after acute lipemia induced by infusion of a 10% sesame oil emulsion or of lipemic plasma [470].

Kapp et al. [446] used the glass bead test [354], and observed a progressive decrease in platelet adhesiveness on Intralipid ® (a 20% emulsion of soyabean oil) infusion (500 ml) to normal fasting volunteers. In vitro addition of the emulsion to citrated blood (10 and 20 g/l blood) induced a dose-dependent increase in platelet adhesiveness. They speculated that the discrepancy in results between in vivo and in vitro administration may be due to the release in vivo of a platelet stickiness reducing agent.

5.2.1.2. Effect of prolonged fat feeding

Frost [271], induced hypercholesterolemia in rabbits by feeding a diet containing 2% cholesterol for two to three weeks, and observed numerous platelets adhering to the wall of the abdominal aorta and of the carotid arteries, by means of the scanning electron microscope. He also saw enhanced endothelial separation and adhesion of drop-like bodies, probably fat droplets. In control animals, these lesions were not found. It is evident from this study that increased thrombogenesis will decrease the average circulation time of platelets. Mustard and Murphy [584] used this concept as early as 1962 for their studies of the effect of dietary fats on the half-life and turnover of circulating platelets in volunteers receiving either a low-fat (21 en% mainly vegetable fat) or a high-fat diet (37–39 en% containing mainly maize oil or animal fats consisting of egg yolk and dairy fats for three weeks. Platelet half-life was shortest and platelet turnover greatest on feeding the high animal fat diet. The high vegetable fat diet gave a shorter platelet half-life than the low vegetable fat diet. Platelet turnover was least on the low fat diet, but the difference with the high-vegetable fat diet was not significant.

Nordøy and Chandler [609], induced intravascular platelet aggregation in rats by injection of ADP into the inferior vena cava and found trombosis in histological sections of lung tissue excised shortly after the injection. Light- and electron microscopy of these thrombi revealed them to consist of aggregated platelets with intact membranes and internal structure. Fibrin was not observed [592]. Feeding rats diets containing 10% saturated fat (hydrogenated coconut oil) and 1% cholesterol, considerably increased thrombosis incidence as compared with feeding a low (unsaturated) fat diet [610]. Daily oral administration of 50 mg linseed oil to the animals on the saturated fat diet did not modify the high incidence of thrombosis. In later experiments [613] with lower ADP doses, the thrombogenicity was compared for diets containing 10% hydrogenated coconut fat (10 CF), 40% hydrogenated coconut fat (40 CF) and 32% hydrogenated coconut fat + 8% cottonseed oil (8 CO) or 8% linseed oil (8 LO). After feeding for one day, thrombosis incidence in all groups was not significantly different. After five to six weeks, however, it was significantly higher in the 40 CF group than in the other groups; the latter did not differ significantly from each other. Electron microscopical investigation showed that in the 10 and 40 CF groups, thrombi contained zones of platelet membrane fusion, which was not observed in the 8 CO and 8 LO groups [593].

Kloeze [457], fed 50 en% ($\approx$ 27 weight %) coconut oil, soyabean oil, maize oil, linseed oil, whale oil or butterfat to rats for one, two or five weeks, and observed no differences in the platelet adhesiveness in whole citrated blood (glass bead test) between the six groups after overnight fasting. Nordøy [612], using the modified glass bead test [355], measured ADP-induced platelet adhesiveness in citrated platelet-rich plasma of rats fed a normal stock diet (control group) or a saturated fat diet containing 10% hydrogenated coconut oil and 1% cholesterol for four months. During the last month, animals on the saturated fat diet were daily administered 80 mg maize oil, linseed oil or water. Platelet adhesiveness was higher in the saturated fat and water groups than in the control group. Maize oil supplementation increased platelet adhesiveness further, whereas linseed oil administration decreased it to nearly the control level. Roughly, the effect of these dietary fats on the formation of experimental venous thrombi [611] was analogous.

Kloeze et al. [459] performed similar experiments in rabbits which were offered diets containing 14% hydrogenated coconut oil, 10% hydrogenated coconut oil + 4% safflower or linseed oil. After 18 and 62 weeks feeding, platelet adhesiveness determined by the modified glass bead test [355] was not significantly different. In an earlier investigation [832], rabbits were fed a 1:1 mixture of maize and coconut oil (15% fat in the diet), while another group was fed these dietary fats separately during alternate periods of ten weeks. After two years feeding, the atheroma index in the alternately fed group was twice as high as that in the group fed the fat mixture. However, no difference in platelet adhesiveness was observed.

Mathues et al. [527] fed rabbits either a stock diet as such or supplemented with 6% coconut oil and 2% cholesterol for three to seven weeks. Platelet adhesiveness determined in native platelet-rich plasma (glass bead test) was significantly higher in the supplemented group than in the control group. No difference was observed in artificial thrombus formation in the Chandler loop. Phosphatidyl serine, infused 30 min prior to blood collection, normalized the high adhesion values in the fat/cholesterol group completely.

McDonald and Edgill [530] showed that the enhanced platelet stickiness (citrated platelet-rich plasma in the rotating bulb) in patients with ischemic heart disease could be decreased by lowering the dietary fat intake. Mustard and Murphy [584] did not find significant effects on the platelet adhesive index (glass wool braid) of diets containing either 21 en% mixed vegetable fats, 37 en% vegetable fats (mainly maize oil) or 39 en% mixed animal fats, fed for four weeks to normal volunteers. Owren et al. [642] showed that maize oil, cod-liver oil and safflower oil in doses of 100 ml/day were rather ineffective in changing the increased platelet adhesiveness in atherosclerotic patients (modified glass bead test [355] while soyabean oil normalised it within three days. Linseed oil was reported to be extremely beneficial in this respect, but this was revoked later [643]. In a clinical trial on patients with coronary heart disease, Borchgrevink et al. [78], using the same technique, did not see any effect of daily doses of 10–30 ml linseed or maize oil on platelet adhesiveness, nor did the mortality and the reinfarction rate differ between the two groups [77]. Bentzen et al. [44] measured the platelet adhesiveness with the glass bead column technique in a group of elderly patients (average age 75) before and after one to five weeks' treatment with one daily dose of 20 ml oil containing either 55% linolenic acid or 52% linoleic acid, the rest being about similar. In the linolenic acid group, they oserved a very significant decrease in platelet retention after one week, but a significant increase after three weeks' treatment. After four weeks, platelet retention was still elevated but after five weeks no difference existed as compared with the pre-experimental value. This 'rebound' phenomenon is not explained. In the linoleic acid group, no significant change was seen after one week, but after three weeks platelet retention had dropped significantly. After four weeks, this drop was even more pronounced, but after five weeks all differences had disappeared.

Geill and Dybkaer [287] treated female patients for two periods of eight weeks with 15 ml of a fatty acid mixture containing 56% linolenic acid, 20% oleic acid, 14% linoleic acid and 10% saturated fatty acid. Platelet adhesion (glass bead columns) was not affected significantly but tended to increase. Nordøy and Rødset [618] gave 20 healthy volunteers diets containing 40% soyabean oil or MCT-oil, and did not observe significant differences in ADP-, collagen and thrombin-induced platelet aggregation (turbidimetric technique; see refs. 82 and 630) as compared with the pre-experimental values; nor did they find dietary effects in platelet electrophoretic mobility. The technique they used for this latter determination [312] fails, however, to discriminate between 'normal' and 'atherosclerotic' platelets, in contrast to the technique used by Hampton and Mitchell [337]. This is probably due to differences in the potential gradients applied [810] and therefore an effect of the dietary fats on this parameter cannot be excluded. Platelet factor 3 (PF-3) activity decreased significantly in the soyabean oil group, while in the MCT group it increased slightly. The same tendency in PF-3 activity was found after exposure of platelets to kaolin, ADP, and freezing and thawing.

5.3.1.3. Conclusion

In sum, it can be stated that in the literature, there is no unanimity as to the effect of dietary fats on in vitro platelet stickiness, regardless whether the fats are administered as a single oral load, by intravenous infusion or by continuous feeding. The conflicting results cannot be ascribed to differences in fatty acid composition but may be due to the different techniques employed, particularly the in vitro platelet studies which may be disturbed by technical artifacts. Moreover, the interpretation of in vitro findings is very difficult. For instance, a low platelet aggregation in vitro does not necessarily imply that all the platelets have a low thrombosis tendency. On the contrary, it is very possible that due to thrombogenesis in vivo, the most active platelets are involved in aggregation and thrombus formation and that only the less active ones remain as single platelets in the circulation. Therefore, the validity of any in vitro technique to measure the thrombosis tendency has to be tested.

5.3.2. *Investigations into the effect of dietary fats on platelet aggregation in vitro*

For most of these experiments we used material from rats fed diets containing antithrombotic sunflowerseed oil (SO, 50 or 60 en%) or thrombogenic hydrogenated coconut oil (HCO, 45 or 55 en%, supplied with 5 en% SO to prevent essential fatty acid deficiency). Apart from a consistent effect on arterial thrombosis tendency (Fig. 5.1), we also noted that the HCO diet invariably caused a higher whole blood platelet count than the SO-diet (Fig. 5.4).

Platelet aggregation in vitro was measured, using the turbidimetric technique as described by Born [82] and O'Brien [630]. To this end, 0.3 ml PRP (obtained as described in section 5.2.) was mixed with 2.3 ml saline and 0.2 ml $CaCl_2$-solution (7.5×10^{-3} mol.l^{-1}) and incubated for 2 min at 37° C while stirring at 1000 rev. min^{-1}. Aggregation was then induced by adding 0.2 ml of the following solutions:
- ADP (disodium salt, ex Sigma) 2.5 and 1.25 μg. ml^{-1} in saline, giving a final concentration of 0.167 and 0.083 μg. ml^{-1}, respectively.

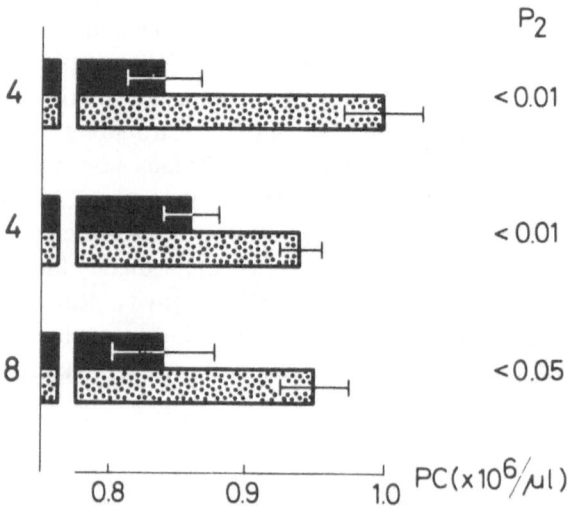

Fig. 5.4. Platelet concentration (PC $\pm$ SEM) in blood of rats fed SO ($\blacksquare$) or HCO ($\blacksquare\!\!\vdots$) diets for four and eight weeks (n = 12–16)

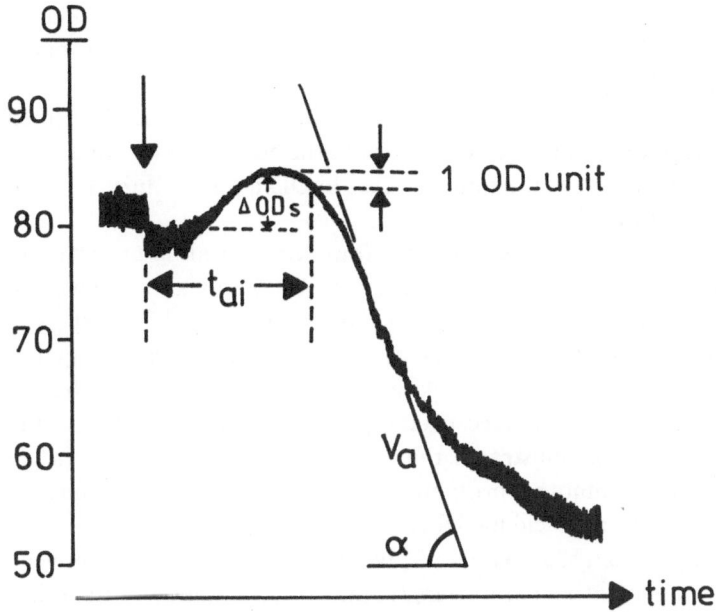

Fig. 5.5. Course of Optical Density (OD) of a platelet suspension after adding collagen to the suspension (arrow). For explanation: see text

- Thrombin (ex Hoffmann-La Roche and Co, Basle, Switzerland) 2.5 and 2 NIH-units per ml in saline, providing a final concentration of 0.17 and 0.13 NIH- units per ml, respectively.
- Collagen (from Achillis tendon, ex Merck, Darmstadt, F.R.G.) prepared as follows: 1 g collagen was suspended in 50 ml saline by intermittent homogenization (Ultra Turrax, Type 45., No. 5202 Janke and Kunkel, A.G.) for 10 min at $0°$ C. Subsequently, the suspension was centrifuged for 10 min at 60 g and $0°$ C. The clear supernatant was decanted, diluted 1:5 with saline, divided into 2.5 ml portions and stored at $-20°$ C until use. For aggregation measurements, this stock was diluted with saline in a ratio of 1:3 and 1:5.

All working solutions were stored in melting ice. The aggregation-induced changes in optical density of the PRP dilutions were recorded with Vitraton® equipment (Dieren, Holland). ADP- and thrombin-induced aggregation was quantified by measuring the maximal change in optical density (ΔOD_{max}). The aggregation induced by collagen proceeds somewhat different from that initiated by ADP and thrombin. Figure 5.5. shows a typical curve. Addition of the collagen suspension (arrow) results in a slight descent of the OD curves, due to dilution of the platelet suspension. The collagen causes the release of ADP to which the platelets react with a shape change, resulting in an OD increase. The OD curve passes through a maximum (OD_{max}), after which platelet aggregation causes a rapid irreversible decrease in OD. From this curve, the following parameters were calculated:

- Aggregation induction time, t_{ai}, being the time (s) lapsing between collagen addition and a decrease by 1 OD-unit (full scale ~ 100 Units) after the curve has passed through OD_{max}.
- Aggregation velocity, V_a, which is the tangent of the angle (α) which is formed by the steepest slope of the aggregation curve and the horizontal ($=$ time) axis.
- Platelet shape change, ΔOD_s, the total increase in OD after administration of the collagen suspension.

Results obtained with ADP and thrombin after four weeks feeding are given in Table 5.4. The differences between the two groups were not significant, which is not in agreement with the results obtained by Renaud and coworkers [685] who showed that thrombosis tendency was positively related to thrombin-induced aggregation and inversely related to ADP-induced aggregation. This discrepancy might be due to the different diets used (see 5.2.2). In recent studies diets more comparable to ours were used with which they demonstrated that hydrogenated coconut oil, when replacing corn oil, slightly promoted thrombin-induced, but not the ADP-induced aggregation. Palmitic and stearic acid increased both thrombin- and ADP-induced aggregation considerably [532, 533]. Table 5.5 gives the results of collagen-induced aggregation. For both aggregation parameters (t_{ai} and V_a), the values for the HCO group indicate a lower platelet aggregation (longer aggregation induction times, lower aggregation velocities). Platelets shape change (ΔOD_s) is significantly more pronounced in the HCO group ($P_2 < 0.01$, Wilcoxon's two-sample test). Because of the (unexpected) tendency of platelets from the thrombogenic HCO group to aggregate to a lesser extent in response to callagen than platelets from animals receiving the antithrombotic SO-diet, a second experiment was performed to collect more data on this point. Again it appeared that, especially in the lower-dose range, collagen induced aggregation is lower in platelets from animals fed the thrombogenic HCO-diet (Fig. 5.6).

This discrepancy between in vitro and in vivo findings indicates that in vitro results should be interpreted with the utmost care. This can also be concluded from a different experiment described in detail in Chapter 6, section 3. Briefly, rats were fed diets known to induce different arterial thrombosis tendencies. After eight weeks, OTs were determined in 50% of the animals where in the other half, collagen-induced aggregation was measured (as well as some other platelet and vessel wall

Table 5.4. ADP- and thrombin-induced aggregation ($\Delta OD_{max} \pm$ SEM) in PRP/saline dilutions of rats fed SO-(n $=$ 12) or HCO-(n $=$ 11) containing diets for four weeks

Compound	Final concentration	SO	HCO	P_2
ADP	0.167 μg.ml^{-1}	27.7 $\pm$ 1.59	28.5 $\pm$ 1.98	>0.10
	0.083 μg.ml^{-1}	12.2 $\pm$ 1.76	8.3 $\pm$ 1.42	>0.10
Thrombin	0.17 NIH-units.ml^{-1}	37.7 $\pm$ 2.94	42.7 $\pm$ 1.94	>0.10
	0.13 NIH-units.ml^{-1}	25.8 $\pm$ 3.38	26.7 $\pm$ 3.45	>0.10

Table 5.5. Platelet aggregation (t_{ai} and V_a) and platelet shape range (ΔOD_s) induced by collagen in PRP/saline dilutions of rats fed SO (n = 11)- or HCO (n = 10)-containing diets for four weeks. Mean $\pm$ SEM

Parameter	Collagen 1:5		Collagen 1:3	
	SO	HCO	SO	HCO
t_{ai} (s)	85 $\pm$ 4.4	112 $\pm$ 12.0	71 $\pm$ 4.7	79 $\pm$ 6.0
(log s)	1.92 $\pm$ 0.02	2.03 $\pm$ 0.04[a]	1.84 $\pm$ 0.03	1.89 $\pm$ 0.03
V_a (tg α)	2.15 $\pm$ 0.26	1.66 $\pm$ 0.28	2.95 $\pm$ 0.26	2.84 $\pm$ 0.14
ΔOD_s	3.12 $\pm$ 0.21	4.75 $\pm$ 0.25[b]	3.45 $\pm$ 2.36	4.76 $\pm$ 0.16[b]

[a] $P_2 < 0.05$
[b] $P_2 < 0.01$

properties, see Chapter 6). As shown in Fig. 5.7, no correlation was found between arterial thrombosis tendency and collagen-induced aggregation. In separate studies (Chapters 6 and 7), similar results were obtained for ADP- and thrombin-induced aggregation measurements. Therefore, the usefulness of in vitro aggregation tests as indicators for the arterial thrombosis tendency, is highly questionable. The lower 'activation grade' of HCO platelets upon collagen-triggering most probably explains the diminished collagen-induced PF3 availability observed in these platelets (see section 5.2.5).

5.3.3. *Platelet aggregation in circulating arterial blood*

The main disadvantage of the aggregation technique used in the previous section is that any short-lived aggregation-affecting substance that might be present in circu-

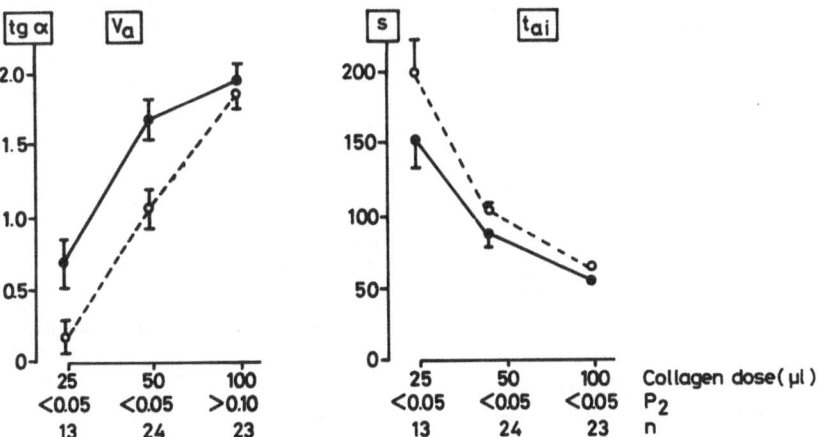

Fig. 5.6. Collagen-induced aggregation velocity V_a, tg$\alpha \pm$SEM) and aggregation induction time (t_{ai}, s$\pm$SEM) of platelets of rats fed SO (— ● —) or HCO (--○--) containing diets for four weeks.

lating blood, will already have been inactivated when aggregation in vitro is ultimately measured. Since the discovery of Thromboxane A_2 and prostacyclin (two unstable substances with very profound effects on platelet function – see Chapter 3), this disadvantage became particularly manifest.

Some time ago we developed a method for measuring platelet aggregation in circulating arterial blood [385] which is based on the screen filtration technique [191, 797]. Since this method does not suffer from the drawback mentioned above, we used it to investigate the dietary fat effect on platelet aggregation.

5.3.3.1. *Method to measure platelet aggregation in circulating arterial rat blood*

A filter system (Fig. 5.8) is connected to the arterial circulation of rats via the so-called aorta loop (see Chapter 4, section 3), which is inserted the day preceding the experiment. Portex vinyl tube no. 4E (internal diameter 2 mm) is used as a connecting tube. Two pressure transducers (Statham, type P23-Db) are connected to the system by glass four-way connection pieces. The blood pressures are recorded by a two-channel recorder. The filter (Veco, Eerbeek, The Netherlands) consists of a round, nickel filter plate (diameter 12 mm, pore width 20 μm), provided with a support screen. By means of two Teflon rings (internal diameter 9 mm), the filter is fitted leak-proof in a metal filter holder (Millipore Swinny Hypodermic Adapter, Cat. No. XX 300 1200). Assembly of the filter is done under water to prevent inclusion or air bubbles. Close to the proximal connection of the filter system to the aorta loop, two thin cannulae (Portex PP 50) are introduced to administer the

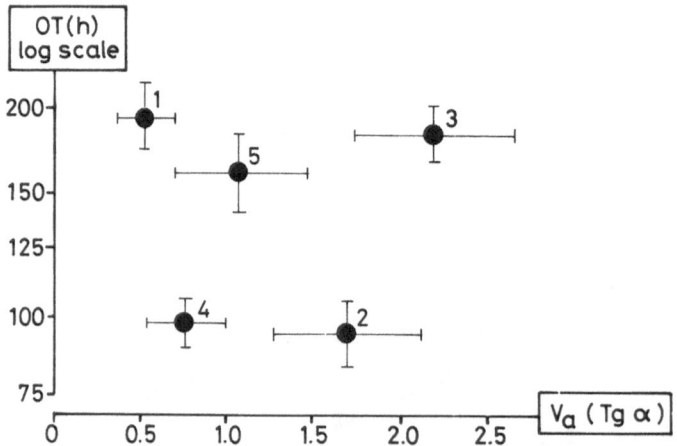

Fig. 5.7. Lack of correlation between collagen-induced aggregation (V_a, tgα $\pm$ SEM) and arterial thrombosis tendency (OT, h $\pm$ SEM, log scale) in rats fed different dietary fats (n = 10–12).
1: 5 en% HCO (essential fatty acid deficient)
2: 5 en% SO (control)
3: 50 en% SO
4: 5 en% SO + 45 en% HCO
5: 5 en% SO + 45 en% LO (linseed oil)

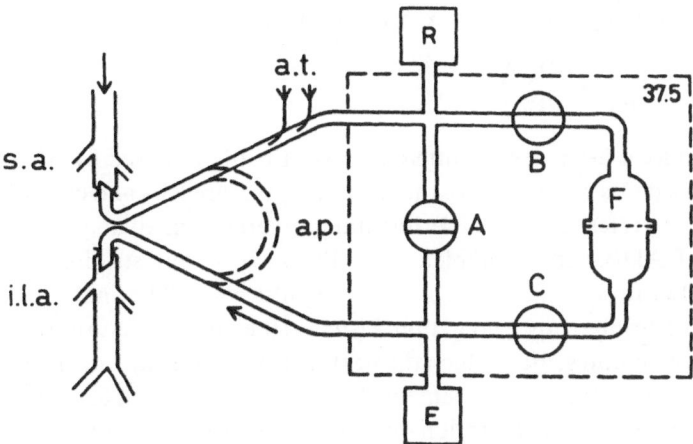

Fig. 5.8. Schematic drawing of apparatus for measuring platelet aggregation in circulating arterial blood. R: recording of reference pressure, E: recording of experimental pressure; A, B, and C: valves; F: filter; s.a.: spermatic arteries; a.p.: aorta loop (cut through); i.l.a.: iliolumbar arteries; a and t: thin cannulae for infusing ADP and substances under investigation.

substances to be investigated. After assembly, the whole system (internal volume ca. 2 ml) is siliconised with Siliclad 1:20 and filled with a 0.9% NaCl-solution containing 500 I.U.ml^{-1} heparin (Vitrum). To prevent the influence of temperature changes on the aggregation process, the system is embedded in a heating block which is kept at 37.5° C by warm water circulation.

After connection of the arterial circulation to the extracorporeal system the blood pressure of the animal drops considerably. In most cases this pressure drop can be prevented by placing an oxygen hood over the animal's head. This device is kept in place during the entire experiment. As a result of the internal resistance of the filter, the pressure before the filter is usually somewhat higher (4-10 mmHg) than behind it. For the rest, the filter has no appreciable influence on the blood circulation for hours. Obstruction as a result of spontaneous aggregation occurs only under certain dietary conditions (Section 5.3.3.3), and is temporary. Therefore, it does not affect the aggregation measurements.

Ten minutes after the filter has been included in the arterial circulation of the rat, the first aggregation measurement can be performed. To this end ADP is administered by means of an infusion device at a rate of 0.1 ml.min^{-1} for 30 s. Depending on the ADP-concentration, more or fewer thrombocytes aggregate, as a result of which the filter is obturated rapidly or slowly, completely or partly, while the blood pressures before and behind the filter change and the pulse wave behind the filter diminishes (Fig. 5.9). The pressure changes consist of an increase in the reference pressure (RP = the systolic blood pressure before the filter) and a fall in the experimental pressure (EP = the systolic blood pressure behind the filter).

For practical purposes an aggregation index A was defined as

$$A = 100 \times \left(1 - \frac{EP_2}{RP_2} \times \frac{RP_1}{EP_1} \right)$$

which is, in fact, the maximum pressure difference over the filter caused by ADP-administration expressed as a percentage of the reference pressure RP_2 and corrected for small variations in reference and experimental pressures immediately before the administration of ADP. After completion of the ADP-administration, the pressure behind the filter rapidly increases, as does the pulse wave. This indicates a cleaning of the filter as a result of disaggregation. Usually, the pressure returns to its initial level within a few minutes, after which the next measurement can take place. The time between two consecutive measurements has been standardised at 10 min, because normalization of the concentration of circulating platelets takes about 6–8 min. When the number of measurements on the same animal is extended, a significant decrease in aggregation index is observed. Most probably, this is not due to thrombocytopenia [385]. Microscopic investigations showed that the material obstructing the filter when ADP is infused consisted mainly of thrombocytes. Moreover, blood smears taken behind the filter during ADP-infusion before the filter, contained fewer and much smaller platelet aggregates than the smears taken simultaneously before the filter. During ADP-administration, the concentration of blood platelets before the filter is also significantly higher than behind it. It is

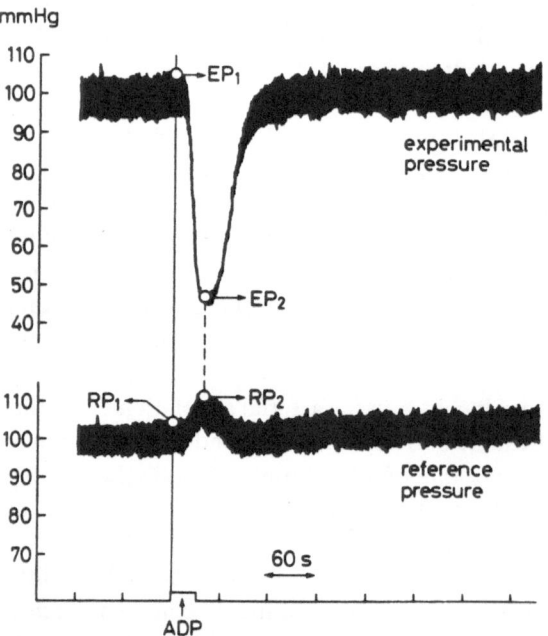

Fig. 5.9. Recording of an aggregation measurement. For explanation of EP_1, EP_2, RP_1 and RP_2, see under section 5.3.3.1.

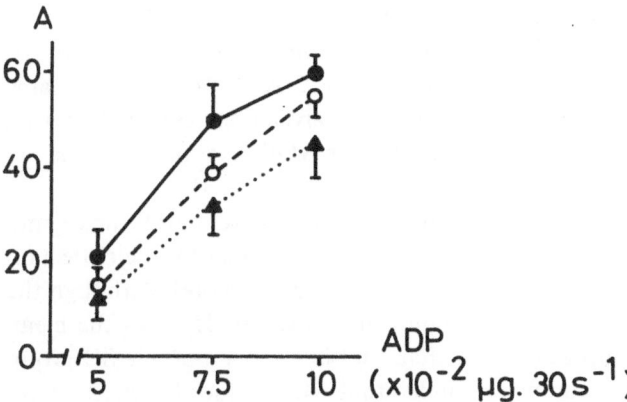

Fig. 5.10. ADP-induced aggregation of blood platelets in circulating arterial blood (A) of rats (n = 18) fed 0.3% w/w Atromid (▲ ... ▲) or given 20 mg Ronicol twice daily (○ --- ○) for three to five weeks. Mean ± SEM. ●———● control group

assumed, therefore, that the changes in pressure before and behind the filter, induced by ADP-administration, are mainly caused by thrombocyte aggregation.

Only substances such as ADP, which induce platelet aggregation immediately can be used to trigger aggregation because the aggregates must have been formed before the reaction mixture passes the filter. Therefore, it appeared impossible to use collagen as an aggregation inducer. The use of thrombin is also impossible, as the animal has to be anti-coagulated to prevent clotting on the filter. Arachidonic acid, however, has been used successfully to trigger aggregation. The filter-loop appeared very useful to measure degree and duration of the platelet aggregation inhibiting effect of prostaglandin E_1 upon parenteral administration [386]. Moreover, we used the technique to demonstrate the platelet aggregation inhibiting effect of two serum lipid lowering drugs, Atromid-S ® [297, 631, 798] and Ronicol® [359, 878] (Fig. 5.10). The filter-loop technique has also been adopted by other investigators, not only for rats [580] but, after minor modifications, also for dogs [100, 414] and monkeys [8]. In these experiments, the technique was successfully used for drug-screening.

Table 5.6. ADP-induced aggregation (A ± SEM) in circulating arterial blood of rats fed diets containing SO or HCO for four weeks (n = 13)

ADP-dose	A ± SEM		
$\mu g.10^{-3}. 30 s^{-1}$	SO	HCO	P_2
25	10.4 ± 2.60	15.1 ± 3.10	>0.10
50	25.8 ± 5.25	49.3 ± 5.53	<0.01

5.3.3.2. *ADP-induced aggregation in rats fed different dietary fats*

In a first experiment with animals fed SO- and HCO-containing diets, respectively, platelet aggregation was measured by administering 2 ADP-doses to the same animal with an interval of 10 min. The lowest dose was given first. As is evident from Table 5.6, HCO feeding causes a significantly higher ADP response than the SO diet.

This experiment has been repeated several times, using different ADP doses and feeding periods. In total, both diets have been compared 16 times for their effect on the ADP-induced platelet aggregation in circulating arterial blood. Although the differences did not always reach the 5% significance level, in 15 cases the mean aggregation in the HCO group was higher than that in the comparable SO group (Sign test: $P_2 < 0.01$). Thus, it can be concluded that ADP-induced platelet aggregation measured in circulating arterial blood is higher on feeding the thrombogenic HCO-diet than when the antithrombotic SO-containing diet is given.

In order to investigate whether arterial thrombosis tendency is correlated with ADP-induced aggregation in circulating arterial blood, six groups of 24 animals were fed diets containing 50 en% of WO, HSO, RO, OO, LO or SO (see Table 4.2.). In 12 animals of each group, arterial thrombosis tendency was measured with the aorta-loop technique (Chapter 4, section 3). In the other animals, aggregation was measured on infusing three different ADP-doses in the same animal with intervals of 10 min. The sequence of the ADP doses varied per 4 animals. The results of the aggregation measurements are given in Table 5.7. From statistical analysis it appeared that, in each dietary group, the ADP dose-response curve did not deviate significantly from rectilinearity. Moreover, all curves ran parallel to each other. The ADP-response in the WO-group was significantly lower ($P_2 < 0.05$) than in all other groups. Platelet aggregation in the group receiving RO was systematically lower than in the groups receiving HSO, OO, LO, and SO ($P_2 < 0.1$). As the ADP-response and the OT were determined in different animals (the OT results have been reported in Chapter 4, section 4.2), no direct relationship between the two parameters could be calculated. However when the mean values within each group were

Table 5.7. ADP-induced aggregation (A ± SEM) in circulating blood of rats fed diets containing 50 en% of different fats for nine weeks (n = 12)

Dietary fat	ADP-dose (ng30 s^{-1})		
(see Table 6.2.)	25	37.5	50
WO	6.3 ± 1.7	13.9 ± 2.8	36.2 ± 6.1
HSO	39.2 ± 6.8	52.2 ± 6.4	68.3 ± 3.4
RO	14.1 ± 2.7	33.3 ± 5.7	50.4 ± 6.3
OO	33.9 ± 5.5	49.0 ± 6.0	64.2 ± 3.7
LO	32.3 ± 5.1	44.8 ± 5.6	64.5 ± 2.4
SO	24.5 ± 3.8	43.5 ± 5.7	63.2 ± 4.4

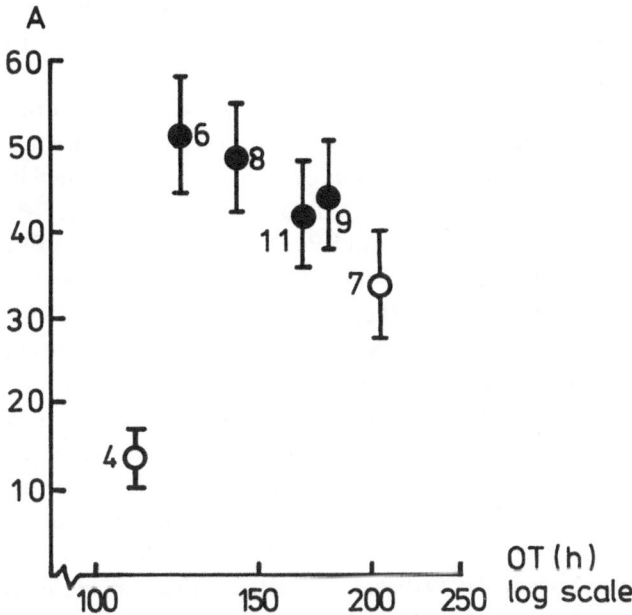

Fig. 5.11. Relationship between arterial thrombosis tendency (OT) and ADP-induced aggregation in circulating blood (A $\pm$ SEM; 37,5 ng ADP in 30 s) of rats fed diets containing 50 en% of different fats for nine weeks. Numbers refer to dietary fats mentioned in Table 4.2.

compared, it appeared that, in general, a high OT value coincides with a low ADP-response (Fig. 5.11). This finding strongly indicates that the dietary fat effect on arterial thrombosis tendency is, at least in part, mediated by changes in platelet aggregability. The deviating behaviour of the WO group will be discussed further in Chapter 7.

5.3.3.3. *Spontaneous platelet aggregation*
To induce aggregation in circulating arterial blood of animals fed a stock diet, ADP has to be infused (section 5.3.3.1.). However, when investigating the effects of SO-

Table 5.8. Frequency (%) and degree (A $\pm$ SEM) of spontaneous aggregation (SA) observed in rats fed SO- and HCO-containing diets for four weeks

Expt.no.	n	SA frequency		SA degree	
		SO	HCO	SO	HCO
1	12	33.3	100[a]	39.2 $\pm$ 17.27	61.2 $\pm$ 6.33
2	13	0	76.9[a]	–	33.9 $\pm$ 5.73

[a] $P_2 < 0.01$

and HCO-feeding, a reversible 'wave' of spontaneous aggregation was sometimes observed immediately after the extracorporeal system had been connected. In retrospect, we observed that spontaneous aggregation occurred more frequently on HCO- than on SO-feeding. In view of this, a prospective study was carried out in which frequency and degree of spontaneous aggregation (SA) were compared in animals fed the SO- and HCO-diets for four weeks. The SA-degree was quantified in the same way as for ADP-induced aggregation (section 5.3.3.1.), except that EP_1 and RP_1 were taken at their minimum difference and EP_2 and RP_2 at minimum EP. Two experiments were performed, the results of which are given in Table 5.8.

The SA frequency was significantly higher in the HCO group than in the SO-fed animals ($P_2 < 0.01$, Student's two-sample test). Because of the great differences in SA-frequency, the differences in SA-degree could not be evaluated statistically. However, there is a distinct tendency that the SA degree is also higher in the HCO group. The same can be concluded after including the retrospective results obtained from the experiments mentioned in section 5.3.2.2. In 103 SO animals, the average SA frequency and SA-degree were 15.5% and 23.8, respectively, whereas in 93 HCO-fed animals, these figures were 77.4% and 35.8. These results allow the conclusion that feeding a thrombogenic HCO diet is associated with a systematically higher frequency and degree of spontaneous aggregation than when an anti-thrombotic SO diet is given.

The SA-inducing mechanism has not yet been elucidated. Since the aorta loop is temporarily clamped immediately before the extracorporeal system is connected, thrombin generation during this stasis period might trigger aggregation. However, the duration of this stasis period was not related to the degree of SA; therefore, this explanation seems rather unlikely. Because spontaneous platelet aggregates were already observed 14 cm proximal to the filter, the filter itself cannot have been the cause of their formation. The extracorporeal system is primed with a rather strong heparin solution and heparin has repeatedly been reported to be an aggregation-inducing substance [224, 373]. The spontaneous aggregation observed might, therefore, be heparin-induced. This suggestion was supported by the observation that the degree of spontaneous aggregation (SA $\pm$ SEM) is significantly higher in the presence (22.8 ± 4.9; n = 24) than in the absence of heparin (9.5 ± 2.9; n = 19, $P_2 < 0.01$, Wilcoxon's two-sample test). However, later experiments demonstrated that heparin stabilises platelet aggregates, resulting in a less rapid break-up when mechanically stressed. Whether this has something to do with the prostacyclin-neutralising effect of heparin which has been reported by several groups [53, 226, 507, 710] and which might be analogous to similar effects of heparin on prostaglandin E_1 [369, 676] remains to be investigated, but seems unlikely (699a).

5.4. POSSIBLE MECHANISMS BY WHICH DIETARY FATS AFFECT PLATELET
AGGREGATION AND ARTERIAL THROMBUS FORMATION

The results presented so far show that the thrombotic or antithrombotic effects of
dietary fats are probably caused by their fatty acid composition. The same has been
reported for atherogenesis: long-chain saturated fats were shown to be atherogenic
whereas linoleic acid had a distinct preventive effect [466, 517, 806, 831]. In the
pathogenesis of atherosclerosis, cholesterol metabolism plays an important role:
hypercholesterolemic diets appear to be atherogenic whereas the hypocholestero-
lemic effect of dietary linoleic acid is associated with a lower incidence of and
mortality from atherosclerotic complications [363, 552, 861, 862]. In rats, the
saturated, thrombogenic HCO diet causes a higher serum cholesterol content than
the linoleic acid-rich antithrombotic SO diet. Since antherosclerosis and arterial
thrombosis are related phenomena (Chapter 1), the dietary fat effects on arterial
thrombosis might also be mediated by the plasma cholesterol content. However,
this appeared highly unlikely, because no significant correlation was observed
between plasma cholesterol content and the OT in animals fed eight different
amounts of linoleic acid-rich SO or five different dietary fats. Similar results were
obtained by Renaud and coworkers [687]. The possible role of platelet cholesterol is
discussed in Chapter 8, section 6.3.

Considering the results presented in Chapter 4, it is tempting to speculate that
linoleic acid causes the antithrombotic effect of sunflowerseed oil, but it should be
realized that other components present in this and other linoleic acid-containing
fats may also play a role. Since it has been reported that the vitamin E content of
vegetable oils increases as their degree of unsaturation rises [422], and since vitamin
E has been suggested to inhibit platelet thrombotic functions [258, 504, 787, 788,
795] and prostaglanoid metabolism [125, 126], at least part of the anti-thrombotic
effect of linoleic acid-rich oils might be due to their relatively high vitamin E content.
This question was investigated by comparing the OTs of animals fed 5, 30 and 60
en% SO with those of rats fed diets containing 5 en% SO and enriched with amounts
of vitamin E equivalent to those present in diets containing 30, 60 and 100 en% SO.
The results of this study (Fig. 5.12) clearly indicate that the antithrombotic effect of
sunflowerseed oil is not due to its vitamin E content because increasing the dietary
amount of vitamin E does not prolong the OT, whereas dietary SO does.

Fibrin formation is an important prerequisite for an arterial thrombus to become
stabilised. This is illustrated by the diminishing effect of heparin on the arterial
thrombosis tendency in rats (Fig. 4.3) as well as by the preventive effect of oral
anticoagulants on myocardial reinfarction in man [16, 199, 417, 540, 760, 876]. So
far, no systematic investigations have been described as to the relative importance of
the fibrinolytic system in the process of arterial thrombosis. It has been reported,
however, that inhibition of fibrinolysis to control haemorrhagic manifestations
resulting from hyperfibrinolysis was followed by multiple arterial thromboses
[591].

88

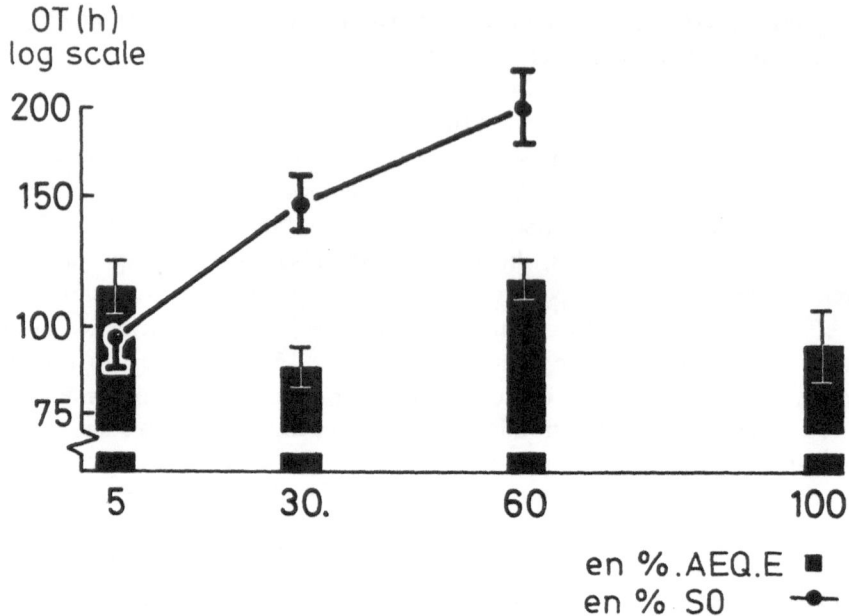

Fig. 5.12. Effect of vitamin E supplementation (bars) and increasing amounts of dietary sunflowerseed oil (dots) on arterial thrombosis tendency in rats (OT ± SEM; n = 12).
Vitamin E was added to a diet containing 5 en% SO in amounts equivalent to those present in 5, 30, 60, and 100 en% SO-containing diets (en% eq.E).

For a long time lipids have been thought to inhibit fibrinolysis, although the literature is rather conflicting on this point, especially as far as the differential effects of saturated and (poly)unsaturated fats are concerned [201, 240–242, 542]. So far it seems rather unlikely that the beneficial effect of linoleic acid rich oils is due to their influence on fibrinolysis [814]. New insights into the biochemistry of fibrinolysis and its regulation [150] are presently leading to the development of new techniques for the measurement of relevant parameters of the fibrinolytic process [709]. Using these techniques, a re-evaluation of the influence of the dietary fat type on fibrinolysis seems appropriate.

Some time ago, the attention was drawn to the possible importance of ADP, derived from damaged erythrocytes or from vascular tissue, for platelet activation, both in vitro [536] as well as in vivo [15, 85–87, 693]. Although no unanimity exists as to the effect of intravascular ADP on platelet aggregation [114, 351] differences in red cell membrane integrity, and thereby in the resistance to haemolysis, are likely to affect thrombus formation [86]. So far, no systematic investigations have been performed as to the effect of dietary fats on haemolysis. No difference was observed, however, in the osmotic resistance of erythrocytes obtained from animals fed either SO- or HCO-containing diets.

Ever since the inhibitory effect of prostaglandin E_1 on platelet aggregation was recognized [458], prostaglandins and related compounds have been implicated in the regulation of platelet function and arterial thrombosis. Since the anti-thrombotic fatty acids (linoleic and α-linolenic acid) are the dietary precursors of the naturally occurring prostanoids, these fatty acids may exert their thrombosis-modulating effect by influencing the prostaglandin production. This was investigated in detail, the results of which are discussed in Chapters 6, 7 and 8.

5.5. SUMMARY

Although diets rich in sunflowerseed oil (SO) or hydrogenated coconut oil (HCO) induce a consistent difference in arterial thrombosis tendency, their effects on blood clotting are only marginal. Whole blood plasma clotting times, APTT and PT, are hardly affected. Moreover, vessel wall induced clotting does not differ significantly. Platelet factor 3 activity and content are also similar in both groups. PF3 availability upon collagen-activation of platelets is, however, significantly depressed in the thrombogenic HCO group compared with that in the antithrombotic SO group. Although it should be realized that the results of measurements performed in systemic blood do not necessarily reflect local processes, it seems rather unlikely that dietary-fat induced differences in blood coagulability, if present, contribute significantly to the differences in arterial thrombosis tendency observed.

In vitro platelet aggregation, induced by adenosine diphosphate (ADP) and thrombin, is similar in both groups and collagen-induced aggregation is even lower in the thrombogenic group. However, collagen-induced shape change of platelets in vitro as well spontaneous and ADP-induced aggregation in circulating arterial blood, are significantly depressed in the antithrombotic group. Moreover, on feeding five different vegetable oils, a close correlation was observed between ADP-induced aggregation in circulating arterial blood and arterial thrombosis tendency. Therefore, it is highly probable that the changes in the thrombotic properties of blood platelets constitute the basis for the dietary-fat induced changes in arterial thrombosis tendency. Plasma cholesterol content and dietary vitamin E concentration are most probably not implicated in the mechanisms by which dietary fats affect arterial thrombosis tendency. From the present studies, it also became evident that the classical in vitro platelet aggregation tests have no indicative value for arterial thrombosis tendency in vivo.

6. THE SIGNIFICANCE OF PROSTANOIDS IN THE DIETARY FAT EFFECT ON ARTERIAL THROMBOGENESIS

6.1. INTRODUCTION

In 1967, Kloeze described that prostaglandins influence the aggregation of blood platelets very effectively. Prostaglandin E_1 (PGE_1) is a strong inhibitor and PGE_2 a week stimulator of platelet aggregation [458]. It was also shown that PGE_1 is able to inhibit arterial thrombus formation (Fig. 4.3). Since linoleic and α-linolenic acid are the ultimate dietary precursors of the prostanoids (Chapter 2), the effect of these essential fatty acids on arterial thrombogenesis might be mediated by prostaglandins and/or related compounds. In order to investigate the possible role of these compounds in arterial thrombus formation, we decided to investigate the effect of essential fatty acid deficiency [391] which is associated with a low PG production in tissues [197, 800].

6.2. ARTERIAL THROMBUS FORMATION IN ESSENTIAL FATTY ACID DEFICIENCY

Essential fatty acid (EFA−) deficiency in animals is caused by feeding them diets lacking essential fatty acids. EFA-deficiency has been observed in a large number of animal species and in man, and found to cause a great variety of deficiency symptoms [1, 375, 538]. We induced EFA-deficiency in newly weaned rats by feeding them a fat-free diet or a diet containing 5 en% hydrogenated coconut oil for at least three months. Control animals received a diet with 5 en% sunflowerseed oil. EFA-deficiency was checked by measuring the water-vapour loss via skin and respiration, which, due to structural changes in the skin, is significantly enhanced in EFA-deficiency. Measurements were carried out according to a method described by Thomassen [805], by which a flow of dry air is blown through a cylinder containing the animals under investigation. Water vapour produced by the animal is taken up by the air, which is fed to a measuring cylinder containing a water absorbent. From the increase in weight of this cylinder the water vapour release of the animal can be calculated. The results, computed per 100 cm² body surface [485] per hour, are about twice as high for EFA-deficient than for control animals.

6.2.1. *Effect of EFA-deficiency on arterial thrombosis*

In the first series of experiments, we repeatedly observed that arterial thrombosis tendency is significantly depressed in EFA-deficient animals. Obstruction times (OTs) of aorta loops (see Chapter 4, section 3) are invariably longer compared with those of control animals (Fig. 6.1). Feeding an EFA-free, thrombogenic diet to EFA-deficient animals does not result in a shortening of their OTs. This is illustrated in Fig. 6.2, where the effect of additional hydrogenated coconut oil (HCO, a thrombogenic fat, see Chapter 4) on the OT of EFA-deficient rats is shown. This demonstrates that the prothrombotic effect of saturated fats is prevented in EFA-deficiency. A small amount of sunflowerseed oil (SO), which cures EFA-deficiency because of its linoleic acid content, quickly normalises arterial thrombosis tendency.

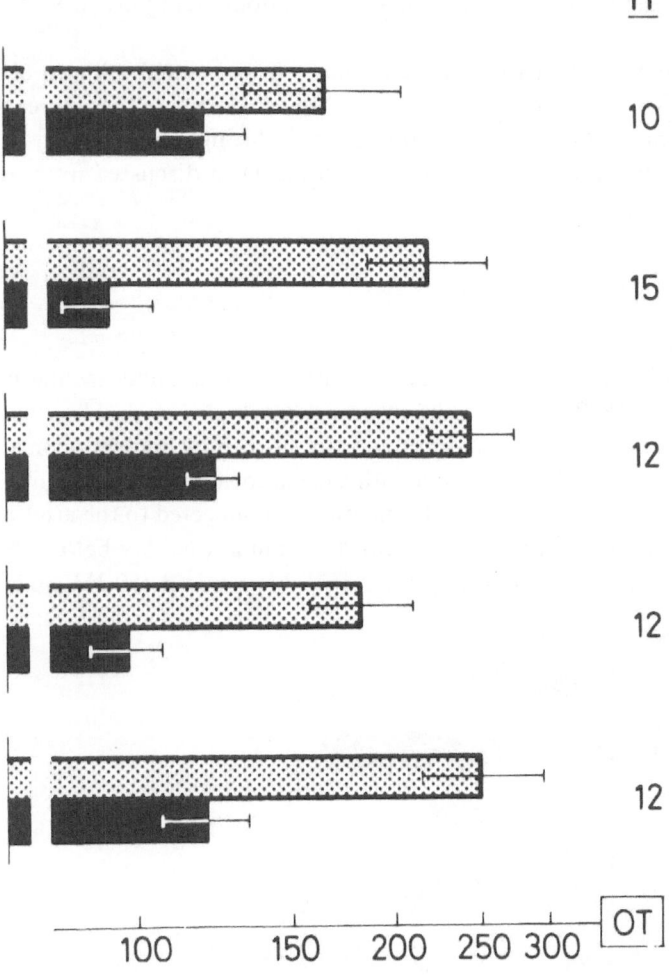

Fig. 6.1. Arterial thrombosis tenency (OT ± SEM, h, log scale) in EFA-deficient (▨) and control (■) rats.

(Fig. 6.2). To find the minimal EFA-requirement for normal thrombogenesis (OT ± 120 h, see Chapter 4), newly weaned rats were fed diets containing 50 en% HCO, which was replaced by increasing amounts of SO. OTs were measured after twelve weeks of feeding. To check EFA-deficiency, water vapour release in vivo was measured after a feeding period of ten weeks. The fatty acid composition of plasma total lipids was also determined (gas-liquid chromatography) approximately two weeks after loop obstruction. Results of OT and water-release measurements are given in Fig. 6.3., from which it can be seen that 0.6–2.5 en% SO (0.4–1.5 en% linoleic acid) is sufficient to prevent EFA-deficiency changes as far as these two criteria are concerned. There was a close inverse relationship between the OT and the plasma arachidonic and linoleic acid contents ($r = -0.92$; $P_2 < 0.01$), whereas the OT was positively related to the plasmatic content of mead acid (20:3(n–9); $r = 0.96$; $P_2 < 0.001$). In EFA-deficiency, this fatty acid replaces arachidonic acid [537] (see also Chapter 2).

From these studies it is evident that EFA-deficiency is associated with an abnormally low arterial thrombosis tendency. It should be recalled here that increasing the dietary SO-content further causes the arterial thrombosis tendency to decrease again. This is indicated in Fig. 6.3 also and has been discussed in more detail in Chapter 4 section 4.1.

6.2.2. *Platelet function in EFA-deficiency*

6.2.2.1. *Platelet adhesion*

Platelet adhesion to a glass surface was measured with a flow-chamber technique devised by Lyman et al. [502] and Friedman and coworkers [262]. The flow-chamber is covered with a microscopic slide, previously cleaned by immersion in an ethanol-ether (1:1) mixture for 48 h, polished with a clean towel, kept overnight in ether and air-dried in a dust-free cylinder. The chamber is connected to the arterial blood circulation via an aorta loop, inserted into the animal one day before the experiment. The extracorporeal system is primed with heparinised (50 IU·ml⁻¹)

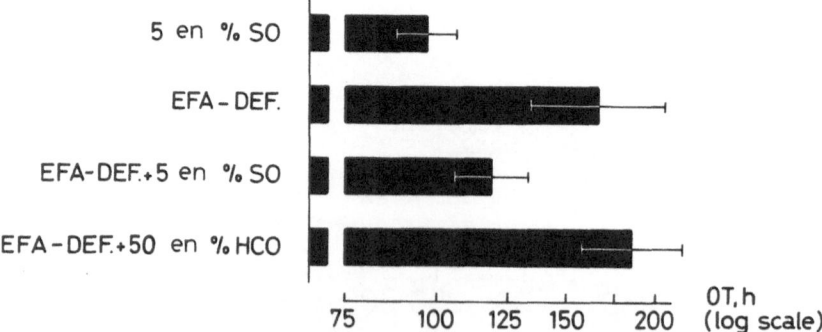

Fig. 6.2. Effect of SO and HCO-containing diets, fed to EFA-deficient animals for four weeks, on arterial thrombosis tendency (OT ± SEM; n = 12).

Table 6.1. Adhesion of EFA-deficient and control rat platelets to a collagen-coated glass rod. Mean ± SEM [118]

Exp. No.	Ht[a] (%)	EFA-deficient		Control		P₂
		n	pl·10^{-3}·mm^{-2}	n	pl·10^{-3}·mm^{-2}	P_2
1	20	15[b]	58.0 ± 4.4	10[b]	110.9 ± 4.9	<0.001
2	20	10[b]	89.5 ± 2.7	10[b]	119.5 ± 5.9	<0.001
3	40	8[c]	66.5 ± 2.5	7[c]	88.5 ± 4.1	<0.001

[a] Obtained by adding washed red cells to platelet suspensions
[b] Experiments were performed n times in pooled platelet suspensions
[c] Each test was performed in quadruplicate in individual platelet suspensions of n rats.

saline. Immediately after connection of the flow-chamber, the blood is allowed to circulate through it for exactly 2 min. During the first 30 s, a blood sample is taken proximally to the flow-chamber for platelet counting. Subsequently, the chamber is disconnected and exactly 1 min. later, the blood is removed by flushing the chamber with 10 ml phosphate-buffered saline (pH 7.4) at a flow-rate of 2 ml·min^{-1}. Finally, the flow-chamber is flushed with 10 ml methanol. After this fixation, the cover slide is removed and air-dried. The adhered cells are stained with Harris' Haematoxilin for 3 min, rinsed in tap water, stained for 30 min with Giemsa-stain (3 drops·ml^{-1})

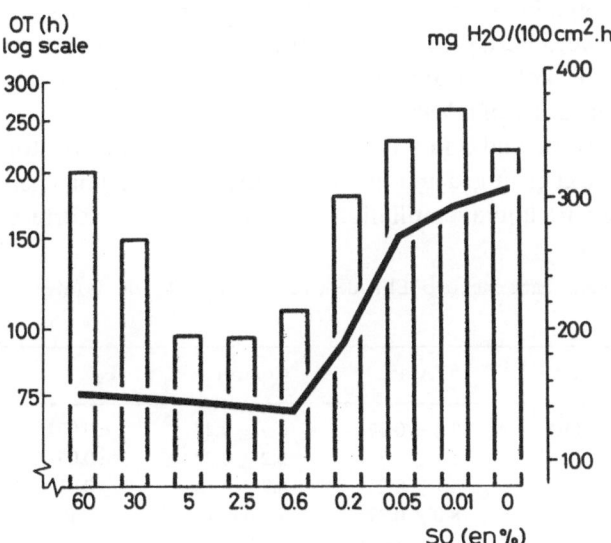

Fig. 6.3. Effect on dietary sunflowerseed oil SO content (en%) on arterial thrombosis tendency (OT, bars) and water-vapour release in vivo (mg H_2O, line). Diets were fed for twelve weeks. Each group comprised 16 animals. EFA-deficiency changes are observed at dietary SO levels below 0.6 en% (~0.4 en% linoleic acid).

rinsed again and air-dried. The number of adhered cells is counted (magn. 1000 x) in seven standardised microscopic fields ($80 \times 80\,\mu m^2$) which are fixed by presettings of the microscope stage. For control animals, 48 ± 14.2 platelets adhered per microscopic field whereas for EFA-deficient animals, this figure was significantly lower: 5 ± 1.3 (mean $\pm$ SEM, n = 12, $P_2 < 0.05$, Wilcoxon's two-sample test). The whole blood platelet count was the same for both groups (0.96 ± 0.07 and $0.95 \pm 0.05 \times 10^6$ platelets$\cdot\mu l^{-1}$).

Platelet adhesion to a collagen-coated glass rod [119, 120] was measured by Dr. J.P. Cazenave. He invariably observed significantly lower adhesion values for EFA-deficient platelets as compared with platelets of control animals (Table 6.1).

6.2.2.2. *Platelet shape change*

When triggered by collagen, the shape change of EFA-deficient platelets is more pronounced than that of control platelets (Table 6.2). This was measured during collagen-induced aggregation in vitro (see Chapter 5, section 3.2).

Using a light-scattering method developed by Michal [548, 549], the ADP-induced shape change was measured also. The results in Table 6.2 clearly show that for EFA-deficient platelets, the ADP-induced shape change is significantly enhanced also in relation to that of control animals.

6.2.2.3. *Platelet aggregation and release*

PRP was prepared as described in Chapter 5, section 2, and incubated at room temperature with 0.2 μCi ^{14}C-serotonin (5HT) per ml PRP (specific activity of ^{14}C-5HT: 58 μCi$\cdot$mmol^{-1}). After 30 min. 5 HT-uptake was almost complete (90–95%) and showed no difference between both groups. Platelets in PRP dilutions (1:10 in saline) were triggered by ADP, collagen and thrombin in the aggregometer as described in Chapter 5, section 3.2.). For release measurements, 0.1 ml samples were taken from the aggregation cuvette and 0.1 ml EDTA (1% w/v) was added to stop the reaction. The samples were centrifuged and the radioactivity of 0.1 ml platelet-free supernatant was measured in a liquid scintillation counter. Values were correct-

Table 6.2. Collagen- and ADP-induced shape change of EFA-deficient and control platelets (Mean $\pm$ SEM, n = 12)

Stimulus		Unit	EFA-def.	Control	$P_2{}^a$
Collagen[b]	0.05 ml	OD	9.6 ± 0.57	6.9 ± 0.47	<0.002
ADP[c]	25 ng$\cdot$ml^{-1}	AU[d]	6.1 ± 0.31	5.2 ± 0.22	<0.05
	75 ng$\cdot$ml^{-1}	AU	8.1 ± 0.25	6.8 ± 0.16	<0.01
	125 ng$\cdot$ml^{-1}	AU	8.0 ± 0.37	7.3 ± 0.24	<0.10

[a] Student's t-test
[b] Added dose
[c] Final concentration
[d] Arbitrary Units.

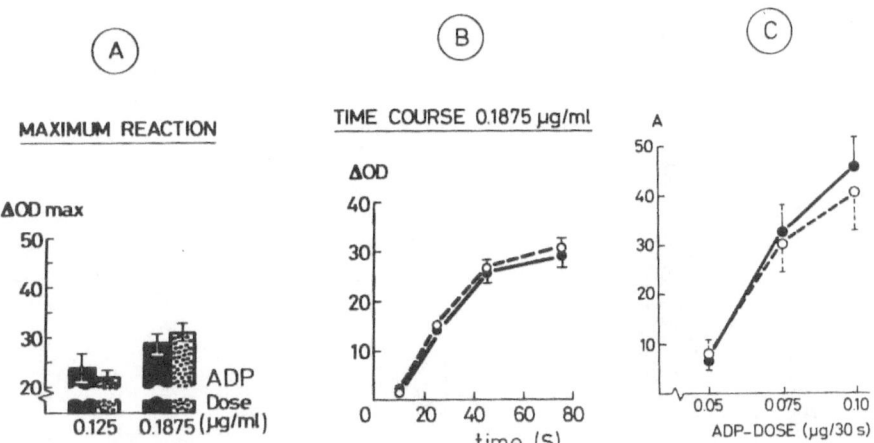

Fig. 6.4. ADP-induced aggregation in vitro (A, B, n = 8) and in circulating arterial blood (C, n = 12) in EFA-deficient (▨ - o -) and control rats (■ - ●-). Mean values ± SEM.

ΔOD: change in optical density (see Chapter 5, section 3.2); A: aggregation index (see Chapter 5, section 3.3.1)

ed for initial radioactivity measured in a sample taken 30 s before adding the aggregating agent. No correction was made for any re-uptake of released 5HT. Platelet aggregation was also measured in circulating arterial blood, as described in Chapter 5, section 3.3.1.

ADP-induced aggregation was not different from normal in EFA-deficiency, neither in vitro nor in circulating arterial blood (Fig. 6.4). McGregor and Renaud [531] observed a lower ADP-induced platelet aggregation in vitro of EFA-deficient

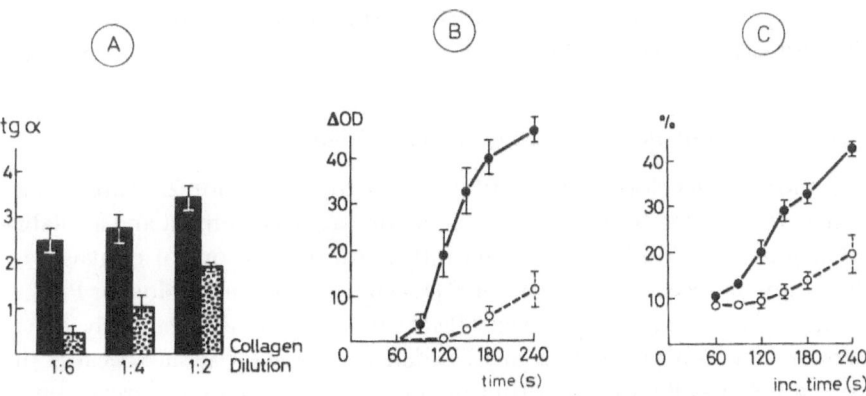

Fig. 6.5. Effect of EFA-deficiency on collagen-induced aggregation and release of blood platelets in vitro. EFA-def.: ▨ - o -; Control: ■ - ●-; Mean values ± SEM; n = 10.

A: Aggregation velocity. For explanation of tgα, see Fig. 5.5.

B: Time course of collagen-induced aggregation. Collagen dilution 1:6. ΔOD = change in optical density.

C: Time course of ^{14}C-5HT release (%). Collagen dilution 1:6.

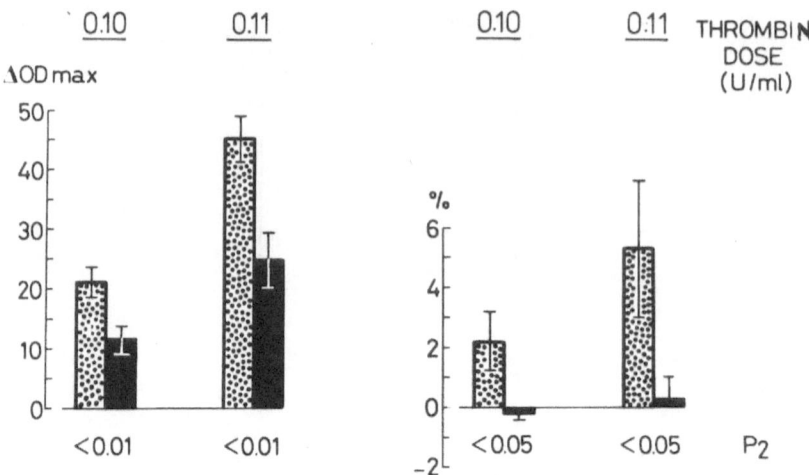

Fig. 6.6. Thrombin-induced aggregation ($\Delta OD_{max} \pm SEM$) and ^{14}C-5HT-release ($\% \pm SEM$) of platelets of EFA-deficient (▨) and control (■) rats. n = 10.

platelets but they used diets with a much higher fat content than were used in our studies (40 vs. 2 w/w%). ADP, in the doses applied by us, did not cause significant 5 HT-release. Collagen-induced aggregation and 5 HT-release were significantly diminished in EFA-deficiency (Fig. 6.5) although later studies showed that this difference largely disappears at a higher trigger strength (Chapter 8, section 3.1). Aggregation and release of EFA-deficient platelets in response to thrombin are enhanced as compared with control platelets (Fig. 6.6). This was also observed by McGregor and Renaud [531, 533] and is thought to be due to the formation of a lipoxygenase product of mead acid (20:3(n − 9)), which appeared to stimulate thrombin-induced aggregation [474].

6.2.3. *Effect of EFA-deficiency on coagulation and platelet factor 3*

Recalcification plasma clotting times (PCT, see Chapter 5, section 2.2.) are normal in EFA-deficient plasma (Fig. 6.7.). Platelet factor 3 activity, content and availability (see Chapter 5, section 2.5.) are significantly lower than in control animals (Fig. 6.8). Vessel wall induced clotting [398, 400] when measured in autologous PRP, is significantly enhanced in EFA-deficiency (Fig. 6.9.A). This is, at least partly, due to the lower prostacyclin production of EFA-deficient vascular tissue, because the difference in vessel wall induced clotting greatly diminishes upon pre-treatment of the vascular tissue with indomethacin (Fig. 6.9.B). When incubated in standard PPP, EFA-deficient aortas causes a more active clotting response than control tissue (Fig. 6.9.C), indicating that EFA-deficient vascular tissue has a stronger clot-promoting effect than normal tissue. No difference were observed when standard tissue was incubated in EFA-deficient or control PPP (Fig. 6.9.D).

6.2.4. *Discrimination between prostanoid-dependent and prostanoid-independent functions of EFA in arterial thrombogenesis*

Columbinic acid, a stero-isomer of γ-linolenic acid, with a *trans* double bond between the 13th and 14th carbon atom (see Chapter 2, section 1) has recently been shown to possess various functions of essential fatty acids [406]. Since columbinic acid is not a prostanoid precursor and in fact inhibits prostaglandin formation considerably this fatty acid can be used to investigate whether the distrubed arterial thrombogenesis and platelet functions observed in EFA-deficiency are the results of a prostanoid-deficiency. This seems rather likely, since EFA-deficient platelets produce only small amounts of TxA_2 upon their activation [107, 395, 828 see also section 3. and Chapter 8, section 3.2.). On the other hand, prostacyclin formation is also depressed in EFA-deficiency [396], which might counteract the effect of a lower platelet TxA_2 production.

Rats were made EFA-deficient by feeding them a 5 en% HCO-containing diet. Control animals received a diet with 5 en% SO. After twelve weeks, the EFA-deficient animals were divided into three groups. One group remained on the EFA-deficient diet. In the diet of the other groups, 3 en% HCO was replaced by the methyl ester of either columbinic acid or linoleic acid. Three weeks later, the water-vapour release in vivo was measured, while after four weeks feeding aorta loops were inserted in all animals to determine thrombosis tendency. After all loops

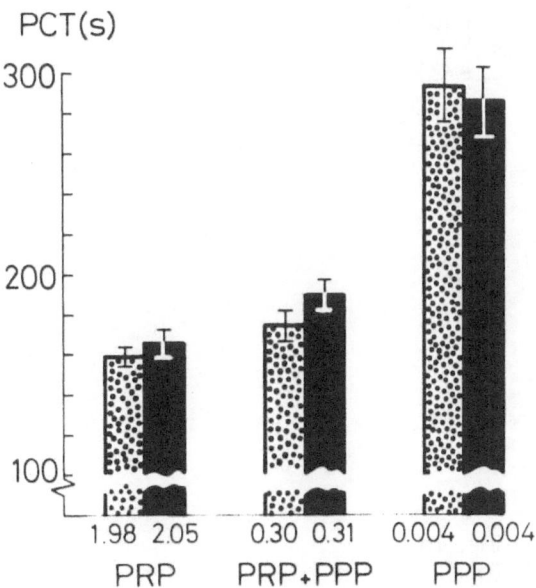

Fig. 6.7. Recalcification plasma clotting time (PCT,s $\pm$ SEM) of EFA-defidient (▨) and control rats (■). Numbers under bars denote platelet concentrations ($\times 10^6 \cdot \mu l^{-1}$). Each group consisted of 14 animals.

98

had been obstructed, the animals were bled by puncturing the aorta just proximal to the loop and PRP was prepared for measuring collagen- and thrombin-induced aggregation. The results are given in Fig. 6.10. With respect to the normalization of the water-vapour release, columbinic acid was equally effective as linoleic acid. The same holds for thrombin-induced aggregation and these functions are, therefore, prostanoid-independent. Dietary linoleic acid but not columbinic acid normalised the arterial thrombosis tendency and the collagen-induced aggregation. Consequently, these functions can be considered prostanoid-dependent.

6.2.5. *Summary*

In EFA-deficient rats, the arterial thrombosis tendency is significantly lower than in control rats. This is associated with a significantly lower platelet factor 3 activity, content and availability. Moreover, platelet adhesion and collagen-induced aggregation and serotonin-release in vitro are significantly depressed. ADP-induced

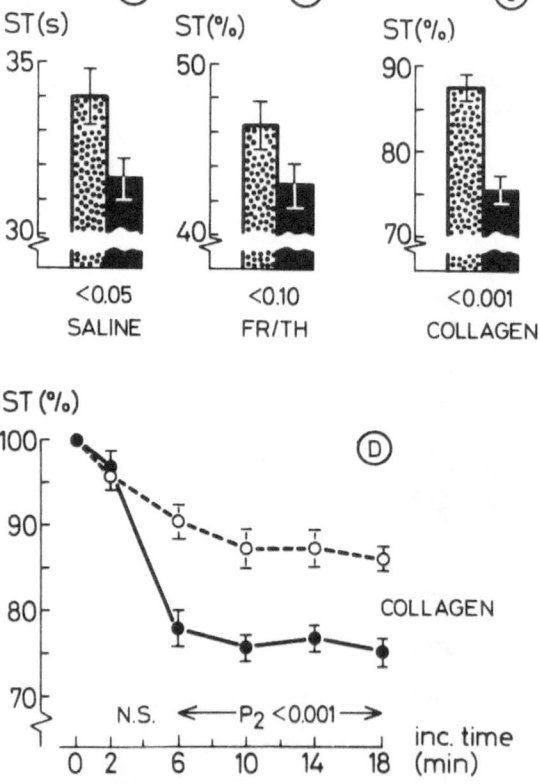

Fig. 6.8. Platelet factor 3 activity (A), content (B) and availability (C and D) of EFA-deficient (▨-o-) and normal (■-•-) blood platelets (mean ± SEM, n = 12).
ST: Stypven time (See Chapter 5, section 2.5); Fr/Th: platelets lysed by 3 times freezing and thawing.

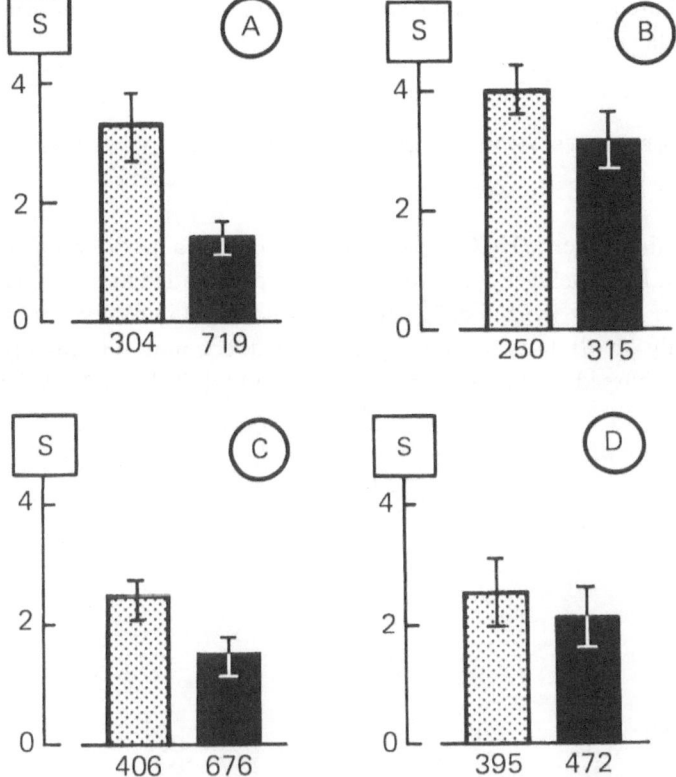

Fig. 6.9. Effect of EFA-deficiency on vessel wall induced clotting (mean ± SEM).

A. non-threated aorta in autologous PRP (n = 10);

B: indomethacin-treated aorta in autologous PRP (n = 12);

C: EFA-deficient and control aortas in reference PPP (n = 7);

D: reference aorta in EFA-deficient and control PPP (n = 12). Figures below bars represent clotting times (s) calculated from mean S values. ▨ EFA-def; ■ control.

Vessel wall induced clotting is indicated by the clotting index S = 1/clotting time (seconds) × 1000.

aggregation, both in vitro and in circulating arterial blood, is not different from normal. Platelet shape change, induced by ADP and collagen in vitro and thrombin induced aggregation and release in vitro are significantly enhanced in EFA-deficiency, as is vessel wall induced clotting. No difference was observed between the recalcification times of platelet-poor and platelet-rich plasma.

Feeding EFA-deficient animals with the methyl ester of columbinic acid which shares the structural effects of essential fatty acids but is not a prostanoid precursor, had no effect on the disturbed arterial thrombosis tendency nor on the collagen-induced aggregation. Therefore, it can be concluded that, in our model, arterial thrombus formation is primarily regulated by prostaglandins and/or thrombo-xanes. This implies that the dietary fat effects on the arterial thrombosis tendency

(Chapter 4) may be mediated by an effect of the various dietary fats on the formation of platelet and/or vascular prostanoids.

6.3. EFFECT OF DIETARY FATS ON PLATELET AND VASCULAR PROSTANOID FORMATION

Rats were fed diets containing 5 en% HCO or SO (control). Due to a lack of linoleic acid, the first diet caused EFA-deficiency. Three other groups included in the study received diets containing, apart from 5 en% sunflowerseed oil, 45 en% of either sunflowerseed oil (maily (n–6) fatty acids), hydrogenated coconut oil (mainly saturated fatty acids) or linseed oil (mainly (n–3) fatty acids) (cf. Table 4.2). After

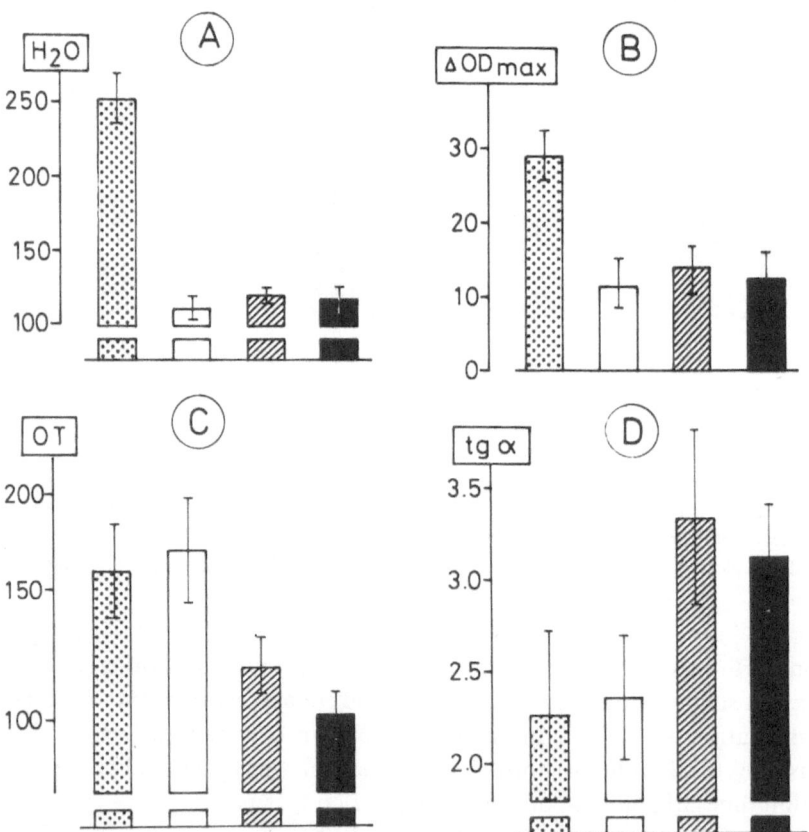

Fig. 6.10. Effect of dietary columbinic acid (□) and linoleic acid (▧) on some EFA-deficiency criteria. ▦ EFA-deficient; ■ Control. Mean ± SEM.

A: Water release in vivo (mg $H_2O \cdot cm^{-2} \cdot h^{-1}$), n = 10.

B: Thrombin-induced platelet aggregation in vitro (ΔOD_{max}), n = 8.

C: Arterial thrombosis tendency (OT, h, log scale), n = 12.

D: Collagen-induced platelet aggregation in vitro (tg α), n = 8.

eight to ten weeks feeding, platelet TxA_2-formation and vascular PGI_2-production were quantified. For this purpose the animals were bled under ether anaesthesia by puncturing the abdominal aorta. PRP was prepared as described in Chapter 5, section 2. After adding EDTA (7.7 mmol·l^{-1} final concentration) the PRP was centrifuged at 600 g for 10 min. PPP was removed and the remaining pellet carefully resuspended in phosphate-buffered saline, pH 7.4, to a concentration of $1-1.5 \times 10^6$ platelets·μl^{-1}. Immediately upon bleeding, aortas were quickly removed, cleaned of adhering tissue, opened longitudinally, divided into two parts and kept in Krebs-Henseleit buffer with or without indomethacin (2 μg·ml^{-1}) at 0°C for at least 60 min.

Platelet TxA_2 was measured as malondialdehyde (MDA), which is formed in equimolar amounts with TxB_2 upon platelet stimulation [54]. MDA, formed upon supramaximal stimulation of the washed platelet suspensions with collagen, was quantified using the spectrophotometric thiobarbituric acid method [639, 767]. Extinctions were corrected for values obtained for non-stimulated platelets and using a standard curve obtained with MDA-bis(di)-ethylacetal, the results were calculated in nmol MDA produced per 10^9 platelets. Vascular prostacyclin formation was measured in two ways. In the first method, a small piece of tissue (diameter 3 mm, dry weight approx. 100 μg) is punched from the aorta and incubated immediately in 200 μl 0.02 M Tris/saline buffer, pH 7.2 in a gently shaking vial at room temperature. After 4 min, 50 μl of the incubation fluid is added to an aggregometer cuvette (Born/Michal, Mark IV) containing 0.9 ml normal rat PRP diluted with saline to a platelet concentration of about 180.000·μl^{-1}, preincubated at 37.5° C for 2.5 min. Thirty seconds after incubate addition, 0.1 ml ADP is added to a final concentration of 2.5×10^{-7} mol·l^{-1} and the aggregation quantified in the usual way. Control measurements are performed using tissue of the same blood vessel pretreated with indomethacin. The inhibition of aggregation caused by the incubate of the non-treated tissue is converted into a PGI_2-concentration by using a standard curve obtained with synthetic PGI_2.

Unfortunately, this method does not take into account possible influences due to physiological factors such as plasma prostacyclin inhibitors/stimulators (see Chapter 3, section 4.2). Moreover, possible differences in platelet prostacyclin sensitivity between the groups are not taken into account either. Therefore, vascular prostacyclin production was also measured in autologous PRP. To this end, a piece of vascular tissue is added to a 1:10 saline dilution of autologous PRP in the aggregometer. Thirty seconds later, a standard amount of ADP is administered and the resulting aggregation quantified by measuring the tangent of the steepest part of the aggregation curve. Due to PGI_2-formation, aggregation in the presence of normal vascular tissue is lower than that obtained on addition of a piece of indomethacin-treated aorta. For this reason, the proportional difference in aggregation induced by ADP in the presence of either a piece of normal aorta or a piece of indomethacin-treated tissue, is taken as a measure of the amount of PGI_2 formed.

At the end of the experiment, it appeared that both methods gave comparable aggregation inhibition values ($r = 0.75$; $n = 45$; $P_2 < 0.001$), indicating that neither plasma factors nor platelet properties interfered with the first measuring technique. Since only the values obtained by this first method could be expressed in PGI_2-equivalents, these results will be reported here. It should be stressed that both the TxA_2-production as well as the PGI_2-formation are measured after stimulation of the platelets (collagen) and the vascular tissue (mechanical stress, see ref. 243) respectively. Therefore, the results (Table 6.3) reflect production potencies rather than actual formation rates. Analysis of variance revealed that platelet MDA-production and vascular PGI_2-formation in the LO- and EFA-deficient groups are significantly depressed ($P_2 < 0.01$) as compared with the other groups the results of which do not differ significantly from each other.

Using a newly devised pulsatingly perfused rat-aorta preparation, Ten Hoor and coworkers [802] have recently demonstrated that in rats vascular prostacyclin production increases with an increasing linoleic acid/saturated fatty acid ratio. Voss and coworkers [835a], however, using the same technique, were unable to reproduce these findings with rabbits. Our results do not confirm Ten Hoor's observation either, since the prostacyclin production by tissue obtained from rats fed a highly saturated diet (HCO) did not differ from that by tissue obtained from animals fed a high linoleic-low saturated fatty acid diet (SO). Not long ago, Galli and coworkers [284] confirmed our data in an experiment with rabbits fed diets contain 8 w/w% corn oil or butter. They even noticed a significantly higher PGI_2-formation in the group fed the saturated (butter) diet.

De Deckere et al. [177], measuring the 'spontaneous' prostacyclin release from isolated rabbit and rat hearts perfused according to a modified Langendorf technique, also noted that saturated fat feeding (35 en% lard and hydrogenated coconut oil) does not coincide with a lower but rather with a higher vascular prostacyclin production.

In Fig. 6.11.A, the mean platelet MDA formation is plotted against the mean arterial thrombosistendency from which is evident that, in general, arterial thrombosis tendency is higher (OT is shorter), the higher the platelet MDA formation. The sunflowerseed oil group seems to be an exception because it shows a low

Table 6.3. Effect of different dietary fats on arterial thrombosis tendency (OT), platelet MDA-formation (MDA) and vascular production of prostacyclin-like material (PGI_2). Mean ± SEM; $n = 10$–12

Group No	Diet	OT		MDA · nmol per 10^9 platelets	PGI_2 · ng per piece per min.
		log h	h		
1	5 en% HCO (EFA def.)	2.29 ± 0.049	195	0.46 ± 0.070	0.26 ± 0.047
2	5 en% SO (control)	1.99 ± 0.054	97	1.20 ± 0.064	0.66 ± 0.055
3	50 en% SO	2.27 ± 0.041	187	1.20 ± 0.074	0.56 ± 0.058
4	45 en% HCO + 5 en% SO	1.99 ± 0.037	98	1.42 ± 0.095	0.62 ± 0.040
5	45 en% LO + 5 en% SO	2.21 ± 0.054	163	0.72 ± 0.034	0.32 ± 0.050

thrombogenicity in combination with a normal MDA production of the activated blood platelets. This exceptional behaviour of animals fed the sunflowerseed oil diet was confirmed in later studies in which another indicator of TxA_2 (HHT) was measured by gas chromatography and mass spectrometry (see Chapter 8, section 3.2).

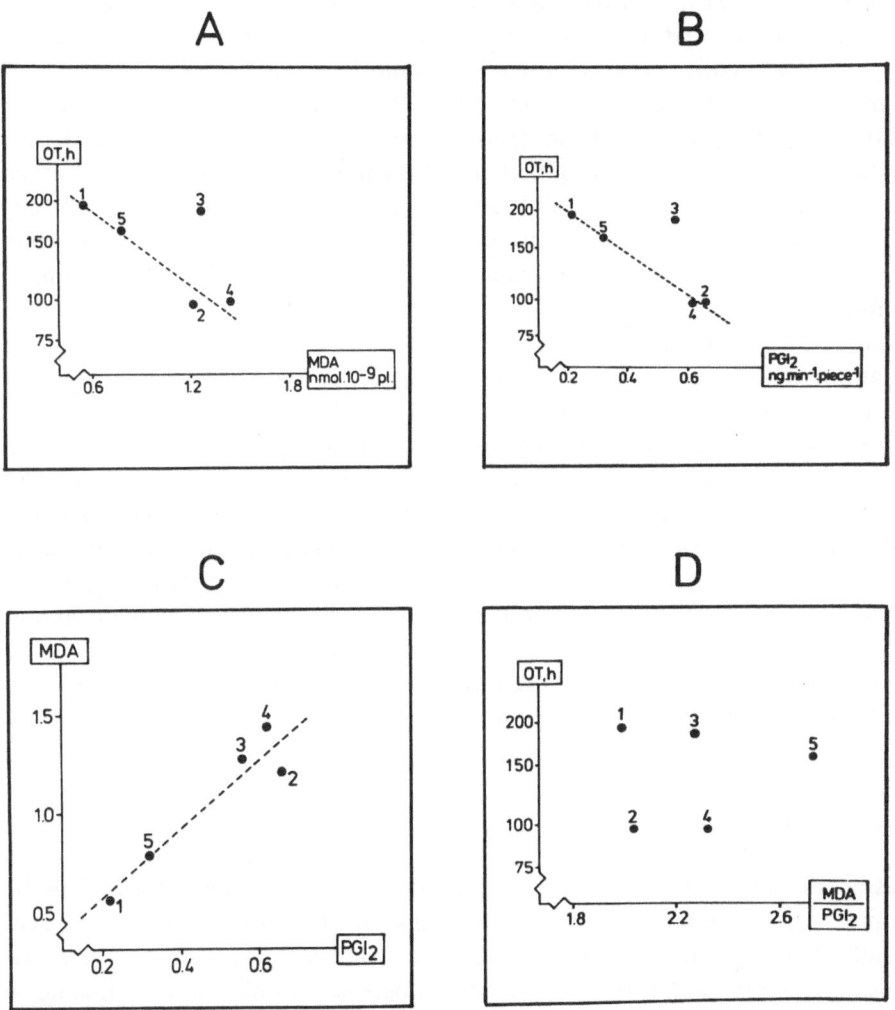

Fig. 6.11. TxA_2/PGI_2 balance in arterial thrombus formation. Each point represents the mean value of 9–11 animals.

Dietary groups: 1, EFA-deficient (5 en% HCO); 2, Control (5 en% SO); 3, Sunflowerseed oil (50 en% SO); 4, Hydrogenated coconut oil (45 en% HCO + 5 en% SO); 5, Linseed oil (45 en% LO + 5 en% SO).

A: Relationship between arterial thrombosis tendency (OT) and MDA formation by activated platelets.

B: Relationship between arterial thrombosis tendency (OT) and vascular PGI_2 formation.

C: Relationship between platelet MDA formation (Y, $nmol \cdot 10^{-9}$ platelets) and vascular PGI_2 production (X, $ng \cdot min^{-1} \cdot piece^{-1}$). $Y = 0.18 + 1.08 X$; $r = 0.59$; $n = 50$; $P_2 < 0.001$.

D: Relationship between arterial thrombosis tendency (OT) and the MDA/PGI ratio.

In Fig. 6.11.B the mean vascular prostacyclin formation is plotted against the mean arterial thrombosis tendency. Surprisingly, the relationship is essentially similar to that between MDA and OT. Here again, the sunflowerseed oil-fed animals behave anomalously. There appeared to be a striking correlation between the MDA production of platelets and the prostacyclin produced by the vessel wall (Fig. 6.11.C), leaving the actual value of the TxA_2/PGI_2 ratio essentially unchanged irrespective of the great differences in arterial thrombosis tendencies between the groups. Consequently, no correlation was found between this ratio and arterial thrombosis tendency (Fig. 6.11.D). This seems to be in contrast with the hypothesis that the TxA_2/PGI_2 ratio determines thrombosis tendency [302, 566]. This balance hypothesis only holds if we accept that, under the present experimental conditions, the prothrombotic effect of platelet TxA_2 is far more important for arterial thrombus formation than the antithrombotic effect of vascular PGI_2. This would be in line with the statement of Ally and Horrobin [6], that, on a molar base TxA_2 is more potent than PGI_2.

Our results strongly indicate that the antithrombotic effect of an EFA-deficient diet and that of a linseed oil-containing diet is due to the diminished potency of platelets to produce TxA_2 upon their activation. On the basis of this platelet property, animals fed a sunflowerseed oil-enriched diet may be expected to have a high thrombosis tendency. However, this is not the case; on the contrary, SO appeared to be an antithrombotic substance (see Figs. 4.4, 4.5, 5.1 and 6.11). Upon SO-feeding, an effective antithrombotic mechanism might, therefore, become operative, which efficiently counteracts the thrombotic properties of the blood platelets. It is possible that the classical prostaglandins from sources other than platelets and vascular tissue play an important role here, because with rats [629] and human subjects [267, 880], urinary PG-excretion was shown to increase dose-dependently with the dietary sunflowerseed oil content (See also Chapter 9, section 6).

6.4. GENERAL SUMMARY

In essential fatty acid deficiency, arterial thrombus formation appeared to be diminished. Normalisation could be obtained with small amounts of linoleic acid but not with columbinic acid, which is able to alleviate the prostanoid-independent deficiency symptoms, but not the prostanoid dependent ones (because it is not a prostanoid precursor). From this finding it was concluded that in our arterial thrombosis model, prostanoids are of primary regulatory importance. Dietary-fat induced changes in arterial thrombosis tendency were not associated with a change in the thromboxane A_2/prostacyclin ratio measured in collagen-activated platelets and mechanically stimulated vascular tissue in vitro. However, large differences in the levels of TxA_2- and PGI_2 formation were observed on feeding different diets, the arterial thrombosis tendency being higher, the more elevated the TxA_2 production of activated platelets. This suggests that for the regulation of arterial thrombus formation, platelet TxA_2 is more important than vascular PGI_2. Moreover, it would explain the antithrombotic effect of an EFA-deficient diet and of a diet containing linseed oil. Dietary sunflowerseed oil, however, does not lower platelet prostanoid formation and yet causes the arterial thrombosis tendency to go down.

7. EFFECT OF FISH OIL FEEDING ON ARTERIAL THROMBOSIS, PLATELET FUNCTION AND BLOOD COAGULATION

7.1. INTRODUCTION

It has been a well-known fact for centuries that Greenland Eskimos have an enhanced bleeding tendency [215]. As early as 1856, and several times thereafter, this condition was suggested to be due to the Eskimo diet [28]. In this respect the observations of Peter Frencken, the Danish arctic explorer, are highly suggestive: 'An extremely frequent disorder ... is the frequent nose-bleeding .... The frequency of nose-bleeding is probably connected with the nutrition which is exclusively of animal origin, because I myself, when living for longer periods as a hunter or travelling on expeditions under which circumstances I never carry bread or other European provisions, get just as frequent nose-bleeding (but not so heavy) as the Eskimos. Under domestic circumstances this has never been the case.' [260]

Mortality from acute myocardial infarction is also very low in Greenland Eskimos [10]. This was confirmed after more valid statistical data became available from which it could also be appreciated that the lifespan of Eskimos living in Greenland is now over 60 years [67, 467, 560]. This low mortality rate from ischaemic heart disease might be related to the plasma lipid and lipoprotein pattern of traditionally living Eskimos: the low and very low density lipoprotein concentrations are significantly lower than in caucasian Danes which also holds for plasma cholesterol and triglyceride levels [25, 26, 212]. Moreover, HDL-concentrations are higher in Eskimo males than in male Danes [25, 212].

When Eskimos adopt a Western way of life, their plasma lipid and fatty acid patterns change towards that of people living in the West [25, 211]. This largely rules out the implication of a genetic factor and strongly suggests that environmental conditions may play an important role in the different lipid and lipoprotein pattern in Eskimos. Diet may be one of these factors because the genuine Eskimo diet is very different from that in Western societies [27, 29]: it is low in carbohydrates and rich in fat from marine animals, the fatty acid composition of which is characterised by a high content of long-chain polyunsaturated fatty acids of the (n − 3) family, whereas the content of (n − 6) fatty acids is usually very low. This diet-hypothesis is supported by various experimental studies showing that feeding fish, fish oils or fish oil concentrates to animals and man results in a plasma lipid and lipoprotein shift towards 'Eskimo values' [217, 289, 344a, 499, 600, 706, 722, 725, 726, 755, 783], although a few negative results have also been reported [102, 706].

Since the fatty acid composition of tissue reflects that of the diet [9, 618, 686] (see also Chapter 8) it was not surprising that in Greenland Eskimos, plasma and platelet arachidonic acid appeared largely replaced with the eicosapentaenoic acid of the (n–3) family, timnodonic acid (TA) [215]. This fatty acid is the precursor of prostanoids of the 3-series [594, 789]. Thromboxane A_3 (TxA_3), possibly formed by activated platelets, has been reported to be less thrombogenic than TxA_2 [594, 598], which later studies showed to be due to the activity of prostaglandin D_3 (PGD_3) formed concomittantly with TxA_3 upon incubation of the endoperoxide PGH_3 with platelet microsomes [315, 851]. PGI_3, possibly produced by the vessel wall is equally antithrombotic as prostacyclin (PGI_2, 603). Therefore, Dyerberg and co-workers suggested [214] that the low thrombosis tendency in Greenland Eskimos is due to a shift in the prostanoid production from the 2- to the 3-series, resulting in a change of the TxA/PGI balance towards a less thrombogenic state. They also advocated a dietary enrichment with (n–3) fatty acids, TA in particular, at the expense of (n–6) fatty acids. This publication had a tremendous impact because it led to the general idea that fish oils prevent myocardial infarction. However, upon feeding linseed oil of rats, causing the incorporation of TA in tissues [159] (see also Chapter 8), we noticed a lower production of vascular PGI_2-like material than in control animals (Chapter 6, section 3), which is not in agreement with Dyerberg's hypothesis.

In our systematic investigations of the effect of dietary fat type on arterial thrombogenesis, we also found that dietary whale oil (containing 10–15% TA) was equally thrombogenic as saturated vegetable fats, although, admittedly, it caused a much lower platelet aggregation tendency (Chapter 5, section 3.3.2). Unfortunately, confirmation of our whale oil results appeared impossible because whale hunting and whale oil trading is now prohibited by law in this country. Therefore, we decided to investigate other marine oils as to their effects on arterial thrombogenesis and some of its underlying processes.

7.2. EFFECT OF DIETARY FISH OIL ON ARTERIAL THROMBUS FORMATION IN RATS

7.2.1. *Comparison of cod-liver oil with sunflowerseed oil*

Rats were fed adequate diets containing 5 en% sunflowerseed oil (SO, control), 50 en% SO or 45 en% cod-liver oil (CLO) + 5 en% SO (to prevent essential fatty acid deficiency). The fatty acid composition of the oils is given in Table 7.1. Since CLO rapidly autoxidises, an anti-oxidant was added to the dietary oils (Santoquin ®, 6-ethoxy-2, 2, 4-trimethyl-1, 2-dihydroquinoline, 0,6 g per kg.)

After 8 weeks feeding, arterial thrombosis tendency was measured in all animals using the aorta-loop model (Chapter 4, section 3). Results are given in Table 7.2. Statistical evaluation (analysis of variance followed by the Newman-Keuls test)

Table 7.1. Fatty acid composition (%) of some marine oils used in our studies (only fractions $\geq$ 1% are mentioned)

Fatty acid	WO	CLO	FO
14:0	8	4	8
16:0	19	10	20
16:1 (n − 7)	12	9	9
17:0	1	1	2
17:1	2		
18:0	4	2	3
18:1 (n − 9)	16	25	17
18:2 (n − 6)	3	2	4
18:3 (n − 3)	1	1	2
20:0		2	2
20:1 (n − 9)	4	12	6
20:5 (n − 3)	10	15	15
22:1 (n − 9/11)	6		2
22:6 (n − 3)	4	10	4
24:0			
24:1	6	1	

WO: Whale oil;
CLO: Cod-liver oil;
FO: Fish oil of unknown origin.

revealed that both the CLO- and the SO-enriched diets prolonged the OTs significantly as compared with the control group (P_2 <0.05). This effect was significantly more pronounced in the CLO than in the SO group (P_2 <0.05). This experiment clearly demonstrates that CLO has a distinct antithrombotic effect in rats.

7.2.2. *Comparison of two different fish oils*

The experiment of the previous section was repeated without adding an anti-oxidant to the dietary fats. Also another fish oil (FO) was included, the composition of which is given in Table 7.1. Autoxidation of the oils was prevented by storing them under nitrogen in a cold (− 5° C) room. Food was prepared daily. Each experimental (SO, CLO and FO) group comprised 28 animals: 16 were used for OT

Table 7.2. Effect of diets containing sunflowerseed oil (SO) or cod-liver oil (CLO) on arterial thrombosis tendency (OT, h)

Diet	n	log OT ± SEM	OT
5 en% SO	16	1.96 ± 0.037	91
50 en% SO	14	2.14 ± 0.057	139
45 en% CLO + 5 en% SO	16	2.45 ± 0.076	279

measurements and 12 for the determination of other parameters, which will be reported in subsequent sections. The control (5 en% SO) group (n = 16) was used for OT measurements only. The OT results are given in Fig. 7.1. Although the mean OTs of the three experimental groups did not differ significantly from one another (analysis of variance), the different diets caused different responses compared with the control group: the FO effect was not significant whereas that of the other diets was (Student's two-sample test). FO contains about twice as many long-chain saturated fatty acids as CLO (see Table 7.1.). Since these fatty acids have been shown to have a prothrombotic effect (Chapter 4) this fact may be responsible for the different results obtained for both fish oils. Another discrepancy between these oils is the difference in cholesterol content: approx. $2.2\,\mathrm{mg}\cdot\mathrm{g}^{-1}$ in CLO and $6.4\,\mathrm{mg}\cdot\mathrm{g}^{-1}$ in FO. Since it is mainly free cholesterol which is readily taken up by platelets [740] and platelet cholesterol content has been implicated in thrombotic platelet functions [740, 742, 791, 874], experiments were repeated with FO, which had been treated with activated alumina to remove free cholesterol [423]. This treatment removes free tocopherols as well. Therefore, the original amount of α-tocopherol was added again afterwards.

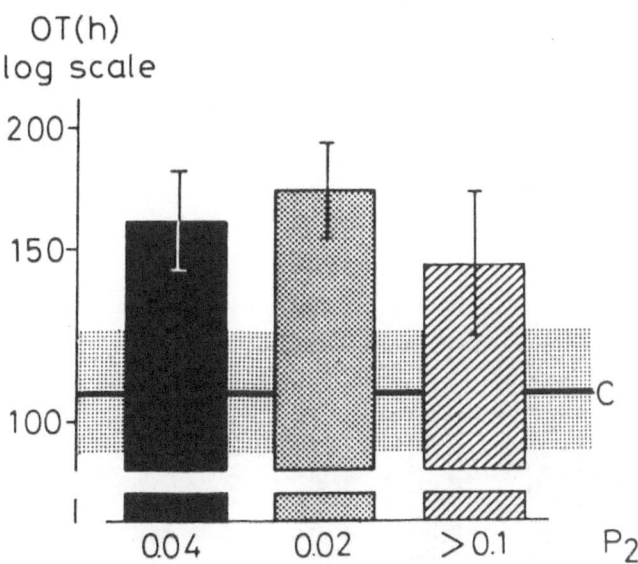

Fig. 7.1. Comparison between dietary sunflowerseed oil (SO), cod-liver oil (CLO) and another fish oil (FO) as to their effect on arterial thrombosis tendency in rats (OT ± SEM; n = 14–16).
C: Control group (5 en% SO);
thick line: mean
shaded area: SEM.;
■ 50 en% SO;
▨ 45 en% CLO + 5 en% SO;
▨ 45 en% FO + 5 en% SO.

110

7.2.3. *Effect of low-cholesterol fish oil*

Rats were fed adequate diets containing 5 (= control) or 50 en% sunflowerseed oil. Five other groups were given diets which contained not only 5 en% SO but also increasing amounts (5–45 en%) of FO, which had been pretreated in order to remove the free cholesterol. Obstruction times were measured after 8 weeks feeding and the results are shown in Fig. 7.2. From statistical evaluation (Student's two-sample test) it was concluded that the 50 en% sunflowerseed oil diet prolonged the OT significantly (P_2 <0.05). None of the FO groups had an OT significantly longer than that of the control group. Even if all FO animals were combined, the mean OT-value (log OT = 2.080 $\pm$ 0.0225 ; OT = 120 h ; n = 79) was not significantly different from that of the control group (log OT = 2.007 $\pm$ 0.048, OT = 102 h ; n = 16)

7.2.4. *Discussion*

Cod-liver oil fed to rats in a concentration of 45 en% lowers arterial thrombosis tendency. Diets containing another fish oil with more saturated fatty acids, less 22:6(n–3) and the same amount of TA as CLO, showed a tendency to prolong the OT only as compared with a standard diet. Therefore, it can be concluded that not all fish oils are equally antithrombotic. Whale oil had no antithrombotic effect at all. (Chapter 4, section 4.2.)

It has been shown that 8 en% menhaden oil, fed to cats for three to four weeks, has some protective effect on focal cerebral infarction, experimentally induced by li-

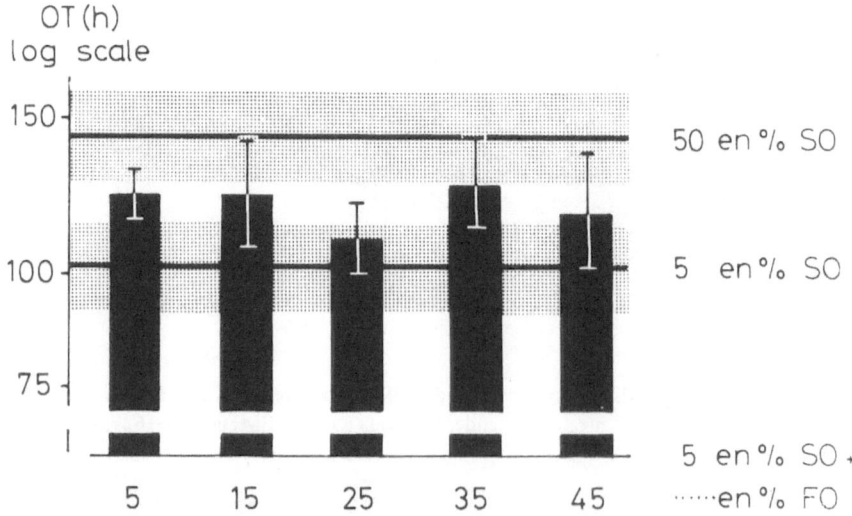

Fig. 7.2. Effect of different amounts of sunflowerseed oil (SO) and fish oil (FO) on arterial thrombosis tendency in rats (OT $\pm$ SEM; n = 16).

gation of the left middle cerebral artery [68]. Moreover, dietary supplementation with menhaden oil (25 en%) six to seven weeks appeared beneficial in reducing myocardial damage associated with coronary artery occlusion in dogs, induced by the intravascular application of a prolonged electrical stimulus [166]. Both experiments may suggest an antithrombotic effect of dietary menhaden oil; the experimental designs as well as some additional findings, however, rather point to an effect of the dietary treatment on the constrictive tone of the microvasculature. Consequently, the anti-thrombotic effect of cod-liver oil as demonstrated in this section has not yet been confirmed by others.

7.3. BLEEDING TIME: COMPARISON BETWEEN THE EFFECT OF DIETARY FISH OILS AND SUNFLOWERSEED OIL

Bleeding times are strikingly prolonged in Eskimos on a marine diet [28, 215]. In order to test the suitability of the rat as a model in thrombosis and hemostasis research, bleeding times were measured upon fish oil feeding and compared with values after feeding sunflowerseed oil. The measurements were performed as follows. Rats were anaesthetised with sodium pentobarbitone (Nembutal ®, $40\,mg\cdot kg^{-1}$ intraperitoneally). The tail was transected at 3 mm from the tip and the distal end (5 cm) of the tail was immersed vertically in saline (NaCl $9\,g\cdot l^{-1}$) at 37.5° C. The period between transection and the moment bleeding stopped was taken as bleeding time. Results after 8 weeks feeding are given in Table 7.3. As compared with the SO-group, both fish oil diets prolonged the bleeding times significantly: $CLO:P_2 = 0.03$; $FO:P_2 = 0.09$, (Student's two-sample test)

These results are in agreement with the prolonged bleeding times observed in traditionally living Eskimos. They also agree with some human studies in which either an Eskimo-type diet was eaten [755], a fish-enriched diet was given [299a, 344a, 808] cod-liver oil was added to the diet [721, 722] or a fish oil concentrate was administered [218]. In this latter case, however, the prolongation of the bleeding time, although statistically significant, was rather small. Moreover, a negative result has been reported [102].

Table 7.3. Effect of different dietary oils on bleeding time (BT,s) in rats, n = 12

Group	BT ± SEM
SO	244 ± 30
CLO	372 ± 44
FO	346 ± 50

SO: 50 en% sunflowerseed oil;
CLO: 45 en% cod-liver oil + 5 en% SO;
FO: 45 en% fish oil (origin unknown) + 5 en% SO.

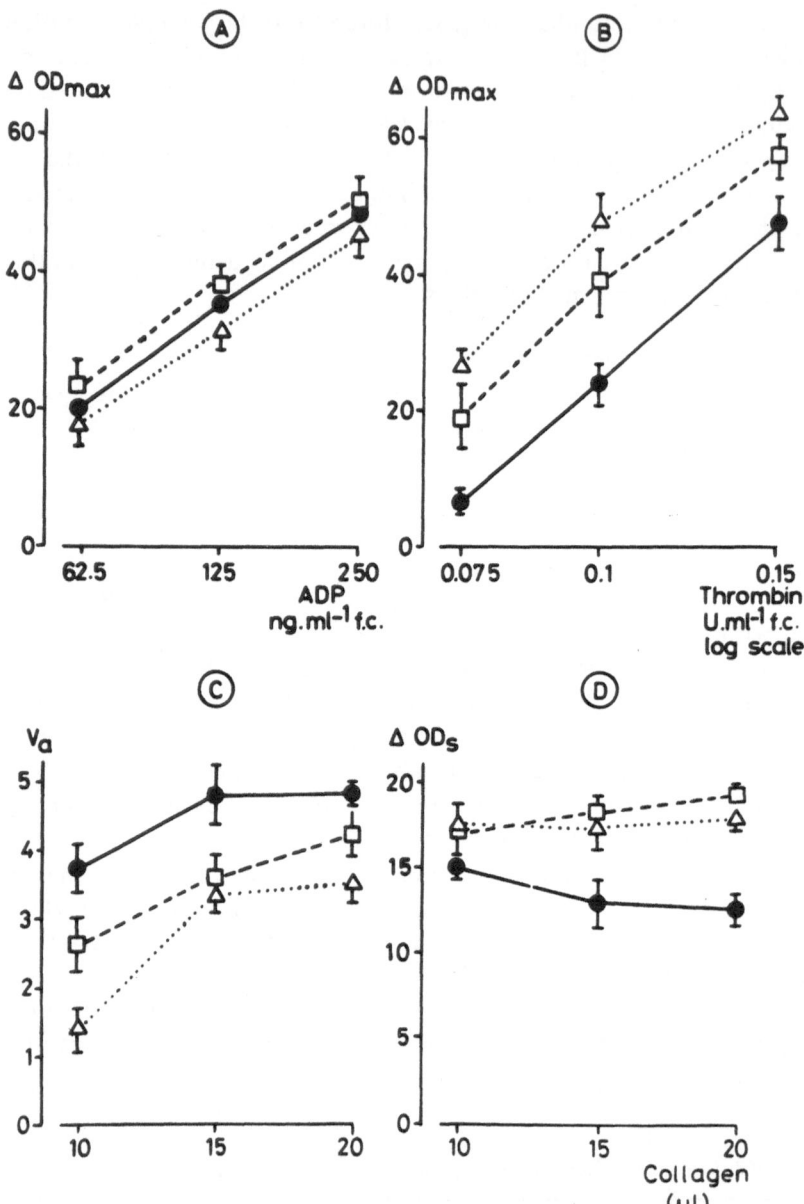

Fig. 7.3. Effect of fish oil feeding on rat platelet aggregation in vitro (mean · SEM; n = 10).

A: ADP-induced aggregation ΔOD_{max}: maximum change in optical density of PRP after ADP-addition.
   f.c. = final concentration in aggregation cuvette.

B: Thrombin-induced aggregation.

C: Collagen-induced aggregation. V_a: aggregation velocity, see Chapter 5, section 3.2 and Fig. 5.5.

D: Collagen-induced shape change. ΔOD_s: total increase in OD after collagen addition.

●— ● 50 en% SO; □---□ 45 en% CLO + 5 en% SO; △...△ 45 en% FO + 5 en% SO.

7.4. EFFECT OF DIETARY FISH OILS ON PLATELET AGGREGATION

From the bleeding time studies it is likely that fish oil feeding lowered the haemo-static effectiveness of the blood platelets. Therefore, we measured platelet aggre-gation, both in PRP in vitro and in circulating arterial blood.

7.4.1. *Platelet aggregation in vitro*

Animals from the experiment mentioned in section 7.2.2 (50 en% SO, 45 en% CLO + 5 en% SO and 45 en% FO + 5 en% SO) were bled under ether anaesthesia by puncturing the abdominal aorta. PRP and PPP were prepared at room temperature, following the procedure described in Chapter 5, section 2. The platelet count of the PRP was 'normalised' to the lowest value of each series by adding the required amount of autologous PPP. Aortas were quickly removed and treated for measure-ment of vascular PGI-production and vessel wall induced clotting. The PRP was partly used for measuring MDA formation upon triggering with collagen as well as for the determination of vessel wall induced clotting. These results will be described in following sections. In the rest of the PRP, platelet aggregation was measured (Chapter 5, section 3.2) in a Chronolog aggregometer, using ADP, thrombin and collagen as aggregation-inducing agents. The results are shown in Fig. 7.3. The ADP-induced aggregation did not differ significantly. Similar results have been reported in dogs, fed 25 en% of menhaden oil for 6–7 weeks [166].

Results of human studies are somewhat contradictory. Dyerberg et al. [215] demonstrated that the ADP threshold concentration for producing secondary ag-gregation is significantly increased in Greenland Eskimos as compared with Danes. This finding could not be reproduced when a fishoil concentrate was fed to human volunteers [218]. This latter treatment, however, did lower the platelet aggregation response at this threshold dose of ADP. Hirai et al. [367] compared the ADP-induced aggregation in 42 inhabitants of a fishing village with that of 43 volunteers, living in a farming village. The ADP dose that produced 50% of maximum aggre-gation was almost 3 times higher (p < 0.001) in the fish-eating group. When human volunteers are fed with 500–800 g of mackerel per day for six days, ADP-induced aggregation in their PRP tends to become lower. However, the average change for 7 volunteers did not reach the level of statistical significance [749]. Brox and co-workers [102] demonstrated that 25 ml of cod-liver oil per day for a period of six weeks does not result in a significant change of the ADP-induced aggregation in human volunteers. However, 20 ml of cod-liver oil per day, given to healthy male subjects was shown by Sanders et al. [722] to increase the ADP-induced aggre-gation after five weeks. The long-term administration of a fish-enriched diet has been claimed to lower the ADP-induced aggregation [808]. However, since aggre-gation did not return to baseline levels after normalization of the diet and no control group had been included in the study, this effect seems rather doubtful. Recently Goodnight et al. [299a] demonstrated that a salmon-enriched diet resulted in a moderate reduction of the ADP-induced aggregation. Results concerning collagen-induced aggregation are much more consistent: in all experiments except two [166, 299a] fish oil feeding reduces collagen-induced aggregation (Fig. 7.3.C. and ref. 102, 215, 218, 749, 808). In our study the effect of FO ($P_2 < 0.01$) was more pronounced than in the CLO-group ($P_2 < 0.05$), indicating that various fish oils may have different effects. The decreased collagen-induced aggregation is most probably the result of the lower platelet arachidonic acid content and, consequently, of the lower TxA_2-formation (see sections 7.6 and 7.7). It has been demonstrated that timnodonic acid (TA), which is one of the major long-chain polyunsaturated fatty acids present in marine oils, when added to a suspension of blood platelets, inhibits platelet aggregation [213, 315, 426]. This might be due to the interference of TA with AA peroxidation by CO [477, 598] or to the fact that TA might block platelet receptors for endoperoxides and thromboxanes [315]. The physiological relevance of these experiments is, however, rather doubtful, because in vivo, TA is mainly present as albumin-bound acid, which is likely to behave quite differently from the sodium salt used in in vitro studies [124].

The collagen-induced shape change is significantly enhanced in the fish oil groups, compared with that in the SO-group (Fig. 7.3.D). However, this only holds for the two higher collagen doses. The shape change in both fish oil groups was not significantly different from each other. Aggregation induced by thrombin was significantly higher in the fish oil groups versus the SO-group ($P_2 = 0.06$ (CLO) and < 0.001 (FO) respectively, Student's two-sample test). Both fish oil groups did not differ significantly from each other. These data have not yet been confirmed in the literature. In fact, thrombin-induced aggregation has been reported to be unaffected by a salmon-enriched diet [299a]. As far as the aggregation/shape change patterns in our study are concerned, there is a striking similarity between platelets of fish oil fed animals and those of EFA-deficient rats. Also in the latter, collagen-induced aggregation is depressed and aggregation brought about by ADP does not differ from normal. Moreover, platelet shape change is enhanced, as is thrombin-induced aggregation (Chapter 6, section 2.2).

The reason for the enhanced platelet response upon stimulation with thrombin is not clear. Platelet prostaglandins and thromboxanes are most probably not involved considering the fact that thrombin-induced aggregation appeared highly independent of this pathway (Chapter 6, section 2.4). Lagarde et al. [474] have recently demonstrated that the lipoxygenase product of Mead acid – 20:3(n-9), the fatty acid accumulating in EFA-deficiency (see Chapter 2, section 2.2), stimulates thrombin-induced aggregation, which might explain the higher thrombin-induced aggregation under this condition. Fish oil feeding leads to the incorporation of timnodonic acid (20:5(n-3), TA) in rat platelets which, upon platelet stimulation, is converted by the platelet lipoxygenase into a monohydroxy acid, HEPE (section 7.7). It might well be that this substance, in analogy to the hydroxy acid formed from mead acid [474], stimulates thrombin-induced aggregation, which would explain the higher values upon fish oil feeding.

Arachidonic acid induced aggregation has been reported to be normal in Eskimos [215], as well as upon fish oil feeding to dogs [166] and man [102, 299a]. No effect of dietary menhaden oil has been observed on the epinephrine-induced aggregation of dog platelets [166] nor did a salmon-enriched diet modulate the epinephrine-induced aggregation [299a]. Finally, platelet retention in a glass bead column appeared depressed upon feeding human volunteers a salmon-enriched diet [344a, 299a].

7.4.2. *Platelet aggregation in flowing arterial blood of rats*

As discussed before (Chapter 5, section 3.3) platelet aggregation, when measured in PRP, is unable to pick up possible differences due to short-lived, platelet aggregation affecting substances such as prostacyclin. Therefore, we decided to measure the effect of fish oil feeding on platelet aggregation in circulating blood, by using the filter loop technique [385] (see also Chapter 5, section 3.3.1). Rats were given diets containing either 50 en% SO or 45 en% CLO + 5 en% SO for three months, after which aorta-loops were inserted. During the insertion procedure, 1 ml of arterial blood was taken for the measurement of 6-keto-PGF$_{1\alpha}$, the results of which will be described in section 7.6.3. One day after loop-insertion the ADP-induced aggregation was measured. The results of these measurements are given in Fig. 7.4 from which it is evident that CLO-feeding causes the ADP-induced aggregation to increase as compared with sunflowerseed oil. The difference was significant only at the lowest ADP-dose (P$_2$ = 0.03) and disappeared gradually upon using higher ADP-doses.

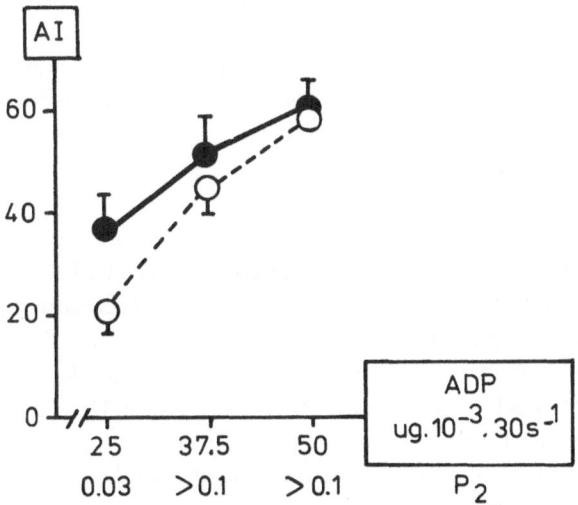

Fig. 7.4. Effect of sunflowerseed oil (50 en% SO) and cod-liver oil (45 en% CLO + 5 SO) fed for twelve weeks on the ADP-induced aggregation of platelets in circulating arterial rat blood.
Mean ± SEM; n = 12
SO: ●   CLO: ○

These results are in striking contrast with the in vitro data obtained by us and most other investigators and are most probably explained by the lower amounts of the anti-aggregatory substance prostacyclin, found in the CLO-blood (section 7.6.3). The higher ADP-induced aggregation in circulating blood is not a generalised effect of dietary marine oils. Thus earlier studies demonstrated whale oil feeding to decrease this type of platelet aggregation (Chapter 5, section 3.3.2). Since the fatty acid composition of whale oil and cod-liver oil are highly different (Table 7.1) the effect of the fatty acid composition of marine oils on ADP-induced aggregation should be further investigated.

7.5. THE EFFECT OF FISH OIL FEEDING ON SOME COAGULATION PARAMETERS

From the in vitro aggregation studies reported so far, it appeared that the fish oil of unknown origin (FO) caused a collagen-induced aggregation significantly lower than that observed upon cod-liver oil (CLO) feeding. (Fig. 7.3.C). Yet, arterial thrombosis tendency was not significantly modified upon FO administrations, whereas it was definitely decreased when CLO was given as a dietary fat (section 7.2). Since thrombin seems to be of primary importance in platelet aggregation upon vessel wall damage [398] as well as after the addition of other stimulants [14, 122] the higher sensitivity of FO-platelets towards thrombin (Fig. 7.3.B) could provide an explanation for this discrepancy. However, this would have physiological implications only if thrombin formation upon FO-feeding is not lower than that after CLO administration. This was investigated with material from the same animals in which we determined arterial thrombus formation and platelet aggregation in vitro. Measurements comprised the clotting process initiated by damaged vascular tissue and some othe, more basic, clotting parameters. Moreover, some human studies will be reported.

7.5.1. *Vessel wall induced clotting*

Vessel wall included clotting (VIC) was measured in an aggregometer at 37° C as described before [398, 400]. PRP and PPP were prepared by differential centrifugation of citrated blood, obtained by puncturing the abdominal aorta of ether-anesthetized animals. After bleeding, the aorta's were quickly removed, cleaned from adhering tissue, opened longitudinally and kept in ice-cold Krebs-Henseleit buffer (KH, see ref. 464). Fifty μl PRP or PPP and 450 μl Ca^{++}-containing saline (final Ca^{++} concentration 1 mmol.l^{-1}) are placed into the cuvette and stirred at 600–700 rev. min^{-1}. After 3 min. a small piece of tissue, 3 mm in diameter, is punched out of the aorta and transferred into the cuvette, while light transmission is recorded continuously. In PPP, fibrin formation is indicated by an initial decrease in light transmission, immediately followed by a rapid increase, when the fibrin fibres become twisted around the stirring bar. In PRP fibrin formation is not always clearly visible, due to the high turbidity of the solution. The subsequent increase in transmission, however, is more pronounced than in PPP, because platelets are trapped in the fibrin strands, twisting around the stirring bar. The time lapse (seconds) between tissue addition and the moment of the sudden increase in light transmission is considered the clotting time (t_c), which, for statistical reasons, is given as the clotting index $S = 1/t_c \times 1000$. S is higher, the higher the clotting tendency of the plasma.

VIC was shown to be of mixed extrinsic and intrinsic origin; it is stimulated by the presence of platelets, especially after their activation, and inhibited by prostacyclin produced by the vascular tissue [398, 400]. This inhibiting effect of prostacyclin is, at least partly, due to the inhibition by PGI_2 of the participation of platelets in the activation of Factor X and the conversion of prothrombin into thrombin [58, 101, 110, 345, 812]. Thrombin, generated as a result of vessel wall induced clotting appeared essential for the aggregation of platelets in response to the damaged tissue;

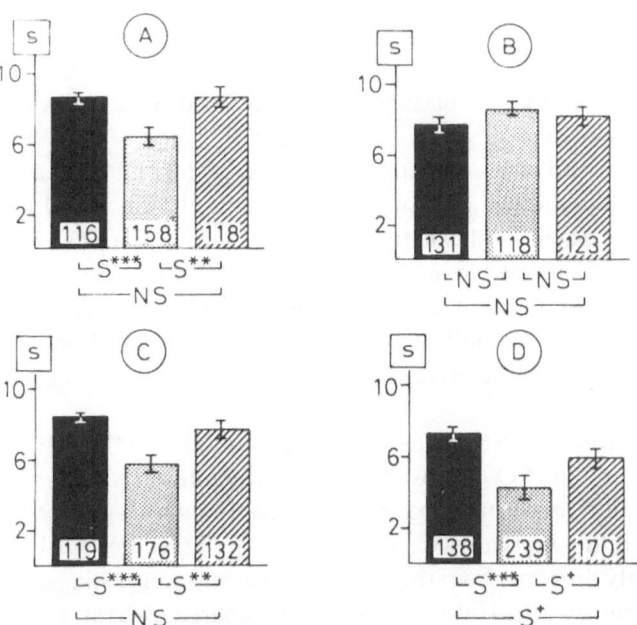

Fig. 7.5. Vessel wall induced clotting measured with vascular tissue, platelet-rich (PRP) and platelet-free (PFP) plasma of animals fed different diets (S ± SEM; n = 10)
■ 50 en% SO ▨ 45 en% CLO + 5 en% SO ▨ 45 en% FO + 5 en% SO. Numbers in bars represent clotting times (seconds) calculated from mean S-values (1/clotting time (s) × 1000)
A. Vascular tissue in autologous PRP.
B. Vascular tissue in PRP of stock animals.
C. Vascular tissue of stock animals in different PRP's
D. Vascular tissue of stock animals in different PFPs.
NS: $P_2 > 0.10$; S*: $P_2 < 0.10$; S**: $0.001 < P_2 < 0.01$; S***: $P_2 < 0.001$.

TxA_2 and ADP were only of secondary importance [398, 400].

In pilot experiments we observed that CLO-feeding caused a significantly lower vessel wall induced clotting response which appeared to be due to some plasma condition [398]. The results of the present experiment are given in Fig. 7.5. Vessel wall induced clotting in autologous PRP is significantly lower in the CLO-group as compared with both other groups, which do not differ significantly (Fig. 7.5.A). This difference disappears when the aortic pieces are placed in PRP obtained from stock animals (Fig. 7.5.B). Therefore, the CLO-effect is located in the PRP and not in the aorta. This was confirmed in an experiment in which pieces of aorta from stock animals were used to activate clotting in the different PRP's: essentially, differences were similar to those observed in the first experiment (Fig. 7.5.C). To find out as to whether the CLO-effect is located in the platelets or in the plasma, the experiment with aortas of stock animals was repeated in platelet-free plasma (Fig. 7.5.D). It then appeared that clotting in the CLO plasma was again lower than in the other group, indicating that the lower clot-promoting effect of vascular tissue, as observed in CLO-fed animals, is located in the plasma.

7.5.2. *Activated partial thromboplastin time (APTT)*

APTTs were measured in platelet free plasma (PFP), obtained as described in Chapter 5, section 2.3 and diluted to 20% with a Tris buffer (10^{-3} mol·l^{-1} in saline) at pH 7.35. The activation mixture consisted of inositin, 50 mg·ml^{-1}, 0.2 ml; kaolin, 100 mg and Tris/saline buffer, 19.8 ml. 0.1 ml plasma dilution and 0.1 ml activation mixture were incubated in plastic tubes placed in a waterbath (37.5° C) and stirred with a siliconised metal bar at 800 r.p.m. After 2 min clotting was initiated by adding 0.1 ml CaCl$_2$ (0.033 mol·l^{-1}) and fibrin formation was checked visually. Each sample was tested in triplicate. Apart from the SO, CLO and FO groups, a control group was included receiving a commercial stock diet (Muracon®, Trouw, Amsterdam).

Results (Fig. 7.6.A) are expressed in S-values (1/clotting time (s) × 1000). APTTs of plasmas from the CLO and the FO groups did not differ significantly from each other but were markedly different from those of the control- and SO-groups (P_2 <0.001), which did not differ mutually. Consequently, APTTs of both fish oil groups are also significantly different from those of the SO group, suggesting a less active intrinsic clotting pathway in fish oil-fed animals as compared with rats fed the SO- or the control diet. Essentially similar results were seen when Actin® (Ex Dade, B-D and Company, Rutherford, New Jersey), an activated cephaloplastin reagent, was used to activate clotting in undiluted PFP and fibrin formation was checked with a small metal hook. In this test system, the clotting response was somewhat higher, which might have been due to the different clotting-inducing reagents, the different way in which the endpoint was determined, the rather long storage time at −15° C between both sets of experiments (approx. one year) and the fact that the plasma had been thawn once before.

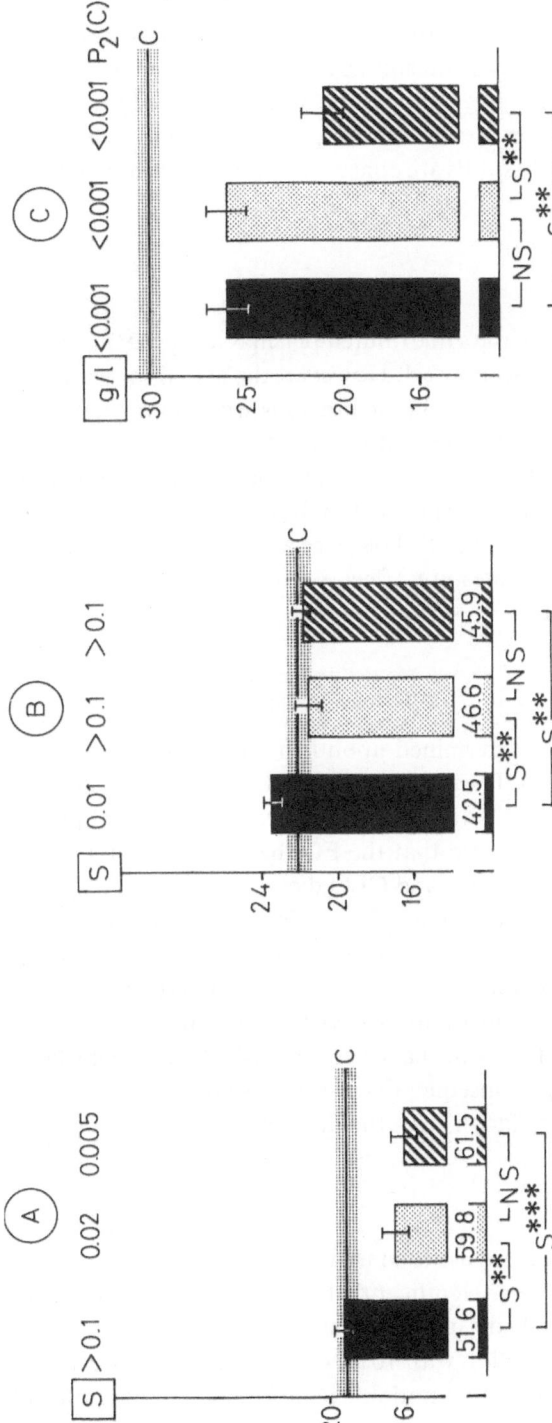

Fig. 7.6. Effect of diets containing sunflowerseed oil (SO), cod-liver oil (CLO) and another fish oil (FO) on intrinsic (A, APTT) and extrinsic (B, PT) clotting and fibrinogen content (C, g.l.$^{-1}$) of rat plasma (Mean ± SEM; n = 10)

S: Clotting index = 1/clotting time (s) × 1000. ■ 50 en% SO; ▨ 45 en% CLO + 5 en% SO; ▒ 45 en% SO; ▨ 45 en% FO + 5 en% SO; C: stock diet. thick line: mean. shaded area: SEM. P_2(C): Significance level compared with control group; NS: $P_2 > 0.10$; S**: $0.001 < P_2 < 0.01$; S***: $P_2 < 0.001$. Numbers in bars represent clotting times (seconds) calculated from mean S-values.

In traditionally living Eskimo's APTT-values did not differ significantly from that of Caucasian Danes [215]. Moreover 10 ml of cod-liver oil, given twice daily to 5 normal volunteers for five weeks did not result in a significant change in APTT [725], nor did a fish-enriched diet given for eleven weeks [808]. Therefore, a significant effect of dietary fish oil on intrinsic clotting is rather unlikely and may occur only when large amounts of these oils are consumed (as was the case in the rat study).

7.5.3. Prothrombin time (PT)

PT measurements were carried out in the same diluted plasmas as the APTTs, using the method described in Chapter 5, section 2.4. However, the actual measurement took place in the stirred system as described in the previous section for APTT. The results are depicted in Fig. 7.6.B. As compared with the control group, PT in the SO-group was significantly shortened (S-value increased, Student's two-sample test). Both fish oils did not differ from the control group, but they did from the SO-group. Epidemiological [215] and experimental [725, 808] (see also section 7.5.6.) human studies indicated that a marine-diet does not affect extrinsic clotting, which is in agreement with our findings in rats.

7.5.4. Fibrinogen

The plasma fibrinogen content was determined upon fish oil feeding according of the method described by Claus [143]. The results are given in Fig. 7.6.C from which it is evident that a high fat diet is associated with a significantly decreased plasma fibrinogen content. Moreover, it appeared that the FO-diet causes a significantly lower plasma fibrinogen level than the SO- and CLO diets.

The fibrinogen content of traditionally living Eskimo's was found to be significantly higher than that in Danes, matched for age and sex [215]. No effect on the plasma fibrinogen content of normal human volunteers was observed when 10 ml cod-liver oil was administered twice daily for five weeks [725] or a fish-enriched diet was given for 11 weeks [808]. Similar results have been described after giving 20 ml cod-liver oil for six weeks [722]. Consequently, the deviating values found in Eskimo's may be due to some other factor than the dietary fat type.

7.5.5. Antithrombin III

Dyerberg et al. [220] have recently demonstrated that immunoreactive antithrombin III (AT-III) and AT-III activity were significantly higher in Greenland Eskimos as compared with age- and sex-matched caucasian Danes. They also demonstrated that a three week dietary supplementation with 10 ml of a cod-liver oil concentrate per day (providing approximately 6 g of timnodonic acid) resulted in a significant increase of the immunoreactive AT-III in blood of normal human volunteers. The change in AT-III activity, however, appeared not significant. These latter findings are in agreement with results obtained by Saynor and Verel [725]: 10 ml of cod-liver oil given twice daily for five weeks did not result in a significant change of AT-III values in 5 normal subjects. Sanders and coworkers [722], however, noticed a decrease in the plasma AT-III content (immunological) upon administration of 20 ml cod-liver oil per day for six weeks. After withdrawal of the supplement the AT-III values remained decreased as compared with the value measured before starting the supplementation period. Since no control group was included in this study, the interpretation of these data is very difficult.

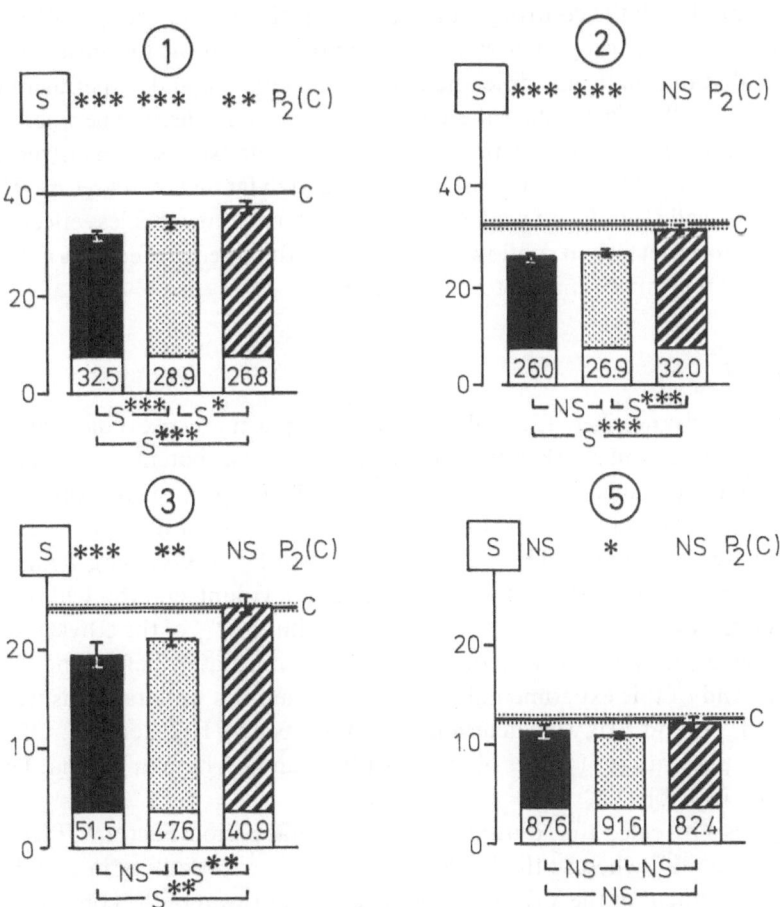

Fig. 7.7. Clotting times (indicated by the clotting index $S = 1000/t_c$) induced by adding fibrinogen to defibrinated rat plasma incubated with thrombin for 1, 2, 3 and 5 min. (Mean $\pm$ SEM, n = 16).
■ 50 en% SO; ▨ 45 en% CLO + 5 en% SO; ▨ 45 en% FO + 5 en% SO.
C: stock diet.   thick line: mean.   shaded area: SEM
P_2(C): Significance level compared with control group
NS: $P_2 > 0.10$; S*: $P_2 < 0.05$; S**: $0.01 < P_2 < 0.05$; S***: $P_2 < 0.001$
Numbers in bars represent clotting times (s) calculated from mean S-values.

In our fish oil study we also measured AT-III activity, using a method originally described by Hensen and Loeliger [361] as modified by V.d. Meer et al. [541]. Briefly, a standard amount of thrombin was incubated with the plasma under investigation, which had been defibrinated beforehand. After varying incubation times clotting times were measured upon the addition of a standard amount of fibrinogen. These thrombin clotting times increased progressively upon prolonged incubation. Therefore, statistical evaluation of the results was performed after transformation of these clotting times into their clotting indices $S = 1000/t_c$. The results after 1, 2, 3 and 5 min of incubation are given in Fig. 7.7. After 1 min of incubation AT-III activities appeared significantly higher for the three experimental groups as compared with the control group. Moreover, the dietary groups differed mutually, AT-III activity being highest in the SO and lowest in the FO-group. On prolonged incubation, first the differences between control and experimental groups decreased, followed by the differences between these three experimental groups. Finally, after 7 min of incubation no difference could be observed anymore (not shown in Fig. 7.7.). These findings indicate that a high fat diet increases AT-III activity in a statistically significant way. A fish oil diet seems somewhat less effective in this respect than a diet rich in sunflowerseed oil. Whether these differences are of any physiological relevance remains to be determined.

7.5.6. *Factor VII*

Recently, Meade and coworkers [539] observed that the plasma level of coagulation factor VII is a 'cardiovascular risk indicator' which is at least as potent as the serum cholesterol content. Hemker et al. [357] demonstrated that part of the plasmatic Factor VII circulates in an activated form and they developed a test for the estimation of activated Factor VII. Through the courtesy of Dr. J. Dyerberg we were able to perform this test in plasma obtained from human volunteers who had been given 10 ml per day of a cod-liver oil concentrate containing 67% of the ethyle ester of timnodonic acid [217] for a period of three weeks. Immediately before and two weeks after the end of this experimental period blood samples were taken as well. Levels of Factor VII and VII$_a$ were determined as described by Hemker et al. [357] and expressed in percentage of values obtained with a standard human plasma. The results are given in Table 7.4.

Statistical analysis revealed that during the experimental period Factor VII levels decreased significantly, whereas the levels of VII$_a$ increased, resulting in a highly significant enhancement of the VII$_a$/VII ratio. After withdrawal of the concentrate all values normalize within two weeks. These findings indicate that the cod-liver oil concentrate causes a considerable increase in the activation level of Factor VII, leading to an enhanced turnover of Factor VII which is not completely compensated for by the synthesis of new Factor VII.

The activated form of clotting factor VII can be considered more hazardous than the non-activated form. This is indicated by the enhanced VII$_a$/VII ratio observed in women on oral contraceptives [356] who have been shown to have a higher risk for arterial thrombotic complications [149, 222, 518–520]. Consequently, our results point to an adverse effect of the cod-liver oil concentrate which severely hampers further research with this material. It should be mentioned, however, that prothrombin times were not affected by administration of the concentrate. Sanders and coworkers [722] measured Factor VII levels before, during and after the daily administration of 20 ml cod-liver oil for 6 weeks to 12 male volunteers. No significant changes were observed.

7.5.7. Discussion

The effect of dietary fish oil on blood coagulation has been investigated only rather superficially, so far. Although no striking differences were seen in Eskimo's in comparison with caucasian Danes [215] – apart from a higher AT-III activity [220] – rat studies indicate that vessel wall induced clotting is significantly depressed upon CLO feeding. This appeared to be due to a plasma condition so that it may have been caused by the significantly lower intrinsic and extrinsic coagulabilities found in CLO fed animals. Rats fed another, more saturated fish oil, however, did not show a significantly depressed vessel wall induced clotting activity although the effect of this fish oil on intrinsic and extrinsic coagulation was comparable to that of CLO. This discrepancy needs further investigation.

Human experimental studies showed no significant effect of dietary fish oil on PT, APTT [808] and the recalcification time of citrated blood [102]. A major difference between the experimental designs of the human and rat studies is the much smaller amount of fish oil given to the human volunteers. This condition may account for the discrepancies observed. Therefore, human studies with larger amounts of fish (oils) are indicated. However, such diets may give rise to unfavourable side effects as observed in our VII_a/VII study. Consequently, these experiments should be conducted with great care.

Table 7.4. Plasma levels of coagulation factors VII (total) and VII_a (activated form only) in 16 human volunteers before (A), during (B) and after (C) the daily oral administration of a cod-liver oil concentrate. Values in percentage of results obtained for standard plasma. Mean $\pm$ SEM

Sampling time	VII	VII_a	VII_a/VII
A	117.6 ± 4.77	66.6 ± 5.08	0.57 ± 0.044
B	105.6 ± 3.22^a	92.2 ± 9.81^a	0.88 ± 0.091^b
C	115.4 ± 5.57	74.6 ± 5.71	0.67 ± 0.069
B - A	-12.2 ± 4.67^a	$+25.6 \pm 10.54^a$	$+0.30 \pm 0.101^b$
C - A	-2.2 ± 8.63	$+8.0 \pm 7.03$	$+0.10 \pm 0.082$

[a] $P_2 < 0.05$
[b] $P_2 < 0.01$

7.6. EFFECT OF FISH OIL FEEDING ON PLATELET THROMBOXANE PRODUCTION AND THE VASCULAR FORMATION OF PROSTACYCLIN-LIKE MATERIAL

The first experiment to be described in this section was performed with animals fed diets containing 50 en% SO, or 45 en% CLO or FO + 5 en% SO. The effect of these diets on arterial thrombosis tendency has been reported in section 7.2.2 and studies concerning platelet functions and coagulation in sections 7.4 and 7.5, respectively. In a second experiment, the effect of the dietary amount of fish oil was investigated in animals used for the OT-measurements reported in section 7.2.3.

Blood for the studies to be described was collected approximately one to two weeks after occlusion of aorta loops (sections 7.6.1 and 7.6.2) or during loop insertion (section 7.6.3). Platelet TxA_2, formed upon triggering with collagen, was measured as its stable metabolite MDA, according to the method described in Chapter 6, section 3. MDA formation reflects total thromboxane production from all three prostanoid precursors: 20:3(n–6), 20:4(n–6) and 20:5(n–3). The formation of vascular prostacyclin-like material was measured with the platelet aggregation bio-assay described in Chapter 6, section 3. It should be emphasized

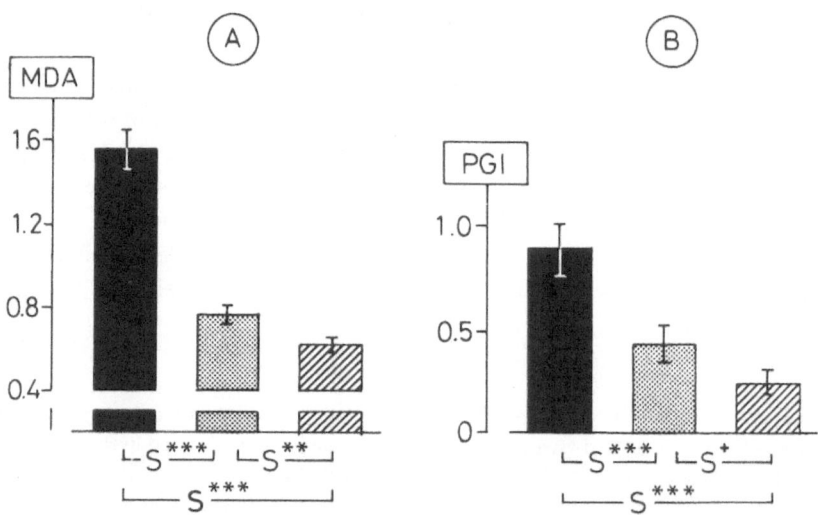

Fig. 7.8. Effect of fish oil feeding on the formation of platelet and vessel wall prostaglandins (Mean ± SEM).
A. Malondialdehyde (MDA, nmol.10^{-9} platelets)-formation by collagen-activated blood platelets (n = 13).
B. Formation of prostacyclin-like material (PGI) by aortic tissue. Results expressed in ng PGI_2-equivalents . min^{-1} . piece of aorta^{-1}. (n = 11 – 12)
S*: $0.10 > P_2 > 0.05$; S**: $0.01 > P_2 > 0.001$; S***: $P_2 < 0.001$.
■ 50 en% sunflowerseed oil (SO); ▨ 45 en% cod-liver oil + 5 en% SO; ▨ 45 en% of another fish oil + 5 en% SO.

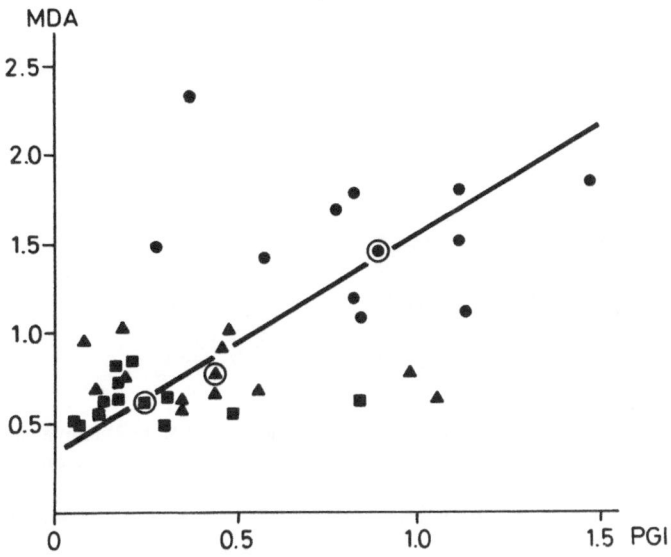

Fig. 7.9. Intra-individual correlation between vascular PGI-production (ng PGI_2-like material.aortic piece^{-1}.min^{-1}) and platelet MDA-formation (nmol MDA.10^{-9} platelets) as influenced by dietary fat type.

● 50 en% sunflowerseed oil (SO); ▲ 45 en% cod-liver oil + 5 en% SO; ■ 45 en% of another fish oil + 5 en% SO.

Encircled symbols represent group means.

that this method measures the production of $PGI_2 + PGI_3$ (PGI_1 is not formed, because PGH_1 is not a substrate for PGI-synthase [418, 597]).

7.6.1. *Effect of fish oil feeding on platelet MDA- and vascular PGI-formation*

MDA and PGI measurements were carried out in material from the same animal and are, therefore, directly comparable. As shown in Fig. 7.8, both CLO- and FO-feeding cause a much lower MDA and PGI formation than a diet rich in SO. The values obtained for the FO group are significantly lower than those measured for the CLO-fed animals. A significant linear correlation was observed between vascular PGI formation (X) and platelet MDA production (Y), which can be characterized by the equation $Y = 0.37 + 1.20 X$ ($r = 0.51$; $n = 35$; $P < 0.01$, see Fig. 7.9).

7.6.2. *Dose–response effect of fish oil on platelet MDA- and vascular PGI-formation*

As shown in Fig. 7.10, the effect of fish oil on platelet MDA and vascular PGI-formation, partly depends on the amount in the diet: the effect increases with the dose up to about 25 en% FO. Another 20 en% increase in the amount of dietary FO

126

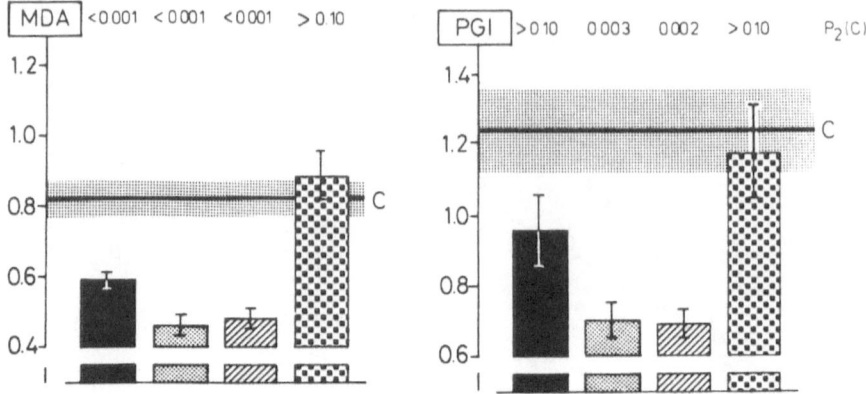

Fig. 7.10. Effect of increasing amounts of dietary fish oil (FO) and sunflowerseed oil (SO) on platelet MDA (nmol.10^{-9} platelets and vascular PGI (ng PGI$_2$-equivalents.min^{-1}.aortic piece^{-1})-formation. (Mean values $\pm$ SEM; n = 10).

P$_2$ (C): Significance level of difference in relation to control group (C, 5 en% SO, fat line: mean, shaded area: SEM).

■ 5 en% SO + 5 en% FO;   ▦ 5 en% SO + 25 en% FO;   ▨ 5 en% SO + 45 en% FO;   ▩ 50 en% SO.

did not affect the parameters under investigation further. Since platelet MSA- and vascular PGI-formations were determined in material from the same animal, they could be compared directly. As was the case in earlier investigations (Chapter 6, section 3; see also section 7.6.1), the dietary fat effect was about similar for both platelet MDA and vascular PGI, leaving the ratio between both parameters essentially unchanged (Table 7.5.)

Measurements were carried out with material obtained from animals used earlier for OT-measurements (section 7.2.3) so that the results could be correlated. However, no significant relationship existed between OT and either platelet MDA-formation or vascular PGI-production. This seems contradictory to the results reported in Chapter 6, section 3 for rats fed different dietary fats. However, it should be emphasized that, in contrast to these earlier results, the OTs measured in the

Table 7.5. Ratio between MDA-formation by collagen-activated platelets (ng MDA/10^{-9} platelets) and vascular PGI-production (ng PGI$_2$-like activity.aortic piece^{-1}.min^{-1}) measured in platelets and aortic tissue of rats fed diets containing various amounts of sunflowerseed oil (SO) or fish oil (FO)

Diet : 5 en% SO +	MDA/PGI-ratio
–	0.73 ± 0.087
5 en% FO	0.70 ± 0.086
25 en% FO	0.70 ± 0.071
45 en% FO	0.73 ± 0.071
45 en% SO	0.83 ± 0.094

FO-groups of the present experiment were not significantly different from that in the control (5 en% SO)-group, thus providing only a small 'response area'. Moreover, it should be noted that in the previous investigation, results obtained with animals fed 50 en% SO did not fit the general relationship. Thus, a significant contribution of the SO group in the present experiment is not to be expected either.

7.6.3. Effect of feeding cod-liver oil on the level of 6-keto-$PGF_{1\alpha}$ in blood of rats

The technique employed so far to measure prostacyclin formation is fairly non-specific and indirect. Moreover, the results reflect the production potency of vascular tissue rather than the circulating amount of prostacyclin. Under normal circumstances the circulating level of 6-keto-$PGF_{1\alpha}$ (the stable metabolite of PGI_2) is likely to be very low (Chapter 3, section 4.2). Under slightly stimulated conditions, however, these levels may be measurable using highly sensitive techniques such as the radioimmunoassay (RIA) [ref. 713].

Therefore, we took blood samples during the insertion of aorta loops into animals who had been fed diets containing either 50 en% SO or 45 en% CLO + 5 en% SO for eight months. One day later these animals were used for measuring ADP-induced platelet aggregation in circulating blood (section 7.4.2). 0.45 ml of blood was collected in 0.05 ml of a mixture of sodium citrate (3.8 w/v%) and indomethacin (10^{-4} mol·l^{-1}) and stored in melting ice. Another 0.45 ml of blood was mixed with 0.05 ml of sodium citrate and kept at 37° C for 15 min. Subsequently, PPP was obtained by high speed centrifugation, stored at $-20°$ C and transported on dry ice to Dr. G. Defreyn, Centre for Thrombosis and Vascular Research, University of Leuven, Belgium, for the measurement of the content of 6-keto-$PGF_{1\alpha}$ by RIA. Results are given in Table 7.6. from which it can be seen that the 6-keto-$PGF_{1\alpha}$ levels are significantly lower upon CLO feeding than when SO is given as a dietary fat. The difference in 6-keto-$PGF_{1\alpha}$ levels between the two series of blood samples is most probably due to PGI_2-formation by white cells during storage of the blood [70]. This value is also lower upon CLO feeding as compared with SO-feeding. These results confirm the lowering effect of dietary CLO on PGI_2-formation as was also

Table 7.6. Concentration of 6-keto-$PGF_{1\alpha}$ (pg·ml^{-1}) in plasma of rats fed diets containing either 50 en% sunflowerseed oil (SO) or 45 en% cod-liver oil (CLO) + 5 en% SO. Blood collected in mixture of citrate and indomethacin (C + I) or citrate only (C) P_2: significance of difference between both dietary groups. Mean ± SEM n = 10.

Sample	SO	CLO	P_2
C + I	371 ± 53.9	76 ± 5.6	<0.001
C	1034 ± 220.8	158 ± 25.3	0.001
Difference	664 ± 243.3	83 ± 22.6	0.03

seen with the platelet aggregation bio-assay and may provide an explanation for the higher ADP-induced aggregation in circulating arterial blood of CLO-fed animals (section 7.4.2).

7.6.4. Discussion

Fish oil feeding results in a generalized depression of the formation of prostanoids of the 2-series, as indicated by the lower platelet MDA-formation, the lower formation of PGI_2-like material by vascular tissue, the lower plasma level of 6-keto-$PGF_{1\alpha}$ and the diminished formation of 6-keto-$PGF_{1\alpha}$ by white blood cells. The lower formation of platelet MDA indicates a depressed production of TxA_2. This is confirmed in later experiments in which another stable metabolite of TxA_2 -HHT- was measured. (Chapter 8, section 3.2). Most other investigators obtained similar results: Sies and coworkers [749] observed a significant decrease in platelet TxB_2 formation (RIA) upon feeding 500–800 g of mackerel per day for 6 days to human volunteers. Brox et al. [102] found the same upon giving human volunteers a small amount (25 ml) of cod-liver oil per day for six weeks. Sinclair [755] went on an Eskimo-type diet for a hundred days (seal, fish and water) and observed that his plasmatic TxB_2-level fell dramatically during this period. He also noticed a lower plasma level of 6-keto-$PGF_{1\alpha}$, which is also in agreement with our results. Finally his seminal prostanoids decreased significantly, which strikingly illustrates the systemic effect of the marine diet. Schoene and coworkers [732] observed that Menhaden oil fed to rats (5 w/w% in the diet for 22 weeks) results in an impairment of the capacity of homogenates of kidney medullae and cortices to form 2-series prostanoids. Goodnight et al. (299a), however, demonstrated that a Salmon-enriched diet resulted in the enhancement of platelet MDA-formation upon activation with n-ethylmaleimide. Unfortunately, it was not investigated whether this change was dependent on cyclo-oxygenase activity or whether it merely reflects non-specific lipid peroxidation.

The generalized depression of the formation of 2-series prostanoids is likely to be connected with the change in the fatty acid composition of tissue phospholipids brought about by fish oil feeding. Thus, in plasma and platelets of Greenland Eskimos, eating a marine diet, arachidonic acid $(20:4(n-6))$ is for a considerable part replaced by timnodonic acid $(20:5(n-3))$ (see ref. 215). As is shown in Table 7.7, this also holds for platelets and vascular tissue of cod-liver oil fed rats. These results, which have partly been confirmed by others [102, 299a, 723, 749, 808], were obtained by gas liquid chromatography of platelet and vessel wall phospholipids. The experimental procedure for platelets will be described in detail in Chapter 8, section 2.4. That for vascular phospholipids is given in ref. 401. Since the formation of prostaglandin-like substances is expected to be a function of the precursor fatty acid content of phospholipids [476, 835] (cf. Chapter 8), a lower production of PGs of the 2-series is most probably caused by the lower content of AA, which will be discussed further in Chapter 8. Moreover, the competition between TA and AA for cyclo-oxygenase (CO) may play a role here: although TA is a poor substrate for CO, especially at low peroxide tone (as is the case in vivo, [165]), it very actively blocks the active site of the enzyme leading to an inhibiting effect on AA-conversion [477, 625]. However, findings to be reported in Chapter 8 make this latter explanation rather unlikely.

The replacement of AA by TA not only occurs in platelets and vascular tissue, but seems to be a systemic effect [282], which is likely to result in a generalized depression of the synthesis of prostanoids and other substances derived from AA such as hydroxy fatty acids [80, 81, 331, 435, 836] and leukotrienes [582, 718]. The physiological implications of these changes need further investigation.

7.7. FISH OIL FEEDING AND FORMATION OF PROSTANOIDS OF THE 3-SERIES

The results reported in the previous section clearly demonstrate that fish-oil feeding decreases the formation of thrombosis influencing platelet and vascular prostanoids. The majority of the techniques employed, measures the products of the arachidonic acid (AA) derived 2-series together with those of the timnodonic acid (TA) derived 3-series. Consequently, if fish-oil feeding indeed results in the formation of 3-series prostanoids, the amounts are insufficient to make up for the decreased formation of the 2-series prostanoids.

Table 7.7. Fatty acid composition (%, minor fatty acid not mentioned) of platelet and aorta phospholipids of rats fed diets containing 50 en% sunflowerseed oil (SO) or 45 en% cod-liver oil (CLO) + 5 en% SO

Fatty acids	Platelets		Aorta	
	SO	CLO	SO	CLO
14:0		1	1	1
16:0	28	29	27	28
16:1 (n − 7)		2	1	2
18:0	16	13	36	28
18:1 (n − 9)	4	9	3	15
18:2 (n − 6)	7	5	7	7
20:1 (n − 9)		2		3
20:4 (n − 6)	21	9	12	5
20:5 (n − 3)	0.5	10	0.4	3
22:0	3	1		
22:1 (n − 9)		2		
22:4 + 22:5 (n − 6)	4		6	2
22:5 + 22:6 (n − 3)		2	2	4
24:0	1	1		
24:1	2	6		
Rest	13.5	8	4.6	2

130

As shown in Table 7.7. fish oil feeding causes a considerable replacement of arachidonic acid by timnodonic acid in platelet and vascular phospholipids. Although TA is a poor substrate for cyclo-oxygenase [334, 598, 761, 789], the presence of considerable amounts of TA in platelets and vascular tissue of CLO-fed animals provides a potential for the generation of PG's of the 3-series. In connection herewith, we investigated the conversion of exogenous and endogenous AA and TA by platelet cyclo-oxygenase (CO) and lipoxygenase (LPO) and the production of PGI_2 and PGI_3 from endogenous precursors by the vessel wall.

In these experiments we used specific physico-chemical methods for measuring the production of the following compounds:
- HHT   : (5Z, 8E, 10E) 12-L-hydroxyheptadecatrienoic acid
- HHTE   : (5Z, 8E, 10E, 14Z) 12-L-hydroxyheptadecatetraenoic acid
- HETE   : (5Z, 8Z, 10E, 14Z) 12-L-hydroxyeicosatetraenoic acid and
- HEPE   : (5Z, 8Z, 10E, 14Z, 17Z) 12-L-hydroxyeicosapentaenoic acid.

HHT and HHTE are stable cyclo-oxygenase products of AA and TA, respectively, and considered to reflect TxA_2 and TxA_3 formation. HETE and HEPE are the lipoxygenase products of AA and TA, respectively. As described in detail elsewhere [401], the hydroxy acids were extracted from the reaction mixture with diethyl ether and determined as their silylated methyl esters by gas chromatography and mass spectrometry. In this way, the sum of HHT + HHTE and that of HETE + HEPE is determined. The HHT : HHTE and HETE : HEPE ratios were obtained by high pressure liquid chromatography (HPLC) of their methyl esters on a LiChrosorb 7 RP 18 (reserved phase) column, using acetonitrile/water (70/30 v/v) and UV absorp-

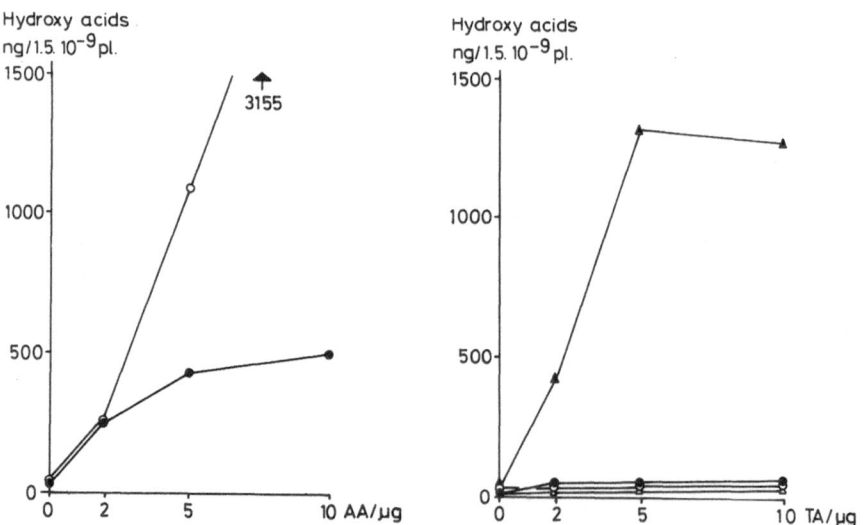

Fig. 7.11. Conversion of added arachidonic acid (AA) and timnodonic acid (TA) into hydroxy acids by rat platelet suspensions.
○ HETE ; ● HHT ; △ HHTE ; ▲ HEPE. (For explanation see section 7.2.1).

tion at 232 nm for detection. The four hydroxy acids are fully separated under these conditions.

PGI$_2$ and PGI$_3$ produced from endogenous precursors by the vessel wall, were measured as their stable metabolites 6-keto-PGF$_{1\alpha}$ and Δ_{17}-6-keto-PGF$_{1\alpha}$, respectively. Twelve pieces of tissue, punched from an aorta (diameter 3 mm, dry weight approx. 100 μg) were incubated in 1 ml phosphate-buffered saline (pH 7.4) for 10 min at room temperature in a shaking vial. After adding 50 ng (ω)-homo-6-keto-PGF$_{1\alpha}$ (see ref 198) as internal standard, the mixture was acidified with citric acid (0.2 mol.l^{-1}) until pH 3–4 and the prostaglandins were extracted twice with 2 ml ethyl acetate. Because the derivatives of 6-keto-PGF$_{1\alpha}$ and Δ_{17}-6-keto-PGF$_{1\alpha}$ (the stable metabolites of PGI$_2$ and PGI$_3$, respectively) do not separate during the gas-chromatographic procedure, prepurification by argentation TLC was carried out [401]. The zones were scraped off, eluted, derivatized into the pentafluoro-benzoxime methyl esters [248] and again purified by TLC. Finally, the products were silylated and analyzed by gaschromatography with electron capture detection [401]. Chemically prepared Δ_{17}-6-keto-PGF$_{1\alpha}$ was used to check the procedure.

7.7.1. Conversion of arachidonic (AA) and timnodonic (TA) acid by platelet cyclo-oxygenase and lipoxygenase

7.7.1.1. Conversion of exogenous fatty acids by platelets
Suspensions of rat platelets were prepared as described in Chapter 6, section 3. In order to measure AA and TA conversions, 0, 2, 5, and 10 μg of fatty acids were incubated for 5 min at 37° C in a stirred cuvette, containing 1 ml phosphate-buffered saline (pH 7.4), 1,5·10^9 platelets of stock animals and EDTA (7.10^{-3} mol·l^{-1}) to prevent platelet aggregation and the liberation of endogenous fatty acids. The results given in Fig. 7.11 show that in contrast to AA, which is readily converted to HHT by platelet CO, TA hardly forms any TxA$_3$ as may be concluded from the extremely small amount of HHTE measured. This confirms earlier observations that TA is a poor substrate for the CO enzyme system [334, 598, 761, 789]. TA appeared to have been converted quite well by platelet LPO (see also ref. 627). Upon incubation with TA, also small amounts of AA-products were detected, indicating that the EDTA, added to the platelet suspensions, did not completely prevent the liberation of some endogenous AA.

7.7.1.2. Conversion of endogenous AA and TA in activated platelets
Rats were fed diets containing 50 en% SO or 45 en% CLO + 5 en% SO. After ten weeks, blood was collected and PRP prepared. One ml portions of PRP (1,5.10^9 platelets · ml^{-1}) were stirred in an aggregometer at 37° C. The platelets were activated by adding 50, 100 or 200 μl of collagen suspension in saline, containing 160 μg protein · ml^{-1}. The reaction was stopped after 5 min by transferring the mixture into 2 ml ethanol and the hydroxy acids were analyzed. Results are shown in Fig. 7.12.

As compared with SO, CLO-platelets produced less than 25% TxA_2 (measured as HHT) and less than 50% of the LPO-product (measured as HETE). No significant amounts of TxA_3 (measured as HHTE) were detected. The production of HEPE, on the other hand, appeared to be quite substantial. These findings confirm the conclusion from the MDA data (Figs. 7.8 and 7.10) that fish oil-feeding coincides with a lower thromboxane formation by blood platelets upon their activation. They also demonstrate that TA liberated from phospholipids upon platelet triggering enters the LPO-pathway but hardly serves as a substrate for platelet CO.

7.7.2. *Prostacyclin- and PGI_3-formation by vascular tissue of rats fed a cod-liver oil containing diet*

On the basis of the results presented in the previous section, it seems that vascular tissue of fish-oil fed rats would be unable to produce PGI_3. However, vessel wall CO may be different from platelet CO, as is shown by its different response towards aspirin [111, 525]. It cannot, therefore, be ruled out that in vascular tissue, TA is converted efficiently into PGH_3 and subsequently into PGI_3. To find this out, we

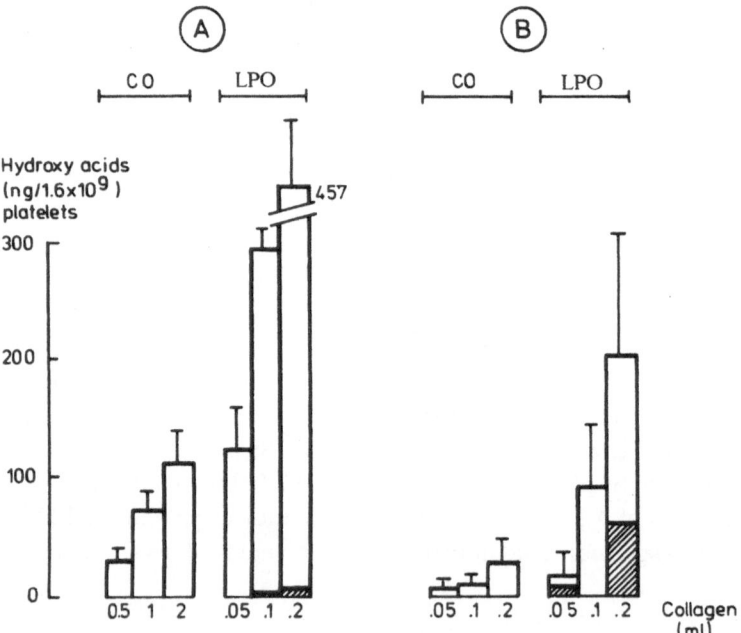

Fig. 7.12. Hydroxy acids formed from endogenously liberated arachidonic acid (AA, open columns) and timnodonic acid (TA, hatched columns) by collagen-activated platelets of rats fed diets containing either 50 en% sunflowerseed oil (SO, A) or 45 en% cod-liver oil + 5 en% SO (B). Mean ± s.d. CO: cyclo-oxygenase products, HHT and HHTE; LPO: lipoxygenase products, HETE and HEPE. Ratios between AA- and TA-derived products determined in separate experiments.

Significance levels of differences between A and B for total hydroxy acid production (Wilcoxon's two-sample test): 0.05 and 0.10 ml collagen: $0.05 < P_2 < 0.10$ (n = 3); 0.20 ml collagen : $P_2 < 0.001$ (n = 7).
* HETE: HEPE ratio not determined

measured the production of 6-keto-PGF$_{1\alpha}$ (stable PGI$_2$ metabolite) and Δ_{17}-6-keto-PGF$_{1\alpha}$ (stable PGI$_3$ metabolite) by pieces of vascular tissue of SO (50 en%) and CLO (45 en% + 5 en% SO)-fed rats upon incubation in phosphate-buffered saline. According to table 7.8, PGI$_2$ poduction by tissue of CLO-fed rats is about 50% lower than that by tissue of rats fed the SO-diet which is in very close agreement with the bio-assay results (Fig. 7.8). No significant formation of PGI$_3$ could be detected.

7.7.3. *Discussion*

Our results strongly indicate that fish oil feeding does not result in the formation of measurable amounts of prostanoids of the 3-series. As is evident from Table 7.7, animals fed a CLO-containing diet, although relatively EFA-deficient, still have appreciable amounts of arachidonic acid (AA, 20:4(n–6)) in their platelet and vessel wall phospholipids (AA/TA ratio is approximately 1). Upon phospholipase activation, except for timnodonic acid (TA, 20:5(n–3)), AA will therefore be released as well. Both fatty acids, AA and TA, compete for the cyclo-oxygenase enzyme system (CO). Since AA is a much better CO substrate than TA [334, 598, 761, 789], TA is expected to be converted to a much lesser extent than AA, even if the latter fatty acid has been partly replaced by the former. This, in fact, is what we found in the previous sections. It might be possible that 3-series prostanoids can be formed if the AA/TA ratio of the tissue phospholipids is $\ll 1$. Moreover the absence of other TA-converting enzymes would be a favourable condition for the formation of 3-series prostanoids, since this would prevent the 'scavenging' of free TA. As shown in section 7.7.1, TA is a reasonable substrate for platelet lipoxygenase. So far no lipoxygenase activity has been demonstrated in the vessel wall, which presents a favourable condition for PGI$_3$-formation.

The observation that exogenous TA incubated with 'exhausted' arterial rings re-activates the tissue to produce an aggregation-inhibiting principle has been taken as evidence that TA, indeed, is converted into PGI$_3$ [214]. An alternative explanation may be, however, that free TA replaces AA from the tissue phospholipids and that this newly released AA serves as substrate for PGI$_2$ formation. This possibility has never been checked but is the more likely since oral administration of TA to rats

Table 7.8. Production of PGI$_2$ and PGI$_3$ (measured as 6-keto-PGF$_{1\alpha}$ and Δ_{17}-6-keto-PGF$_{1\alpha}$ respectively by vascular tissue of rats fed diets containing 50 en% sunflowerseed oil (SO) or 45 en% cod-liver oil (CLO) + 5 en% SO. Mean ± SEM; n = 6.

Diet	ng per piece of aorta	
	6-keto-PGF$_{1\alpha}$	Δ_{17}-6-keto-PGF$_{1\alpha}$
SO	5.9 ± 0.86	<0.2
CLO	2.9 ± 0.82[a]	<0.2

[a] P$_2$ <0.05, Wilcoxon's two-sample test.

results in the stimulation of the aortic formation of the stable metabolite of PGI_2, 6-keto-$PGF_{1\alpha}$ (RIA) [328, 329]. Recently Dyerberg [219] repeated the incubation experiments and using two-dimensional argentation TLC he observed that human (but not rat) vascular tissue is able to convert added TA into a substance that co-migrates with Δ_{17}-6-keto-$PGF_{1\alpha}$, the stable degradation product of PGI_3. Although, so far, mass spectrometry has failed to proof this spot to be Δ_{17}-6-keto-$PGF_{1\alpha}$ [210], this is nonetheless a strong indication that some free TA has, indeed, been converted into PGI_3. It should be emphasised, however, that exogenous TA might be handled by the tissue in a different way than endogenously liberated TA. Moreover the TA conversion rate appeared to be low, so that the diminished PGI_2-production is unlikely to be compensated for by endogenously formed PGI_3. This is also indicated by the fact that with Eskimo women menstruation is usually described as rather scarce and of short duration [28]. Since prostacyclin seems implicated in the regulation of menstrual bleeding [299, 772], this observation is in line with the concept that PGI_2-formation in Eskimos is diminished and is not made up for by the production of PGI_3. Finally Sinclair, eating the Eskimo diet for 100 days, noticed that 'in seminal fluid the total amount of prostaglandins decreased significantly and small amounts of the 3-series appeared' [755]. It is striking, that rat vascular tissue seems unable to convert exogenous TA into Δ_{17}-6-keto-$PGF_{1\alpha}$, [210, 328] indicating that 'rat vascular cyclooxygenase is more specific in its requirement for AA than the human enzyme' [219].

Nonetheless, as demonstrated by Ferretti and coworkers [245], rat medullary tissue is able to produce PGE_3, indicating that rat CO can use endogenous TA for prostanoid formation. The endogenous formation of PGE_3 by the kidneys of menhaden oil fed animals appeared, however, too low to be detectable in the urine [732]. In conclusion, it can be stated that if fish oil feeding results in the formation of 3-series prostanoids at all, the amounts will be highly insufficient to make up for the decreased production of the 2-series prostanoids. Consequently, a major thrombo-regulatory role for 3-series prostanoids as suggested by Dyerberg et al. [214] is unsubstantiated by our work.

7.8. GENERAL DISCUSSION

Cod-liver oil (CLO) fed to rats, has a distinct antithrombotic effect. Another fish oil (FO) containing twice as much long-chain saturated fatty acids, equal amounts of TA but half as much 22:6(n-3), does not affect arterial thrombosis tendency significantly. Earlier experiments with whale oil, the composition of which is comparable to that of FO, also revealed no antithrombotic effect, although platelet aggregation in circulating blood was greatly reduced (Chapters 4 and 5). This finding indicates that in arterial thrombogenesis, apart from platelet aggregation, other processes play an important regulatory role as well. Moreover, our findings again point to the prothrombotic effect of saturated fatty acids. The results presented suggest that the antithrombotic effect of CLO results from a combination of at least two processes. Due to their low AA content, platelets of CLO-fed animals cannot produce sufficient thromboxanes to maintain the platelet aggregation reaction after the initial stimulus has disappeared. As a result of this low aggregation tendency of the platelets, the reduced production of vascular PGI_2-like material has no consequences for the thrombosis tendency. In connection with the lower degree of vessel wall-induced clotting, formation of thrombin at the site of thrombosis will be reduced which may result in a lower contribution of clotting to thrombus formation and thrombus reinforcement by fibrin (see Chapter 3, section 1).

Bleeding time is prolonged on fish-oil feeding, which may be due to the lower platelet aggregability in response to collagen [632, 844, 845, 881]. However, in EFA-deficient rats the platelet collagen reaction is also diminished (Chapter 6, section 2.2.3), whereas bleeding times in these animals are normal. This strongly indicates that the bleeding time may be determined by another factor than platelet aggregability in response to collagen. It is tempting to speculate that vessel wall induced clotting plays a role here: in EFA-deficiency it is enhanced (Chapter 6, section 2.3), thereby possibly counteracting the effect of the lower collagen-induced aggregation, especially so because the thrombin sensitivity of platelets is strikingly increased. Upon CLO-feeding, vessel wall induced clotting is reduced, whereby the effect of the diminished collagen-induced aggregation is possibly potentiated. In FO-fed rats, vessel wall-induced clotting is not different from that in animals after SO feeding and bleeding times in FO-fed rats take an intermediate position between those after CLO- and SO-feeding (Table 7.3). In view of this, it is very likely that the bleeding time is not only determined by the platelet/collagen interaction, but also by the presence of thrombin, generated as a result of vessel wall induced clotting.

It is tempting to speculate that the difference between CLO and FO as to their effects on vessel wall induced clotting may also form an explanation for the finding that only CLO- and not FO feeding causes arterial thrombosis to decrease significantly. Such an explanation is the more likely, since FO and CLO feeding cause similar effects on platelet function and platelet and vascular prostanoid formation. Because of their antithrombotic effect, some fish oils could be important in dietary thrombosis prevention. However, the rapid autoxidation of the highly unsaturated oils constitutes a serious problem because of the general toxicity of peroxides [195], and also because lipid peroxides inhibit prostacyclin synthase [313], which may have prothrombotic consequences and may promote atherogenesis [181]. Moreover, the rapid development of rancidity will be a great drawback to the applicability of fish oils as important dietary constituents. Finally, the potentially harmful effects of marine-type diets should not be overlooked, especially as far as cardiac necrosis and decreased stress tolerance are concerned [317–319]. In addition, a large intake of long-chain polyenoic fatty acids of the (n–3) family is held responsible for yellow-fat disease, a generalised disorder of fatty depots observed in a wide variety of animals [169, 434, 465]. Finally, an excessive intake of salmon and salmon oil was recently demonstrated to be associated with a significant drop in the platelet count [299a].

Another disadvantage of a diet rich in (n–3) fatty acids may be the concomitant consumption of relatively large amounts of some accompanying long-chain mono-enoic fatty acids, e.g. cetoleic acid (22:1(n-11)). As pointed out by Sinclair [756] this fatty acid, as its isomer erucic acid 22:1(n–9), is toxic to lower animals, mainly because muscle mitochondria cannot oxidise it so that it accumulates and causes myocardial fibrosis [37, 830]. However, evidence has now been obtained that extrapolation of the dramatic effect of 22:1 fatty acids in the rat to man is not warranted [2]. Nevertheless, care should be taken when carrying out experiments in which human beings are given large amounts of fish oil type fatty acids in their diet.

Toxicity problems, possibly associated with the intake of anti-thrombotic amounts of timnodonic acid, may be circumvented by using oils, rich in α-linolenic acid, the dietary precursor of timnodonic acid (Chapter 2, section 2). In the rat α-linolenic acid is actively elongated and desaturated to form timnodonic acid (Chapter 8, section 4.3), but the efficiency of these metabolic reactions in man has been questioned [216, 719]. Recently, however, Galli observed a considerable accumulation of 22:6 fatty acids not only in rats [282] but also in human brain lipids of individuals, receiving diets high in acids of the linolenic acid series [826]. Moreover, Beitz et al. [39] gave 11 volunteers 30 ml linseed oil (approx. 50% α-linolenic acid) per day for four weeks and noticed within one week a doubling of the content of 20:5 (n − 3) and 22:6(n − 3) in serum phospholipids. These results were confirmed and extended to platelet phospholipids by Sanders and Younger [723]. Beitz and coworkers noticed, however, that the changes were not accompanied by a significant fall in the arachidonic acid content, which indicate that linseed oil is less effective than certain fish oils in lowering platelet thrombotic properties in man. Moreover, recent studies by Scherhag et al. [726a] demonstrated that linseed oil (and cod-liver oil) feeding to rats resulted in a significant rise in systolic blood pressure. Therefore, and because of its unpleasant taste, linseed oil 'is better employed for protecting cricket bats' [720].

Dose-response studies showed that 5 en% FO had a significant lowering effect on platelet MDA-formation. Such a low dose is unlikely to cause any pathological effects. Sunflowerseed oil-enriched diets cause a low arterial thrombosis tendency although platelet TxA_2 formation remains normal. It seems worthwhile investigating whether a further lowering of arterial thrombosis tendency can be obtained if, in these animals, the potency of platelets to produce TxA_2 is reduced by adding some FO to the high-sunflowerseed oil diet.

7.9. SUMMARY

Cod-liver oil (CLO) fed to rats, has an antithrombotic effect which is at least as pronounced as that of sunflowerseed oil. Whale oil does not change arterial thrombosis tendency significantly, whereas a fish oil of unknown origin (FO) does so to some extent. The effects of FO and CLO on platelet function and plasma clotting are almost similar. Vessel wall induced clotting, however, is depressed in CLO but normal in FO, which might be one of the reasons why FO is less antithrombotic. Fish-oil feeding leads to partial replacement of platelet and vessel wall arachidonic acid (20:4(n–6)) by timnodonic acid (20:5(n–3)), so that platelets produce less TxA_2 upon their activation. TxA_3 is not formed in measurable amounts. Vascular PGI_2-formation is also reduced, which is not compensated for by the formation of PGI_3. Our conclusion is that the antithrombotic effect of cod-liver oil is caused by a lower TxA_2-formation by activated platelets, combined with a reduced vessel wall induced clotting. These results have, in part, been confirmed by other investigators using other animal models or working with human volunteers. Together with the well-documented blood-lipid lowering effect of dietary fish oils, these results may provide a rationale for the use of marine oils in the dietary prevention of coronary artery disease. However, a large intake of long-chain polyunsaturated fatty acids of the (n–3) family, which are abundant in these oils, has been reported to have rather severe pathological consequences. Since the fish oil effect on platelet TxA_2-formation becomes already noticeable when given in relatively small doses, small amounts of certain fish oils could possibly add to the antithrombotic effect of oils rich in linoleic acid.

8. RELATIONSHIP BETWEEN DIETARY FAT TYPE, PLATELET FATTY ACID COMPOSITION AND EICOSANOID FORMATION BY ACTIVATED PLATELETS

8.1. INTRODUCTION

From the previous chapters it can be concluded that the type of dietary fat significantly affects arterial thrombosis tendency in rats, most probably via a change in platelet aggregability. The dietary fat type also influences platelet thromboxane A_2 (TxA_2) and vascular prostacyclin (prostaglandin I_2, PGI_2) production in a strikingly similar way: although the *amounts* of the different compounds produced were greatly affected by the type of dietary fat, the *ratio* between both products remained the same. This suggests that the type of dietary fat affects a common factor, which is as important for TxA_2- as it is for PGI_2-formation.

For all enzymatic reactions, product formation is directly dependent upon enzyme activity and substrate availability. In the process of TxA_2- and PGI_2-formation, only the last step, conversion of the endoperoxide PGH_2, requires a different enzyme. Consequently, the common factor is most likely to be found before this particular step and will, therefore, be involved in the formation of PGH_2 from arachidonic acid.

The formation of thromboxane A_2 and prostacyclin occurs for the greater part in two strictly separate compartments: platelets and vessel wall respectively (see Chapter 3). Since the type of dietary fat has repeatedly been shown to influence tissue lipid composition, including platelet lipids [9, 425, 613, 618, 637, 660, 686, 749], it seems justified to suggest that a change in platelet and vessel wall arachidonic acid (AA) content constitutes the basis for the dietary fat induced changes in prostanoid formation. Recently reported data [283, 526, 780] and the fish oil experiment described in Chapter 7, section 6 suggest the same conclusion.

The results presented in Chapter 6 suggest that the potency of platelets to produce TxA_2 is of primary importance for arterial thrombus formation. In order to investigate whether platelet TxA_2 formation is indeed correlated with the AA content of platelet phospholipids, we decided to measure the effect of the type of dietary fat on platelet arachidonate content and TxA_2 production. We concentrated our fatty acid studies on the phopspholipids because these compounds were shown to be the fatty acid donors for PG-synthesis [476, 835]. It is now fairly well established that AA-peroxidation by the cyclo-oxygenase enzyme system is a membrane- bound process [293, 773]. However, since the fatty acid composition of platelet membrane phospholipids appeared to be strikingly similar to that of whole platelet phospholipids [521] and because we did not want to sacrifice more animals than absolutely necessary, we confined our investigations to the phospholipids of whole platelets.

TxA_2 formation was measured upon platelet activation with collagen. Since TxA_2 is a highly unstable compound, we measured one of its stable metabolites, HHT (12-hydroxyheptadecatrienenoic acid [675]). Recently, the platelet lipoxygenase (LPO) pathway was suggested to be functionally important in platelet aggregation [207, 208]. Therefore, we also measured the final product of this pathway, HETE (12-hydroxyeicosatetraenoic acid). The easiest way to measure these compounds is to incorporate some radioactive arachidonic acid into the platelet phospholipids, extract and separate the reaction products and quantify their amounts by liquid scintillation counting [65]. However, the distribution of newly incorporated AA in the various phopholipid classes is very much different from that of endogenous AA [65, 66]. Consequently, its metabolism might be different as well and would not reflect the normal situation [186]. This is the reason why we decided to measure the formation of endogenously formed compounds using gas chromatography combined with mass spectometry, which is the most specific technique available today.

8.2. EXPERIMENTAL PROCEDURE

Six groups of 24 five-week-old male Wistar rats were fed an adequate diet (Table 4.1) containing the following dietary fats (see Tables 4.2 and 7.1 for fatty acid compositions):

Group 1: 5 en% sunflowerseed oil (SO). This is the control group.

Group 2: 50 en% SO. This diet is rich in linoleic acid (18:2(n–6)).

Group 3: 5 en% SO (to prevent essential fatty acid deficiency) + 45 en% hydrogenated coconut oil (HCO), which is rich in saturated fatty acids.

Group 4: 5 en% SO + 45 en% linseed oil (LO). This diet is rich in α-linolenic acid (18:3(n–3).

Group 5: 5 en% SO + 45 en% cod-liver oil (CLO), providing the diet with considerably amounts of long-chain, polyunsaturated fatty acids of the (n–3) family (20:5(n–3) and 22:6(n–3)).

Group 6: 5 en% HCO, which contains no essential fatty acids (EFA) and causes, therefore, essential fatty acid deficiency.

The diets were fed ad libitum for fifteen weeks. Then, after an overnight fast, the ether-anaesthetized animals were bled by puncturing the abdominal aorta and citrated PRP and PPP were prepared by differential centrifugation and pooled per 4 animals. Of each pooled sample, the platelet count was determined (Coulter Counter) and some PRP was diluted with autologous PPP to obtain well over 4 ml PRP with a platelet count of 10^6 platelets $\cdot \mu l^{-1}$. The rest of the PRP was centrifuged (10 min at 600 g) to produce a platelet pellet, which was carefully resuspended in phosphate-buffered saline (pH 7.41) containing EDTA 7.7 mmol $\cdot 1^{-1}$, final concentration). Platelet loss appeared to be negligible. Of these suspensions, the protein content was determined according to the Lowry technique [500]. The suspensions were stored under nitrogen at $-70°$ C until analysis.

Platelet arachidonate peroxidation products formed upon activation with collagen were measured as described earlier [401]. To this end one ml PRP, platelet count approximately $10^6 \cdot \mu l^{-1}$, was transferred into an aggregometer cuvette (Born/Michal MK IV) and pre-incubated for 3 min at $37.5°$ C and a stirring rate of 1200 rev. min^{-1}. The platelets were activated by adding 50, 75, 100 or 200 μl of a collagen suspension in saline (prepared as described in Chapter 5, section 3.2) containing 160 μg protein $\cdot ml^{-1}$. Aggregation was monitored by continuous recording of the change in optical density. After 5 min, the aggregated PRP was transferred into another tube, after which 2 ml ethanol was added, containing 195 ng deuterated HHT and 185 ng deuterated HETE as internal standards. The reaction mixture was then acidified to pH $4-5$ with 0.5 ml citric acid ($0.2 mol \cdot 1^{-1}$) after which 0.5 ml distilled water was added. Following thorough mixing, the hydroxy acids were extracted with 5 ml dichloromethane, purified, methylated, silylated and quantified by gaschromatography combined with mass spectrometry (GC/MS) [401]. This method allows the reliable measurement of hydroxy acid levels as low as 10 ng $\cdot ml^{-1}$. Unfortunately, it does not allow for discrimination between hydroxy acids derived from arachidonic acid and timnodonic acid, respectively.

Platelet phospholipid analyses were carried out in the frozen platelet suspensions (usually $2.5-3.5$ ml, containing $10-30 \times 10^9$ platelets) to wich 2 ml 2% (w/v) EDTA solution was added after which they were allowed to thaw slowly with repeated mixing. This procedure was followed to minimize platelet phospholipase activation by Ca^{++}, possibly released upon platelet lysis due to a temperature shock. After complete thawing, the diluted suspensions were homogenised by vigorous mixing after which 4–5 ml were extracted according to Bligh and Dyer [71], using a mixture of redistilled chloroform and methanol to which BHT ($0.05‰$ (w/v)) had been added to prevent oxidation of the polyunsaturated fatty acids. The rest of the suspensions was used to measure the protein content (Lowry's method). The lipid residue was taken up in 10 ml chloroform after which two 0.5 ml samples were taken for measuring total phospholipid and cholesterol contents. The rest of the chloroform was evaporated and the residue dried over P_2O_5 under vacuum for at least one night. Phospholipid-class separation was performed by two-dimensional TLC using the method of Broekhuyse [97] which was slightly modified to attain optimum resolution.

For phospholipid class determination, the spots were visualized with iodine vapour, scrapped off and collected in glass tubes. Half a ml $HClO_4$, 70% (w/v), was added and the phospholipids were destructed for 45 min at $180°$ C to obtain inorganic phosphorus (P), which was quantified according the method described by Böttcher et al [88]. Using methyl-PA as an internal standard, phospholipid recovery by the TLC procedure applied was between 70 and 90%. Starting from a mixture of known amounts of PC, PE, PS, PI and SPH, recovery variations were similar for all phospholipid classes. Therefore, variation in recovery did not interfere with phospholipid class dstribution measurements. For the determination of the fatty acid composition of the separate phospholipid classes, the spots were visualized by spraying the TLC plates with Rhodamine 6G (0.01% (w/v) in methanol), marked under UV-light (254 mm), scraped off and collected in glass tubes. An amount of 0.5 ml boron trifluoride (BF_3, 14% (w/v) in methanol) was added to each tube which were than screw-capped under a stream of nitrogen. Phospholipids (see Table 2.1) were hydrolyzed and the fatty acids methylated by heating the tubes at 100° C for 15 min (PE, PS and PI), 30 min (PC) or 90 min (SPH) as described by Morrison and Smith [577].

After cooling, 0.5 ml H_2O was added and the fatty acid methyl esters were extracted three times with 1 ml pentane (+ BHT, 0.05‰ w/v). The extracts were combined, evaporated under N_2 and stored at $-15°$ C until analysis by GLC, for which a Perkin Elmer F17 unit with two glass columns (5% DEGS, 0.2 × 180 cm) and flame ionisation detection was used. The injection temperature was 210° C and the detector temperature 250° C. The analyses were performed using temperature programming, which had been optimised with a reference mixture containing most of the fatty acid methyl esters of interest. This mixture was also used to identify the peaks. The samples to be analysed were taken up in 25–100 μl isooctane containing a known amount of 15:0 as an internal standard. The content of each fatty acid in the mixtures was calculated on the basis of peak height and width.

Simultaneously with each series of 6 samples, a blank (2 ml redistilled water + 2 ml EDTA) was extracted; all results were corrected for the blank values. Previously all glassware had been carefully cleaned in chromosulphuric acid (Merck). After adjustment with respect to the 15:0 peak and correction for the blank samples, the proportional composition of the mixtures was calculated.

8.3. HHT AND HETE PRODUCTION OF COLLAGEN-ACTIVATED BLOOD PLATELETS

8.3.1. *Collagen-induced aggregation*

Platelet aggregation induced by various collagen doses, is given in Fig. 8.1. Statistical analysis (analysis of variance with Newman-Keuls continuation) allowed the following conclusions: aggregation induced by the lowest collagen dose was significantly ($P_2 \langle 0.05$) enhanced in the SO-group, indicating that the platelet-collagen 'activation threshold' is very low after feeding a diet enriched with sunflowerseed oil. However, once this threshold has been exceeded, SO platelets no longer behave differently from the control platelets. Except for the lowest collagen dose, aggregation in the EFA-deficient group is significantly ($P_2 \langle 0.05$) lower than in the other groups, which confirms earlier results obtained with PRP-saline dilutions (Chapter

6, section 2.2.3). Aggregation of HCO platelets is clearly depressed as compered with that of the other high-fat and control platelets. As demonstrated in Chapter 5, section 3.2, this difference is also observed when aggregation is measured in a PRP-saline dilution. Using the latter system, the collagen-induced aggregation of CLO platelets was shown to be significantly lower than that of SO platelets (Chapter 7, section 4.1), but this does not hold for the present situation where aggregation is measured in undiluted PRP. Although for all collagen doses, aggregation is lower in the CLO than in the SO group, the difference is only significant at the lowest dose.

8.3.2. *HHT production*

The effect of dietary composition on the production of HHT by platelets activated with four different collagen doses is illustrated in Fig. 8.2. The values obtained for platelets from EFA-deficient animals were mostly below the levels of reliable quantification ($10 \, ng \cdot ml^{-1}$) but always clearly above zero. For the other groups, analysis of variance showed that increasing collagen doses caused platelet HHT production to increase dose-dependently. The dose–response relationships were not significantly different from rectilinearity, but the various slopes differed significantly ($P_2 < 0.001$). HHT production is highest in the SO group, followed by the control, HCO, LO, CLO and EFA-deficient groups in the order indicated.

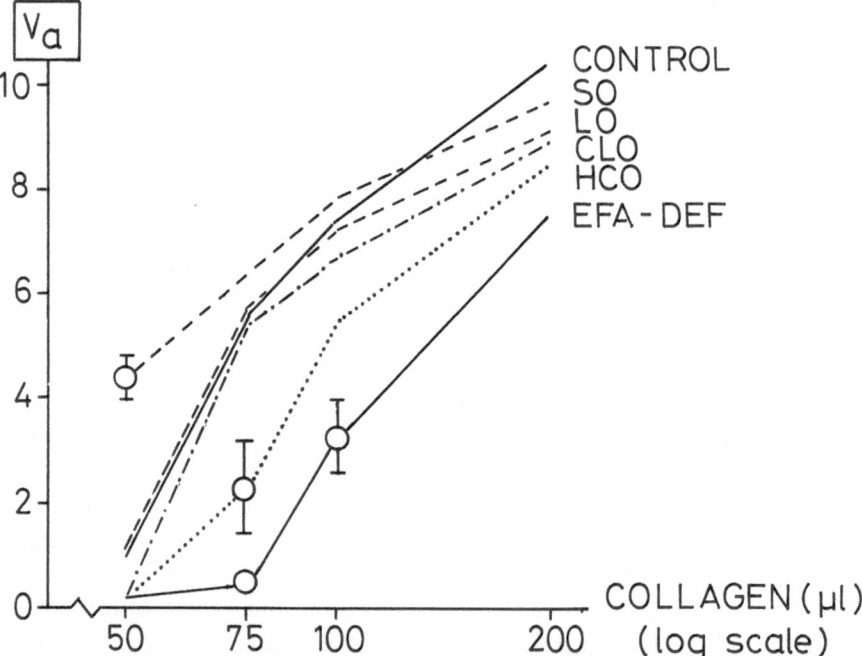

Fig. 8.1. Collagen-induced aggregation (tgα, see Chapter 5, section 3.2) in PRP of rats fed different dietary fats. n = 6 pools of 4 animals. ○ values ± SEM significantly different from those in other groups.

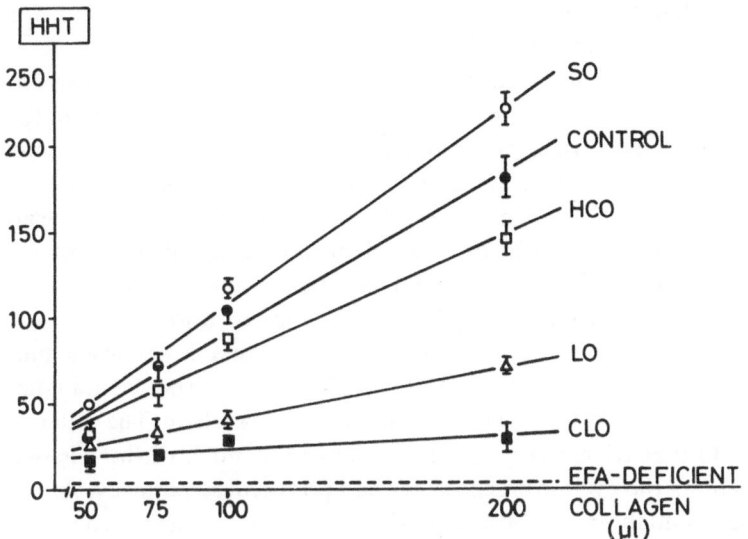

Fig. 8.2. Effect of different dietary fats on the HHT production (ng· 10⁻⁹ platelets) by collagen-activated blood platelets. Each point represents mean ± SEM of six determinations carried out in PRP-pools each obtained from 4 animals. Regression equations for the various groups:

SO: $Y = -6.99 + 1.155\, X\ (\bigcirc)$;
Control: $Y = -1.18 + 0.938\, X\ (\bullet)$;
HCO: $Y = 3.98 + 0.730\, X\ (\square)$;
LO: $Y = 10.09 + 0.310\, X\ (\triangle)$;
CLO: $Y = 14.51 + 0.088\, X\ (\blacksquare)$.

8.3.3. *HETE production*

Figure 8.3 shows the HETE production of collagen-activated blood platelets. As was also the case for HHT, HETE formation increased significantly ($P_2 < 0.001$) with increasing collagen dose (analysis of variance). For the control and SO groups, but not for the HCO, LO and CLO groups, the dose–response curves differed significantly from rectilinearity ($P_2 < 0.05$). HETE production in the EFA-deficient group was below the level of reliable quantification. Analysis of the regression slopes (Student-Newman-Keuls test) revealed no difference between the LO and CLO groups. These slopes were significantly ($P_2 < 0.05$) less steep than those for the other groups, which, most probably, did not differ mutually, although HETE production in the SO group is higher than that in the control and HCO groups. In general, the dietary effect on platelet-HETE formation is qualitatively similar to that observed for HHT production.

8.3.4. *Relationship between HHT and HETE formation*

The ratio between HETE and HHT produced by activated platelets depends on the reaction time: immediately after platelet triggering, more HHT than HETE is produced; after 5 min, the production of both substances is about equal, whereas after 20 min, the HETE/HHT ratio is about 2 [628]. These different time courses for HETE and HHT formation probably explains the different ratios reported in the literature [193, 331, 332, 472]. In our experiment, the HETE/HHT ratio not only differs for the different groups but for the various collagen doses as well (Table 8.1). This collagen effect is difficult to explain, especially so because there seems to be an interaction with the type of diet. Platelet prostanoid formation depends on substrate availability and, consequently, the increased HHT formation at increasing collagen doses indicates that a higher trigger strength results in the liberation of more AA. Since the HHT/HETE ratio has been demonstrated to become lower when substrate availability increases [793a], a lower HHT/HETE ratio is expected at higher amounts of collagen. However, this does not seem to be the case here. The collagen effect might indicate that trigger strength determines how much of the released arachidonic acid enters the cyclo-oxygenase or the lipoxygenase pathway. An alternative explantation might be a 're-routing' of endoperoxides determined by the trigger strength: a higher HETE/HHT ratio might indicate that more PGH_2 is used for the formation of 'classical' prostaglandins so that less PGH_2 is available for HHT production. Finally, a trigger strength-dependent shift in PGH_2 metabolism

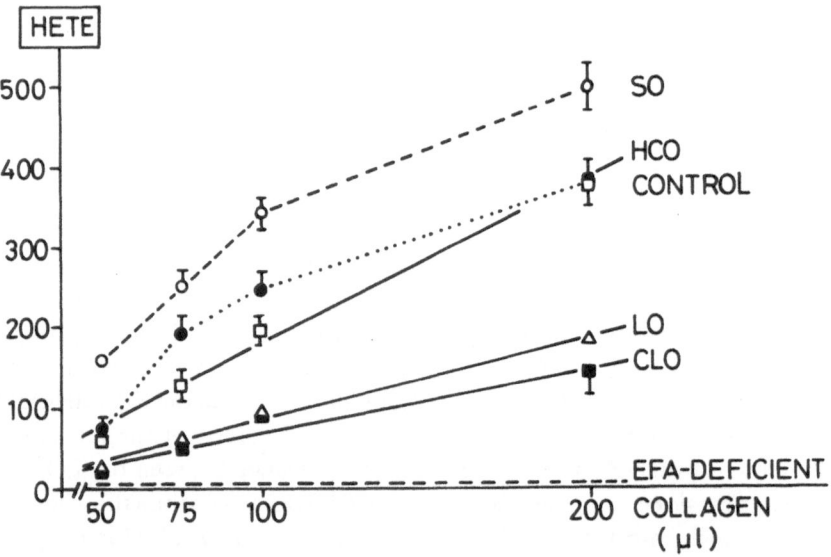

Fig. 8.3. Effect of different dietary fats on the HETE production (ng·10^{-9} platelets) by collagen-activated blood platelets. Each point represents mean ± SEM of 6 determinations carried out in PRP-pools, each obtained from 4 animals. Regression equations for the various groups:

SO:	curvilinear (○);
Control:	curvilinear (●);
HCO:	$Y = -29.3 + 2.07\,X$ (□);
LO:	$Y = -13.5 + 0.99\,Y$ (△);
CLO:	$Y = -6.0 + 0.77\,X$ (■);

towards TxB_2 instead of to HHT + MDA (see Fig. 3.1) might account for a lower HHT production, resulting in a higher HETE/HHT ratio. A detailed analysis of all arachidonic acid products formed upon collagen activation will be necessary to find the final answer.

The most obvious dietary fat effect on the HETE/HHT ratio is that caused by CLO-feeding. It is very likely that this is due to the fact that the GC/MS procedure is unable to discriminate between products derived from arachidonic acid (the 2-series eicosanoids) and those derived from timnodonic acid (the 3-series) and, consequently, measures the sum of HHT + HHTE and of HETE + HEPE. As shown in Chapter 7, section 7, collagen activation of CLO platelets causes the release of endogenous timnodonic acid, which enters the lipoxygenase pathway to form HEPE. Moreover, timnodonic acid does not serve as a substrate for the cyclooxygenase, but may inhibit the conversion of arachidonic acid. This combined effect: the production of HEPE – measured as HETE – and the inhibition of HHT formation, results in an increase in the HETE/HHT ratio.

The results, detailed in Table 8.1, and the explanation for the high HETE/HHT ratio in the CLO group mentioned above, strongly suggest that timnodonic acid is liberated from platelet phospholipids only at a high trigger strength because at lower collagen doses, the HETE/HHT ratio does no longer differ from that in the other groups. Although platelets of animals fed the LO diet also contain a considerable amount of timnodonic acid (see under section 8.4.3), their HETE/HHT ratios do not differ from those in the control group and are therefore lower than those for CLO platelets. This is a strong indication that timnodonic acid has not been liberated upon activation of the LO platelets, which suggests that only a certain pool of timnodonic acid is released on platelet activation, whereas another, earlier 'filled' pool is not (or less readily so).

8.3.5. Relationship between platelet HHT formation and collagen-induced aggregation

Platelets from the SO-group were shown to be very sensitive to a low dose of

Table 8.1. Effect of different dietary fats and trigger strengths on HETE/HHT ratio (mean ± SEM) of collagen-activated blood platelets (n = 6 pools of 4 animals)

Group	Collagen dose (μl)			
	50	75	100	200
Control	2.2 ± 0.23	2.8 ± 0.25	2.4 ± 0.25	2.1 ± 0.06
SO	3.2 ± 0.15	3.6 ± 0.47	2.9 ± 0.20	2.2 ± 0.13
HCO	1.9 ± 0.12	2.3 ± 0.20	2.3 ± 0.21	2.6 ± 0.14
LO	1.5 ± 0.36	2.4 ± 0.57	2.2 ± 0.12	2.6 ± 0.11
CLO	1.6 ± 0.63	2.6 ± 0.35	3.5 ± 0.24	5.2 ± 0.89

collagen: their aggregation response as well as their HHT production are signficantly higher than those in the other groups. This observation supports the concept that collagen-induced aggregation is mediated by cyclo-oxygenase products of arachidonic acid [332]. As can be seen from Fig. 8.4, the type of dietary fat greatly affects the relationship between aggregation and HHT production: in the EFA-deficient, the CLO and the LO groups, the collagen-induced aggregation is almost independent of HHT formation, whereas in the control, SO and HCO groups, there is a pronounced, although mutually different relationship between both parameters. As will be shown in more detail later (section 8.5.), HHT formation depends on the platelet arachidonic acid (AA) content and it is striking to note that collagen-induced aggregation is the more HHT-dependent, the higher the AA content of platelet phospholipids. Thus, it seems highly probable that in the case of a diminished AA-peroxidation by cyclo-oxygenase, an alternative, AA-independent aggregation-mediating pathway takes over.

This aspect was investigated in more detail with platelets of another group of EFA-deficient rats in which MDA formation and ^{14}C-5HT release were measured upon triggering with collagen. Results were compared with those obtained from control platelets (5 en% SO). In a first series of experiments, a supramaximal dose of collagen was used and the reaction was interrupted after exposure times varying between 10 s and 3 min. A second series was performed with different submaximal doses of collagen at a standard reaction time of 3 min. If arachidonate peroxidation governs the release reaction, the relationship between ^{14}C-5HT release and MDA

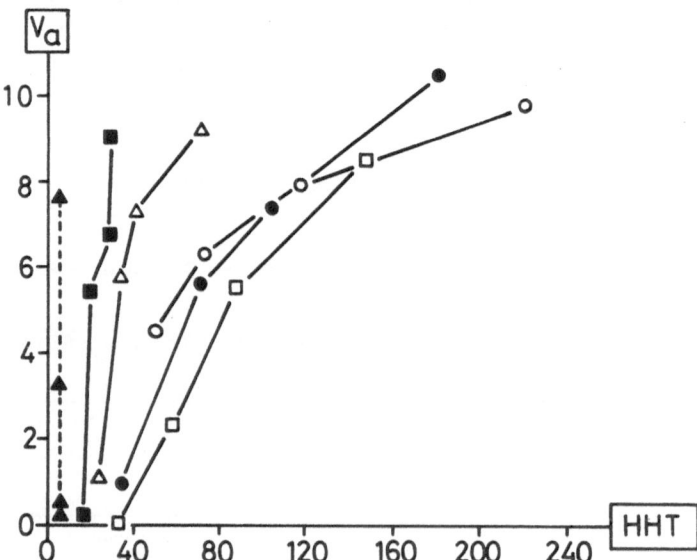

Fig. 8.4. Relationship between collagen-induced platelet HHT formation (ng $\cdot$ 10^{-9} platelets) and platelet aggregation (V$_a$, see Fig. 5.5). Each point represents the mean of 6 determinations carried out in PRP-pools, each obtained from 4 animals.
—○— SO; — ●— Control; —□— HCO; —△— LO; —■— CLO; --▲-- EFA-deficient.

formation should be the same in both the EFA-deficient and the control group. This was not so: in EFA-deficient platelets, the same degree of release coincides with a lower MDA formation than in control platelets [395]. Therefore, in EFA-deficient rat platelets, there must be an additional release mechanism independent of the arachidonate pathway. Bult and Bonta [107] arrived at the same conclusion.

Essentially similar results have been reported when blocking AA-peroxidation with aspirin: although it irreversibly inactivates platelet cyclo-oxygenase (CO) by acetylation [703, 704] and, as a result, inhibits secondary and collagen-induced aggregation [632, 845, 881], aggregation inhibition can simply be overcome by increasing the trigger strength [881] without reactivation of CO-mediated AA peroxidation [273]. Collagen-induced aggregation of platelets of LO- and CLO-fed animals is slightly lower than that of control animals (section 8.3.1, Fig. 8.1), whereas their HHT production is greatly depressed (Fig. 8.2). This finding strongly indicates that these diets enhance the activity of an (the?) AA-independent release and aggregation mechanism possibly by increasing the platelet sensitivity towards collagen, resulting in an effect analogous to that occurring upon increasing the trigger strength in aspirinated platelets.

In the case of EFA-deficiency, platelet HHT production and collagen-induced aggregation are reduced, indicating that the compensatory platelet-sensitivity increase observed for platelets of the LO and CLO groups, does not take place here. This might be ascribed to the diminished platelet-to-collagen adhesion, demonstrated in EFA-deficiency (Chapter 6, section 2.2.1.) which may be connected with a higher saturation level of platelet membrane fatty acids (see section 8.6.2).

In het HCO group, triggering of platelets with collagen gives rise to a 'normal' HHT production in relation to the platelet AA content (see section 8.5). Platelet aggregation, however, is definitely depressed, which strongly indicates that the sensitivity of HCO-platelets towards the aggregating effect of TxA_2 is diminished. This suggestion is also indicated by the results presented in Fig. 8.1. The present finding also suggests that the lower PF_3 availability, observed with HCO platelets upon triggering with collagen (Chapter 5, section 2.5), is not due to a disturbance of the initial platelet–collagen interaction but to some secondary phenomenon. This suggestion is also obtained from the observation that the collagen-induced shape change of platelets from HCO-fed animals is significantly more pronounced than that of other platelets (see Chapter 5, section 3.2; also observed in the present experiment).

Nothing is known yet about the alternative, AA-independent aggregation-mediating pathway, possibly implicated in the aggregation of LO-, CLO- and EFA-deficient platelets. It is unlikely that the platelet-activating factor (PAF) [see refs. 45, 46, 121, 138, 183, 362, 635, 657] plays a part here, since rat platelets seem to be refractory to PAF [824a].

8.4. PLATELET PHOSPHOLIPID ANALYSIS

8.4.1. *Platelet phospholipid content*

Protein determinations were carried out in suspensions diluted with EDTA immediately before extraction (section 8.2). This enables us to report platelet analyses in relation to platelet protein (cf. Table 8.2). No significant differences were observed between the groups. As compared to human platelets (0.20–0.30 μmol lipid-P $\cdot$ mg^{-1} platelet protein [521, 614, 618, 619, 728]), the values for rat platelets are rather high. The same holds for the platelet cholesterol values (Table 8.11) and is most probably due to the low protein content of the platelet suspensions, measured immediately before lipid extraction. It is highly likely that the EDTA added to prevent phospholipase activity, interfered with the Lowry -technique used for the measurement of the platelet protein content [653].

8.4.2. *Platelet phospholipid class distribution*

Table 8.3 gives the platelet phospholipid class distribution. These results are in good agreement with literature data [9, 521, 614, 618, 728]. The slight amount of LPE found in the platelet phospholipids means that only a minor activation of the platelets took place during preparation of the platelet suspensions. In pilot experiments, in which platelets had been washed twice, a considerable PE-hydrolysis was observed so that in the present experiment, we washed them only once.

As to the phospholipid class distribution, significant differences between the groups were observed for LPC only; this compound was considerably diminished in the EFA-deficient and CLO groups ($P_2 < 0.05$). Whether this difference has any functional significance is difficult to establish. LPC has been reported to be implicated in the regulation of platelet function by several investigators. Besterman and Gillet observed that LPC inhibits serotonin- and collagen-induced aggregation, whereas the second phase of ADP- and adrenaline-induced aggregation is also

Table 8.2. Total phospholipid content of platelets (mean $\pm$ SEM) obtained from animals fed different dietary fats

Diet	Platelet phospholipid (μmol lipid-P. mg protein^{-1})
Control	0.44 $\pm$ 0.022
SO	0.42 $\pm$ 0.042
HCO	0.40 $\pm$ 0.060
LO	0.43 $\pm$ 0.018
CLO	0.50 $\pm$ 0.047
EFA-def.	0.44 $\pm$ 0.033

n = 4 pools of 4 animals.

Table 8.3. Phospholipid class distribution (% of total phospholipids ± SEM) of platelets obtained from rats fed different dietary fats

Phospholipid class	Dietary groups					
	Control	SO	HCO	LO	CLO	EFA-def.
LPE	0.4 ± 0.18	0.4 ± 0.21	0.2 ± 0.20	0.3 ± 0.14	0.5 ± 0.25	0.2 ± 0.12
LPC	4.0 ± 0.26	4.6 ± 0.28	4.3 ± 0.33	3.9 ± 0.17	3.0 ± 0.17	2.8 ± 0.18
SPH	13.1 ± 0.55	13.5 ± 0.48	13.1 ± 0.14	13.3 ± 0.10	13.6 ± 0.38	12.9 ± 0.32
PS	10.1 ± 0.54	10.3 ± 0.39	10.8 ± 0.66	11.1 ± 1.40	10.0 ± 0.42	9.4 ± 0.42
PI	3.7 ± 0.22	3.6 ± 0.14	3.6 ± 0.18	3.4 ± 0.31	4.2 ± 0.27	4.0 ± 0.55
PE	28.1 ± 1.02	27.3 ± 0.45	27.0 ± 0.77	27.5 ± 0.24	28.2 ± 0.83	28.5 ± 0.69
PC	40.4 ± 0.49	40.2 ± 0.94	37.5 ± 1.77	40.3 ± 1.25	40.7 ± 1.71	41.9 ± 1.43

n = 3 pools of 4 animals

inhibited [56, 57]. Joist and coworkers [432] also observed a dose-dependent inhibition of PRP aggregation induced by ADP, adrenaline, collagen and thrombin, which might be the result of a direct membrane-disturbing effect of LPC, which has deterging properties [678] and is reported to alter membrane structure [663]. LPC was shown to be taken up by platelets very efficiently [431]; therefore, its effect might also be caused by an intracellular process. It inhibits stimulation of the adenyl cyclase system in various cell types and stimulates guanyl cyclase, possibly leading to enhancement of the cytoplasmatic Ca^{++} level and, consequently, to phospholipase activation [49]. However, it might well be that LPC serves a function in trapping free arachidonic acid before this AA can be converted to TxA_2 so that the

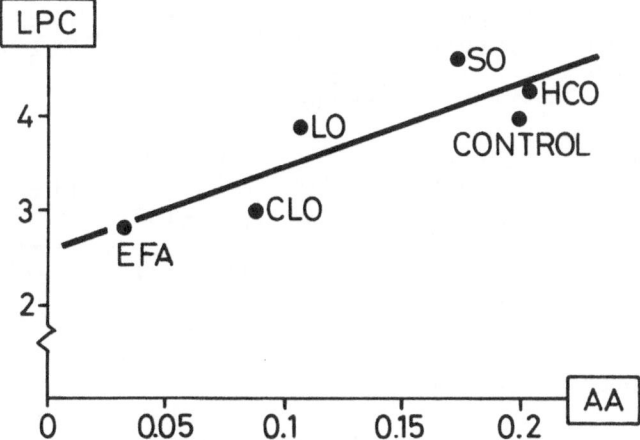

Fig. 8.5. Relationship between platelet arachidonic acid content (AA, μmol · mg protein^{-1}) and the amount of lysolecithin in platelets (LPC, μmol · mg protein^{-1}). Data calculated from the results given in Tables 8.2., 8.3. and 8.9.
Y = 2.56 + 9.01 X ; r = 0.87; P < 0.05.

net result of a change in platelet LPC is uncertain. The observation that platelet LPC increased with the platelet AA content (Fig. 8.5), may be explained by assuming that a high AA content in the phospholipids creates a possible risk of free AA and hence needs a high concentration of an effective free AA scavenger. Further investigations into the role of platelet LPC seems justified.

Our TLC procedure did not discriminate between PE and PPE (plasmalogen form of PE, see Chapter 2, section 5.2). A pilot study indicated that about 40% of PE was in the plasmalogen form. Moreover, LPE found upon repeated platelet washing appeared to be due to PPE-breakdown.

8.4.3. *Fatty acid composition of platelet phospholipids*

The fatty acid composition of the different phospholipid classes is given in Tables 8.4–8.8. From these results and those reported in Table 8.3 (phospholipid class distribution), the total phospholipid fatty acid composition was calculated (see Table 8.9). Apart from SPH, which has a very peculiar fatty acid composition (vide infra), the differences between the groups with regard to the fatty acid composition of total phospholipids, are a reflection of those between the various phospholipid

Table 8.4. Platelet PI fatty acid composition ($\% \pm$ SEM) of animals fed different dietary fats. n = 3 pools animals. Only fractions $\geq 1\%$ are mentioned.

Fatty acid	Control	SO	HCO	LO	CLO	EFA-def.
16:0	4.4 ± 0.55	3.9 ± 0.73	3.7 ± 0.15	3.1 ± 0.64	3.4 ± 0.53	4.3 ± 0.9!
(75)[a]		1.4 ± 0.18	1.3 ± 0.48	1.8 ± 1.13		1.2 ± 0.1?
18:0	36.2 ± 0.27	35.5 ± 2.27	39.6 ± 0.55	37.3 ± 0.65	36.4 ± 0.37	34.6 ± 0.8?
18:1(n–9)	5.5 ± 0.39	3.8 ± 0.46	2.9 ± 0.57	4.2 ± 0.29	6.6 ± 0.28	6.9 ± 0.6!
18:2(n–6)	1.1 ± 0.15	3.5 ± 0.14		1.3 ± 0.07	1.1 ± 0.08	
18:3(n–3)				1.6 ± 0.09		
20:0						
20:1(n–9)		1.3 ± 0.95			1.8 ± 0.00	
(133)		1.2 ± 0.38	1.4 ± 0.41	1.3 ± 0.50		1.1 ± 0.3!
(146)			1.1 ± 0.07	1.5 ± 0.06	1.2 ± 0.12	
20:3(n–9)						38.4 ± 0.9?
20:4(n–6)	44.2 ± 1.07	39.0 ± 2.92	42.4 ± 0.80	34.7 ± 1.79	23.8 ± 0.57	5.5 ± 0.2?
22:0			1.3 ± 0.28			
22.1:1(n–9/11)					1.2 ± 0.33	
20:5(n–3)				6.0 ± 0.40	17.0 ± 1.39	
22:4(n–6)	2.4 ± 0.14	2.1 ± 0.13	2.4 ± 0.18			
22:3(n–9)[b]						2.5 ± 0.5(
22:5(n–3)				2.1 ± 0.20	2.0 ± 0.16	
22:6(n–3)					1.2 ± 0.12	

[a] Numbers in parenthesis refer to retention times (arbitrary units) of unidentified compounds
[b] Tentative identification

Table 8.5. Platelet PS fatty acid composition (% ± SEM) of animals fed different dietary fats. n = 3 pools of 4 animals. Only fractions ≥ 1% are given.

Fatty acid	Control	SO	HCO	LO	CLO	EFA-def.
18:0	36.3 ± 0.18	38.0 ± 0.35	40.0 ± 0.86	39.5 ± 0.90	33.0 ± 0.55	32.3 ± 0.70
18:1(n–9)	6.6 ± 0.57	4.3 ± 0.40	2.4 ± 0.45	10.3 ± 3.67	11.3 ± 0.58	14.6 ± 0.49
18:2(n–6)	2.0 ± 0.18	4.8 ± 0.12	1.8 ± 0.33	8.7 ± 0.24	7.3 ± 0.40	
20:0	1.3 ± 0.22	1.5 ± 0.22	1.7 ± 0.29	1.8 ± 0.41		1.1 ± 0.07
20:1(n–9)				1.0 ± 0.81	2.9 ± 0.21	1.4 ± 0.09
(139)[a]		1.5 ± 0.23				
20:3(n–9)						24.0 ± 0.49
(146)			1.1 ± 0.18	1.9 ± 0.49	2.1 ± 0.13	
20:4(n–6)	37.5 ± 2.33	35.4 ± 1.47	41.7 ± 1.71	20.8 ± 3.71	15.9 ± 0.98	8.2 ± 0.65
22:0	2.5 ± 0.27	3.6 ± 0.29	2.5 ± 0.50	2.4 ± 0.04	1.3 ± 0.46	1.4 ± 0.20
22:1(n–9/11)	1.9 ± 0.12	1.0 ± 0.06		2.0 ± 0.41	10.2 ± 0.32	1.8 ± 0.07
20:5(n–3)				3.4 ± 0.37	7.6 ± 0.70	
22:3(n–9)[b]						7.1 ± 0.32
22:4(n–6)	3.6 ± 0.44	3.2 ± 0.27	2.9 ± 0.32	1.0 ± 0.00		
(191)	1.4 ± 0.09		1.2 ± 0.03		1.0 ± 0.09	
22:5(n–3)				2.5 ± 1.22	1.9 ± 0.29	
22:6(n–3)				1.0 ± 0.24		

[a] Numbers in parenthesis refer to retention times (arbitrary units) of unidentified compounds
[b] Tentative identification

classes. The most prominent changes are observed with the long-chain polyunsaturated fatty acids. The arachidonic acid (20:4 (4-6)) content is almost similar in the control, SO and HCO groups, whereas it is significantly reduced in the LO, CLO and EFA-deficient groups. As to the latter group, this finding is not surprising because the dietary AA-precursor, linoleic acid (18:2 (n–6), LA) is lacking. In the LO and CLO groups, however, LA is fed in the same amounts as in the control group, so a (relative) precursor deficiency cannot be the reason for the reduced AA content observed in these groups. The most likely explanation is the inhibition of LA-desaturation (the key-step in AA biosynthesis, see Chapter 2, section 2.2) by α-linolenic acid (18:3 (n–3), αLA) in the LO-diet and by 20:5 (n–3) and 22:5 and 6 (n–3) in the CLO diet (Tables 4.2 and 7.1). Due to this inhibition of the LA metabolism, the LA content is somewhat enhanced in the LO and CLO groups. The higher LA content in the SO group is most probably due to the large amount of LA in the SO diet.

Timnodonic acid (20:5 (n–3), TA) and 22:5 (n–3) are increased in the LO group, which will be the result of the active desaturation and chain elongation of α-LA present in the LO diet. The enhanced concentrations of TA and 22:6 (n–3) observed in the platelet phospholipids of CLO-fed animals are caused by the rather high content of these fatty acids in cod-liver oil (see Table 7.1).

In EFA-deficiency, lack of LA and α-LA enables oleic acid to become desaturated and elongated, thus giving rise to the formation of mead acid (MA, 20:3(n–9), see

Table 8.6. Platelet PE fatty acid composition (% ± SEM) of animals fed different dietary fats. n = 3 pools of 4 animals. Only fractions ≥ 1% are given.

Fatty acid	Control	SO	HCO	LO	CLO	EFA-def.
16:0 dma[b]	4.5 ± 1.24	4.2 ± 0.04	6.6 ± 0.14	3.6 ± 0.95	4.1 ± 0.87	5.6 ± 0.61
16:0	6.5 ± 0.98	5.4 ± 0.84	2.5 ± 0.40	5.1 ± 0.75	5.1 ± 0.77	5.2 ± 0.41
16:1(n–7)	1.5 ± 0.84			1.3 ± 0.93	1.4 ± 0.46	1.4 ± 0.45
18:0 dma[b]	3.3 ± 1.21	4.1 ± 1.26	9.4 ± 0.58	4.7 ± 1.55	4.2 ± 0.83	3.8 ± 0.61
18:1 dma[b]	3.2 ± 1.22	2.0 ± 0.61	1.8 ± 0.03	2.9 ± 0.89	4.0 ± 1.04	5.8 ± 1.14
18:0	13.2 ± 0.35	16.2 ± 0.09	12.4 ± 0.37	15.8 ± 0.52	12.7 ± 0.42	11.3 ± 0.33
18:1	5.2 ± 0.35	3.5 ± 0.09	1.8 ± 0.31	5.0 ± 0.03	6.3 ± 0.29	8.2 ± 0.12
18:2(n–6)	1.8 ± 0.20	5.9 ± 0.64	1.4 ± 0.18	6.8 ± 0.40	4.3 ± 0.13	
18:3(n–3				1.8 ± 0.03		
20:1(n–9)					2.1 ± 0.10	
(139)[a]		1.6 ± 0.07				
20:3(n–9)						37.8 ± 0.41
(146)				1.2 ± 0.00	1.1 ± 0.06	
20:4(n–6)	44.0 ± 0.82	41.3 ± 2.00	46.9 ± 1.38	27.3 ± 1.13	19.3 ± 0.27	6.8 ± 0.12
22:1(n–9/11)					1.8 ± 0.09	
20:5(n–3)				13.2 ± 0.94	25.1 ± 1.30	
22:3(n–9)[b]						7.4 ± 0.20
22:4(n–6)	10.9 ± 1.22	10.8 ± 0.89	12.5 ± 1.16	1.4 ± 0.22		
(191)	1.4 ± 0.10	1.0 ± 0.12	1.9 ± 0.18			
22:5(n–3)				5.1 ± 1.10	3.4 ± 0.35	
22:6(n–3)					2.1 ± 0.10	

[a] Numbers in parenthesis refer to retention times (arbitrary units) of unidentified compounds.
[b] Tentative identification. dma: dimethylacetal.

Chapter 2, section 2.2). Most probably, 22:3 (n–9) is synthesized as well. The higher contents of 14:0 and 18:0 observed in the HCO group are connected with the rather high dietary concentrations of these fatty acids. The lower 16:0 content of the platelet phospholipids in this group cannot be explained from a dietary composition. Why this low platelet 16:0 level is not compensated for by a higher content of fatty acids of the (n–7) family, cannot yet be accounted for.

In general, the fatty acid compositions of the different phospholipid classes are in agreement with those mentioned in the literature [9, 521, 613, 618, 619, 660, 686, 749]: the AA content (or that of its 'replacers' TA and MA) is highest in PI, PS and PE, where PE is the main phospholipid class of the long-chain (>20 C-atoms) polyunsaturated fatty acids and of the dimethylacetals (mainly originating from PPE). The fatty acid composition of SPH is greatly influenced by that of the diet. The diet-induced changes are only observed in the very long-chain fatty acids 24:0 (increased in the HCO and LO groups and decreased in the CLO and EFA-deficient groups) and 24:1 (strikingly enhanced in EFA-deficiency and in the CLO group and considerably decreased upon SO- and HCO-feeding). SO-feeding also causes a

Table 8.7. Fatty acid composition (% ± SEM) of platelet PC of animals fed different dietary fats. n = 3 pools of 4 animals. Only fractions ≥ 1% are stated.

Fatty acid	Control	SO	HCO	LO	CLO	EFA-def.
14:0	1.5 ± 0.09	1.1 ± 0.07	6.1 ± 0.36	1.0 ± 0.09	2.1 ± 0.18	2.3 ± 0.15
16:0	57.9 ± 0.44	54.1 ± 1.92	45.1 ± 0.68	55.2 ± 1.74	55.5 ± 0.83	54.4 ± 1.37
16:1(n-7)	2.1 ± 0.09	1.1 ± 0.07	1.0 ± 0.06		3.6 ± 0.21	4.3 ± 0.15
(75)[a]						1.0 ± 0.14
18:0	6.8 ± 0.15	11.2 ± 0.37	12.7 ± 0.18	10.0 ± 0.55	6.7 ± 0.10	5.9 ± 0.22
18:1(n-9)	9.7 ± 0.35	3.7 ± 0.18	5.4 ± 0.27	6.4 ± 0.12	10.4 ± 0.53	16.7 ± 0.40
18:2(n-6)	4.7 ± 0.28	11.6 ± 0.32	6.5 ± 0.17	12.8 ± 0.97	6.7 ± 0.83	
18.3(n-3)				2.3 ± 0.09		
20:1(n-9)					2.0 ± 0.12	
(139)		1.8 ± 0.09				
20:3(n-9)						9.0 ± 1.32
(146)			1.1 ± 0.03			
20:4(n-6)	12.8 ± 0.68	11.3 ± 0.49	18.3 ± 0.36	4.6 ± 0.33	2.9 ± 0.38	2.0 ± 0.21
22:1(n-9/11)					1.8 ± 0.09	
20.5(n-3)				2.1 ± 0.07	3.9 ± 0.48	
22:4(n-6)			1.1 ± 0.12			

[a] Numbers in parenthesis refer to retention times (arbitrary units) of unidentified compounds.

Table 8.8. Platelet SPH fatty acid composition (% ± SEM) of animals fed different dietary fats. n = 3 pools of 4 animals. Only fractions ≥ 1% are given.

Fatty acids[a]	Control	SO	HCO	LO	CLO	EFA-def.
14:0			1.0 ± 0.52			
16:0	29.2 ± 0.24	27.2 ± 0.87	28.2 ± 1.66	27.3 ± 0.54	27.4 ± 0.34	32.2 ± 2.48
(75)[a]						1.1 ± 0.44
18:0	6.8 ± 0.94	6.3 ± 0.86	9.0 ± 0.65	6.8 ± 0.87	3.6 ± 1.69	6.1 ± 1.04
18:1(n-9)	1.1 ± 0.57			1.0 ± 0.72		
20:0	2.3 ± 0.16	2.5 ± 0.15	3.2 ± 0.07	2.4 ± 0.09	1.7 ± 0.14	2.3 ± 0.29
20:1(n-9)				1.1 ± 0.38		
(133)			1.0 ± 0.52			
20:4(n-6)	1.4 ± 0.37	1.2 ± 0.35	1.5 ± 0.20			
22:0	9.4 ± 0.08	10.8 ± 0.22	16.0 ± 0.84	10.2 ± 0.23	5.5 ± 0.24	8.6 ± 0.58
22:1(n-9/11)	1.8 ± 0.12				1.4 ± 0.07	2.8 ± 0.35
(170)	1.0 ± 0.04	1.8 ± 0.03	1.4 ± 0.09	1.3 ± 0.03	1.1 ± 0.07	1.0 ± 0.14
(180)						1.7 ± 0.10
24:0	10.6 ± 0.04	9.7 ± 0.21	15.7 ± 0.97	14.4 ± 0.55	6.4 ± 0.30	7.7 ± 0.68
24:1	24.5 ± 1.39	14.5 ± 0.54	13.3 ± 0.84	22.2 ± 0.77	42.5 ± 0.75	30.1 ± 0.32
(205)	7.8 ± 0.16	21.5 ± 0.87	5.7 ± 0.35	5.5 ± 0.29	2.2 ± 0.07	
(225)				3.2 ± 0.27		

[a] Numbers in parenthesis refer to retention times (arbitrary units) of unidentified compounds.

154

distinct increase in the content of an unidentified compound (retention time 205 arbitrary units) the functional role of which has not yet been investigated. It is possible that this compound is a 24:2 fatty acid as earlier observed by Pitas and coworkers [659].

8.5. RELATIONSHIP BETWEEN THE ARACHIDONIC ACID CONTENT OF PLATELET PHOSPHOLIPIDS AND THE HHT PRODUCTION OF ACTIVATED PLATELETS

8.5.1. *Absolute AA content*

Starting from the platelet phospholipid content (μmol$\cdot$mg^{-1} platelet protein), the phospholipid class distribution (% of total phospholipids), the fact that 1 μmol

Table 8.9. Fatty acid composition (%) of platelet total phospholipids. Only fractions $\geq 1\%$ are mentioned.

Fatty acid[a]	Dietary groups					
	Control	SO	HCO	LO	CLO	EFA-def.
14:0	1.0		2.6		1.0	1.0
16:0	31.9	29.3	25.2	29.7	29.8	31.3
16:1(n–7)	1.3				1.9	2.3
(75)[a]						1.0
18:0	13.9	16.9	19.2	17.0	13.3	12.4
18:1(n–9)	7.6	3.8	3.5	6.4	8.8	13.1
18:2(n–6)	2.8	7.3	3.3	8.4	4.9	
18:3(n–3)				1.5		
20:0		1.0				
20:1(n–9)					1.8	
20:3(n–9)						18.9
(146)		1.0				
20:4(n–6)	24.3	22.2	27.6	13.4	9.5	3.9
22:0	1.6	3.5	2.6	1.7	1.0	1.3
22:1(n–9/11)					2.6	1.0
20:5(n–3)				5.3	10.0	
22:3(n–9)[b]						2.5
22:4(n–6)	3.7	4.0	4.5			
24:0	1.5	1.0	2.2	2.0	1.0	1.0
24:1	3.9	2.4	2.3	3.0	6.0	4.0
22:5(n–3)				1.8	1.3	
(205)	1.1	3.0	1.0	1.0		
22:6(n–3)					1.0	

[a] Numbers in parenthesis refer to retention times (arbitrary units) of unidentified compounds.
[b] Tentative identification.

phospholipid equals 2 μmol fatty acids (except for SPH, see Chapter 2, section 5.2) and from the fatty acid composition of the different phospholipid classes, it is possible to estimate the platelet phospholipid fatty acid composition (nmol $\cdot$ mg^{-1} platelet protein). Results obtained in this way for arachidonic acid were plotted against the HHT production (ng $\cdot$ 10^9 platelets) of activated platelets to establish a possible relationschip between these two parameters. HHT production of platelets of the EFA-deficient group which was too low for reliable quantitation was taken as 5 ng $\cdot$ 10^{-9} platelets. Fig. 8.6 A-D show this relationship for the AA content of total platelet phospholipids and the HHT productions of these platelets upon their activation with four different collagen doses. From these figures it is evident that, in general, HHT production is higher, the larger the amount of arachidonic acid in platelet phospholipids. However, this relationship is not absolute, because platelets from the SO group produce more HHT than might be expected from the relationships observed for the other groups. This is particularly clear at the lowest

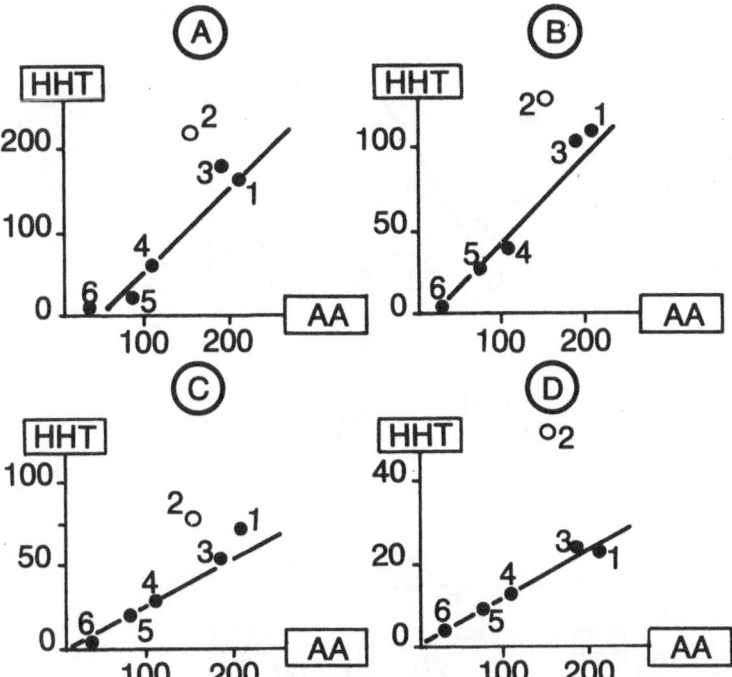

Fig. 8.6. Relationship between arachidonic acid content of platelet total phospholipids (AA, nmol $\cdot$ mg platelet protein^{-1}) and HHT production (ng $\cdot$ 10^{-9} platelets) of platelets activated with different amounts of collagen. Each point represents the mean of 2-3 platelets pools, each obtained from 4 animals.
A: 200 μl collagen;   Y = -42   + 1.0   X;   r = 0.92;   n = 11
B: 100μl collagen;   Y = -17   + 0.6   X;   r = 0.95;   n = 11
C: 75μl collagen;   Y = -   6.9 + 0.33 X;   r = 0.85;   n = 11
D: 50 μl collagen;   Y =   1.1 + 0.11 X;   r = 0.95;   n = 10
Explanation of group code: 1: Control; 2: SO; 3: HCO; 4: LO; 5: CLO; 6: EFA-deficient.
SO group (Group 2) not included for calculation of correlation.

156

collagen dose. Figs. 8.7 A-D show a qualitatively similar relationship between platelet HHT production upon activation with 100 μl collagen and the AA content of the various AA-containing phospholipid classes. This is not surprising because there is a fairly close correlation between the AA contents of total phospholipids and those of the different phopholipid classes: any increase in the AA content of total phospholipids in proportionally distributed over the various PL classes, although there is a tendency for PI to become 'saturated' first and PC last (Fig. 8.8).

8.5.2. Relative AA content

Several long-chain polyunsaturated fatty acids have been shown to compete with

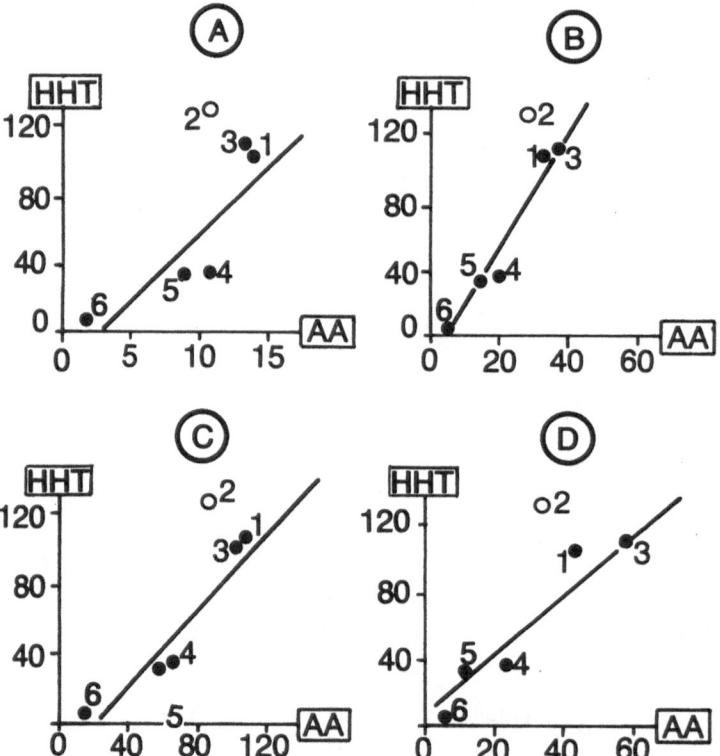

Fig. 8.7. Relationship between the arachidonic acid content of the various phospholipid classes (AA, nmol·mg platelet protein^{-1}) and the HHT production (ng·10^{-9} platelets) of platelets activated with 100 μl collagen. Each point represents the mean of 2–3 platelet pools, each obtained from 4 animals.
A: PI; Y = −22.7 + 8.10 X; r = 0.87; n = 14.
B: PS; Y = −17.7 + 3.49 X; r = 0.95; n = 14.
C: PE; Y = −23.0 + 1.13 X; r = 0.91; n = 14.
D: PC; Y =   6.8 + 1.77 X; r = 0.87; n = 15.
Group 2 (SO) not included for calculation of correlations. For explanation of group codes, see legend of Fig. 8.6.

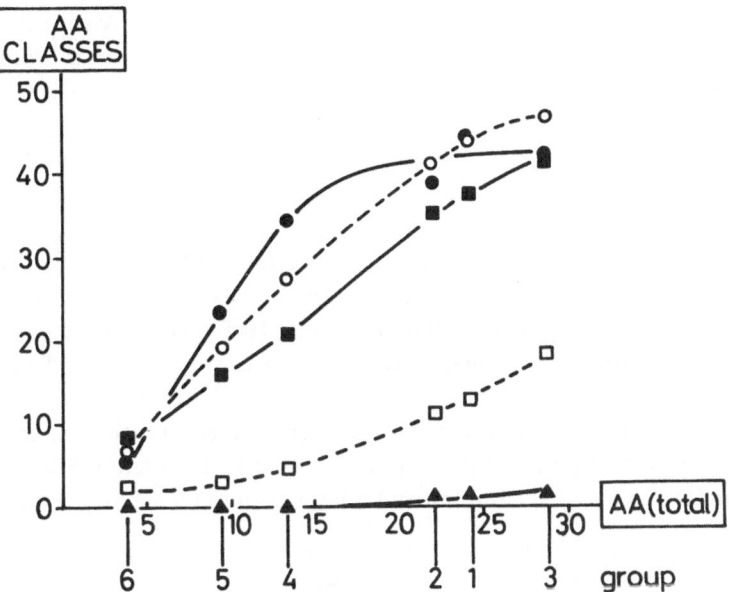

Fig. 8.8. Relationship between the AA-content (% of total fatty acids) of platelet total phospholipids (AA(total)) and that of the various phospholipid classes (AA classes). For explanation of group code, see legend of Fig. 8.6.
— ●—PI; ---□---PC; —■—PS; —▲—SPH; ---○---PE.

AA for the CO-enzyme system so that they inhibit AA conversion [236, 477, 598, 625]. Since these competitors are also located at the 2-position of phospholipids, and platelet phospholipase activity does not seem to be AA-specific [64, 64a] (see also Chapter 7, section 7.1.2), these fatty acids might be expected to become released simultaneously with AA. The following fatty acids are likely to affect AA conversion by CO: 22:6(n–3); 22:5(n–3); 20:5(n–3); 18:3(n–3); 22:4(n–6); 18:2 (n–6); 22:3(n–9) and 20:3(n–9).

No detailed information is available on the mutual differences in affinity for the CO enzyme system. Moreover, for most of these fatty acids the inhibition characteristics of AA oxygenation have not been determined. Therefore, it is supposed, as a first approximation, that for all fatty acids, the CO affinity is similar to that for AA and that all competitors are equally effective as inhibitors of AA oxygenation. On the basis of these presumptions, a relative AA content of platelet phospholipids can be calculated according the equation:

$$\text{relative AA content} = \frac{\%\text{AA}}{\%\text{AA} + \sum\% \text{ competitors}}$$

Figures 8.9 and 8.10 A-D demonstrate the relationship between the relative AA content (AA(rel)) of platelet phospholipids and the HHT production of these platelets following activation with collagen. In essence, the results are similar to those obtained for the uncorrected AA contents (Figs. 8.6 and 8.7). Also in the present case is a good linear correlation observed between both parameters for total phospholipids as well as for the various phospholipid classes. Again, the values obtained for the SO group do not fit this relationship satisfactorily.

8.5.3. Discussion

Platelet prostanoid formation appears to be determined largely by the amount of precursor fatty acid available: a positive linear relationship was observed between the AA-content of rat platelet phospholipids and the HHT-formation of these platelets upon their activation with collagen (Figs. 8.6, 8.7, 8.9 and 8.10). These results are in agreement with findings reported by others. Thus Seyberth and coworkers [637, 739] demonstrated that enrichment of the diet with the prostaglandin precursor fatty acids dihomo-γ-linolenic acid (rabbit) and arachidonic acid (man) causes these fatty acids to accumulate in tissue phospholipids and coincides

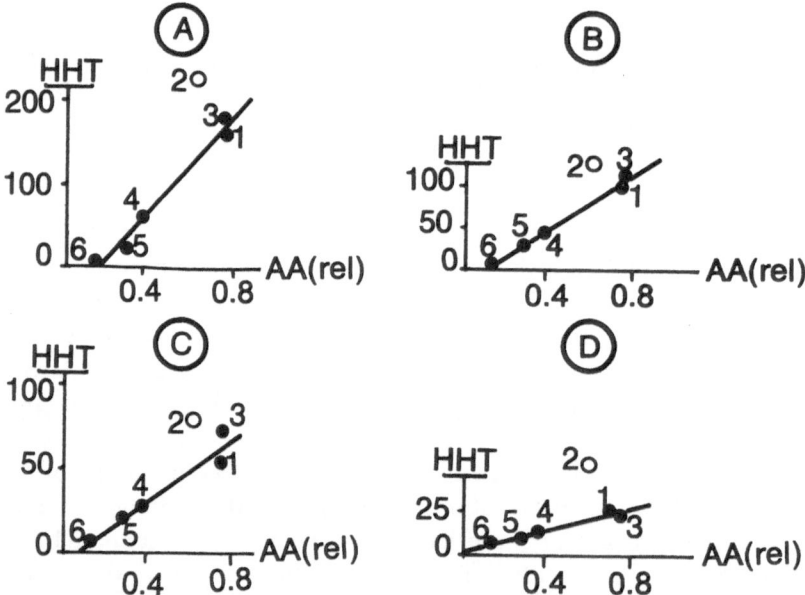

Fig. 8.9. Relationship between the relative arachidonic acid content of platelet total phospholipids (AA(rel), see text section 8.5.2.) and HHT production (ng · 10^{-9} platelets) of platelets activated with different amounts of collagen. Each point represents the mean of 2-3 platelet pools, each obtained from 4 animals.

A: 200 μl collagen; Y = −46 + 290.4 X; r = 0.94; n = 11.
B: 100 μl collagen; Y = −17 + 163.6 X; r = 0.95; n = 11.
C: 75 μl collagen; Y = − 6.6 + 90.1 X; r = 0.84; n = 11.
D: 50 μl collagen; Y = 0.9 + 30.7 X; r = 0.95; n = 10.

SO-group (Group 2) not included for calculation of correlations. For explanation of group code, see legend of Fig. 8.6.

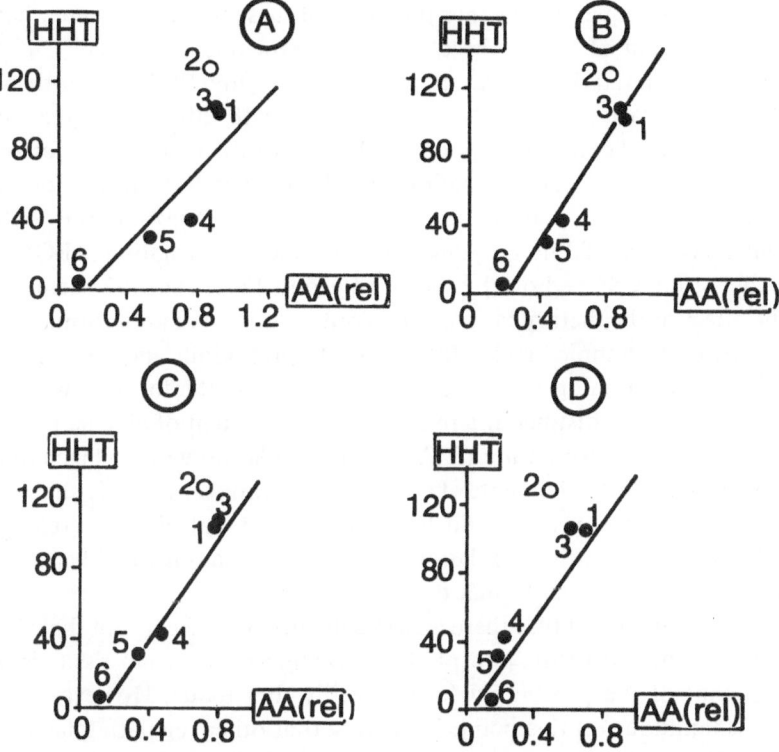

Fig. 8.10. Relationship between the relative arachidonic acid content (AA(rel), see text section 8.5.2) of the various platelet phospholipid classes and the HHT production (ng $\cdot$ 10^{-9} platelets) of platelets activated with 100 μl collagen. Each point represents the mean of 2–3 platelet pools, each obtained from 4 animals. For explanation of group code, see legend of Fig. 8.6.

A: PI ; Y = $-18.5 + 114.2 \, X$; r = 0.85; n = 14.
B: PS; Y = $-34.1 + 157.5 \, X$; r = 0.95; n = 13.
C: PE; Y = $-22.1 + 152.3 \, X$; r = 0.90; n = 14.
D: PC; Y = $- 2.9 + 146.7 \, X$; r = 0.91; n = 15.
Group 2 (SO) not included for calculation of correlations.

with an enhanced prostanoid turnover as reflected by an increased urinary excretion of PGE-metabolites. Friedman and Fröhlich [268] observed that the parenteral administration of Intralipid ®, a fat emulsion rich in linoleic acid, caused a reduction of human tissue arachidonic acid content which was associated with the reduced excretion of PGE-metabolites. Hwang and Kinsella [411, 412, 454] inhibited the linoleic-arachidonic acid conversion by feeding trans-linoleic acid to rats [377]. This treatment resulted in a marked decrease in serum-levels of precursor acids and their respective prostaglandins, synthesised during blood clotting. Later, similar experiments were performed using α-linolenic acid to inhibit the conversion of linoleic acid into arachidonic acid. In this study the earlier results were confirmed and extended [413]. Unfortunately, the composition of the platelet phospholipids was not determined; consequently, the interpretation of these findings is somewhat difficult, especially in light of the results obtained by Fine and coworkers [246]. These investigators measured the formation of PGE_1, PGE_2 and $PGF_{2\alpha}$ in serum of rats that had been fed various amounts of dietary fats with different degrees of unsaturation. Although platelet phospholipids showed distinct differences as to their arachidonic acid contents, no correlation was observed with the formation of PGE_2 and $PGF_{2\alpha}$ upon blood clotting. A slight correlation, however, was seen between the platelet content of dihomo-γ-linolenic acid and the formation of PGE_1. These and further studies carried out by the same group [204, 786, 792] demonstrated that the effect of the dietary fat type and content on prostanoid formation during blood clotting is complex and difficult to interpret. Galli and coworkers [284] fed rabbits diets containing 25 en% of either corn oil or butter for three weeks. These regimens resulted in a distinct difference in the AA-content of platelet phospholipids, but platelet TxB_2-formation (RIA) upon stimulation with collagen did not differ significantly. The AA-contents of aortic phospholipids were only slightly different, whereas the aortic prostacyclin formation (bioassay) differed greatly. Therefore, in this study no consistent relationship could be demonstrated between tissue AA-content and prostanoid formation.

In conclusion it can be stated that there is firm evidence for the concept that the precursor fatty acid content of the phospholipid fraction of a certain tissue is a primary determinant of the prostanoid formation by that tissue. However, the literature is not unanimous on this point, indicating that other regulating factors can be superimposed.

The relationship between the phospholipid AA-content of blood platelets and the formation of prostanoids by these platelets does not seem to be affected by other endogenous long-chain polyunsaturated fatty acids. From the correlation coefficients, r, given in the legends to Figs. 8.6, 8.7, 8.9 and 8.10, the coefficient of determination (r^2) can be calculated, which is a measure of the fit of the regression calculated: the higher the r^2, the better the fit. Using this parameter, it appeared that correction of the AA content of platelet phospholipids for the presence of fatty acids competing with AA for the CO enzyme system, does not systematically improve the relationship with platelet HHT production. Even at the strongest platelet stimulus (200 μl collagen), this correction had no effect although, under these conditions, competitors are the most likely to become liberated from the phospholipids (see section 8.3.4). This lack of improvement might be due to the fact that there is a strong inverse relationship between the amounts of AA and its competitors in the platelet phospholipids (Fig. 8.11). In fact, the various dietary treatments resulted in a partial replacement of platelet AA by the various competitors of the (n–3) and the (n–9) families. Only for PC, the relationship is not significant and it is only for this phospholipid class that correction of platelet AA for the presence of competitors results in a moderate improvement of this relationship.

In vitro, exogenous TA is a potent inhibitor of the conversion of AA by the cyclo-oxygenase enzyme system [334, 598, 761, 789]. Upon platelet stimulation TA is liberated from membrane phospholipids (Chapter 7, section 7.1.2). If this endogenous TA inhibits the conversion of the available AA also, HHT formation will be lower than might be expected on the basis of the AA-content of platelet phospholipids. However, this appeared not to be the case: although platelets of LO- and CLO-fed animals contain appreciable amounts of TA, the AA/HHT ratios found for these platelets perfectly fit the AA–HHT relationship observed for the other groups (SO excluded). This strongly suggest that endogenously liberated TA does not interfere with the conversion of AA by the cyclo-oxygenase, possibly because the free TA is scavenged by the platelet lipoxygenase.

8.6. POSSIBLE CONSEQUENCES OF PLATELET LIPID PROFILE AND FATTY ACID COMPOSITION FOR MEMBRANE FLUIDITY

The extracellular platelet–collagen interaction results in an intracellular series of events, leading to the formation of TxA_2. This implies that a message from the platelet exterior is transmitted towards the platelet interior. A higher collagen dose is likely to initiate a stronger transmembranal message because it results in the

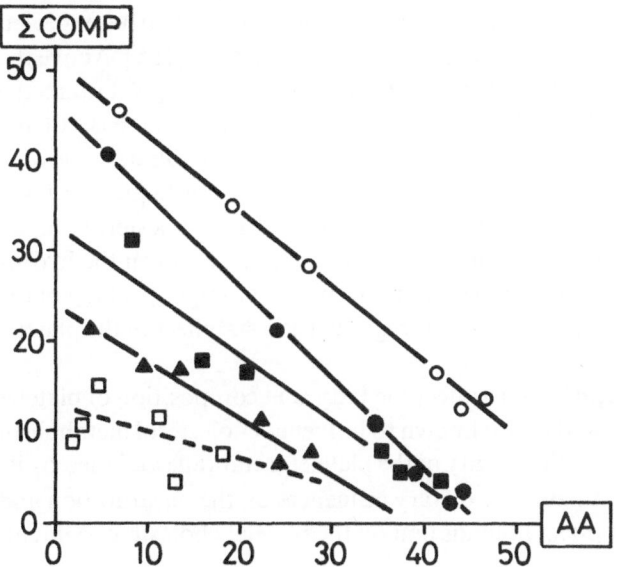

Fig. 8.11. Relationship between the amounts (% of total fatty acids) of AA and its competitors for cyclo-oxygenase in platelet phospholipids.

—O—   PI ; $Y = 45.9 - 1.01 X$; $r = 0.99$
—●—   PS : $Y = 33.1 - 0.72 X$; $r = 0.96$
—■—   PE ; $Y = 50.6 - 0.82 X$; $r = 0.99$
---□---   PC ; no significant correlation ; $r = 0.51$
—▲—   Total phospholipids ; $Y = 23.9 - 0.62 X$; $r = 0.97$

formation of more TxA_2 (measured as HHT, see section 8.3). At a given trigger strength, however, TxA_2-formation might also be expected to be modulated as a result of changes in the efficiency with which the message is transmitted across the membrane. There is ample evidence that the efficiency of such membrane-located processes is, at least in part, determined by membrane fluidity (see Chapter 2, section 8.1).

In previous sections it was demonstrated that platelets of animals fed the SO-enriched diet are very sensitive to the aggregating effect of a low dose of collagen as compared to platelets of other animals. This coincides with and is probably caused by an enhanced TxA_2-formation (measured as HHT), which could not be explained on the basis of platelet AA-content. Therefore, a more efficient transmembranal message might be implicated, which may, for instance, result from an enhanced membrane fluidity.

As discussed in Chapter 2, biomembranes are composed of proteins, cholesterol and a mixture of phospholipids. These latter compounds contain a great variety of fatty acids as a result of which membranes do not show a sharp phase transition at a distinct temperature, as observed for pure phospholipid species, but a broad phase transition profile over a wide temperature range. Because of their low phase transition temperatures, unsaturated fatty acids are likely to change this profile and, by affecting the ultimate state of the membrane, they may increase membrane fluidity thereby affecting membrane function. Similar but opposite effects may be expected when increasing the saturated fatty acid content of biomembranes [155]. Above the phase transition temperature, the presence of cholesterol strikingly lowers the mobility of phospholipid-hydrocarbon groups as a result of an increase of the viscosity of their micro-environment. Under this condition, cholesterol lowers membrane fluidity, which has been shown to have functional consequences [740, 741, 758, 791, 874]. Below the phase transition temperature, cholesterol has an opposite effect since it decreases the hydrophobic interactions between the hydrocarbon groups of membrane phospholipids and thus prevents a tight packing of the lipid molecules. Therefore, cholesterol may be regarded as a stabilizer of the plasticity of biomembranes.

Since the dietary fat type appeared to affect the fatty acid composition of platelet phospholipids (section 8.4.3) and is also known to influence cholesterol metabolism [419], it may, as a result, change the fluidity of the platelet membrane and thereby its function. Therefore, we investigated the dietary influences on the unsaturation and saturation indices of platelet phospholipids and on the platelet cholesterol content.

8.6.1. Unsaturation index

The unsaturation index (U.I.) of the platelet phospholipids was calculated from table 8.9 according to the equation:

$$\sum_{a=1}^{k} \text{(number of double bounds in a)} \times (\% \text{ occurrence of a})$$

for each fatty acid of k fatty acids [855]. This parameter relates to the classical chemico-biochemical term known as iodine value and can be taken as an indicator of membrane fluidity [238]. The results (Table 8.10.) indicate that, as compared to the control group, only the EFA-deficient group shows a distinct deviation, the U.I. being considerably depressed. Platelets obtained from animals fed the fat-enriched diets show only small differences.

8.6.2. Saturation index

A saturation index was calculated by taking the sum of the proportional amounts of saturated fatty acids in platelet total phospholipids given in Table 8.9 ($\sum$ SAFA) and correcting it for the degree of unsaturation indicated by the U.I., so that:

$$\text{S.I.} = \frac{\sum \text{SAFA}}{\text{U.I.}}$$

The results are given in Table 8.10, which again indicates that only platelets of the EFA-deficient animals show a considerable difference with respect to the control group. Platelets obtained from animals fed the fat-enriched diets show hardly any difference. The relative results (% of control group) remained essentially similar after taking into account the chain length of the fatty acids.

8.6.3. Cholesterol–phospholipid ratio

Increasing the cholesterol-phospholipid (C/P) molar ratio of platelet membranes to values above normal results in an increased membrane microviscosity (as calculated from fluorescence probe analysis [746, 824]. This condition is associated with an

Table 8.10. Effect of different dietary fats on the unsaturation and saturation indices of platelet phospholipids. For methodological details: see section 8.6)

Group	Unsaturation index		Saturation index	
	index	% of control	index	% of control
Control	130.4	100	0.38	100
SO	125.6	96.3	0.40	105.3
HCO	140.8	108.0	0.38	100.0
LO	119.8	91.9	0.42	110.5
CLO	131.4	100.8	0.35	92.1
EFA-def.	100.2	76.8	0.47	123.7

increase in platelet aggregability [740, 874], in a resistance to the aggregation inhibitor PGE_1 [758] and in an enhancement of TxB_2 formation following standardised platelet activation [791]. We calculated the C/P ratio for the various dietary groups using the platelet phospholipid values of Table 8.2. and the results of cholesterol determinations (Catalase method) both measured in platelet total lipid extracts. The data obtained are given in Table 8.11 and although the value for the EFA-deficient group tends to be somewhat diminished, the difference between the groups was not significant ($P_2 > 0.20$).

8.6.4. Discussion

As previously stated our measurements were performed with lipid extracts of whole platelets and not with extracts of platelet membranes; therefore, the relevance of our findings to platelet physiology might be doubted. However, Marcus et al. [521] showed that, at least for human platelets, there are only minor differences between whole platelets and their membranes as far as the phospholipid fatty acid composition is concerned. Moreover, our C/P ratio data (Table 8.11) are in good agreement with those obtained by others for platelet membranes [742], which strongly suggests that also as regards the lipid profile, there are only minor differences between whole platelet lipids and membrane lipids.

Neither the degree of (un)saturation of the fatty acids of platelet total phospholipids nor their cholesterol/phospholipid molar ratio are considerably changed by the type of dietary fat. Only for EFA-deficient platelets do changes in fatty acid composition indicate a decreased membrane fluidity. In EFA-deficiency, the cooperativity of various membrane-bound allosteric enzymes is significantly affected [238]. Moreover, the activity of the sarcoplasmic calcium pump is diminished [736]. Since these enzyme functions are likely to be regulated by membrane fluidity [155] the changes in platelet phospholipid (un)saturation as observed for EFA-deficient platelets, may indeed have certain implications in regard to their function. Moreover, the diminished adhesion to collagen, observed for EFA deficient platelets may

Table 8.11. Effect of different dietary fats on platelet cholesterol content (μmol $\cdot$ mg protein^{-1}) and the cholesterol-phospholipid molar ratio (C/P) of platelet total lipids. Values are the mean $\pm$ SEM of four platelet pools, each prepared from 4 animals.

Group	Platelet cholesterol (μmol $\cdot$ mg protein^{-1})	C/P ratio
Control	0.239 ± 0.0201	0.54 ± 0.052
SO	0.224 ± 0.0251	0.54 ± 0.031
HCO	0.223 ± 0.0204	0.60 ± 0.099
LO	0.240 ± 0.0094	0.57 ± 0.046
CLO	0.271 ± 0.0150	0.53 ± 0.066
EFA-def.	0.202 ± 0.0104	0.46 ± 0.047

be connected with these changes. This seems the more likely since it was demonstrated that platelets only adhere to fluid and not to crystalline phospholipid membranes [524].

Considering the other results, it seems rather unlikely that the dietary fat-induced changes in collagen-sensitivity of the blood platelets can be explained on the basis of changes in membrane fluidity as far as could be ascertained by our measurements. However, it should be realised that the parameters we determined only concern overall fluidity at best. Consequently, local changes, e.g. as result of a redistribution of certain lipid domains [447], would not have been detected. Therefore, our negative findings do not necessarily imply that the changes in collagen sensitivity, as induced by the unsaturated fat-enriched diets, did not result from changes in membrane microviscosity. Only a more direct measurement of this parameter, e.g. by fluorescence probe analysis [51], electron spin resonance or nuclear magnetic resonance techniques, will give the final answer.

8.7. SUMMARY

Feeding rats different dietary fats did not cause major changes in platelet total phospholipid content and total phospholipid class distribution. The fatty acid composition of the platelet phospholipids reflect that of the diet. Major changes were observed for the polyunsaturated fatty acids of the (n–6) and (n–3) families, which could be explained on the basis of the metabolic interactions between the dietary fatty acids of these families. Platelets from SO-fed animals showed a marked quantitative increase of an unidentified fatty acid in SPH. In general, there was a close relationship between the diet-induced changes in fatty acid composition of the total phospholipids and those of the various phospholipid classes. A strikin, positive correlation was found between the LPC and AA-content of blood platelets, which suggests a functional interaction between these two parameters. There was also a highly significant, positive correlation between the AA-content of platelet phospholipids and the TxA_2 production by these platelets (measured as HHT) upon collagen activation. Platelets from SO-fed animals did not fit this relationship because their HHT-production was too high. The relationships observed did not change when taking into account the presence of other long-chain poly-unsaturated fatty acids, known to compete with AA for the CO enzyme system.

Notwithstanding the great differences between the fatty acid compositions of platelet phospholipids caused by feeding different dietary fats, the average degree of unsaturation of the phospholipids did not change. Only for EFA-deficient platelets was the degree of unsaturation considerably depressed as compared to that of control platelets. Changes in the cholesterol/phospholipid molar ratio of the platelets did not take place upon feeding different dietary fats, so that, except for the EFA-deficient group, changes in membrane fluidity may not have occurred either. However, more appropriate techniques are required to establish whether changes in membrane fluidity account for the explanation of the diet-induced differences in platelet functions, which, in the present experiment, were reflected by the significant differences observed in the collagen-induced platelet aggregation in PRP. This collagen-induced aggregation appeared to depend on platelet TxA_2 production only if the AA content of platelet phospholipids was within a normal range (20–30% of the total fatty acids). At lower AA levels, a TxA_2-independent release and aggregation pathway takes over. In EFA-deficient platelets, however, this mechanism is less efficient, possibly because of the diminished platelet-to-collagen adhesion. Evidence obtained indicates that diets high in unsaturated fatty acids, cause an enhancement of the collagen sensitivity of platelets. Platelets from animals fed a saturated fat-containing diet show a collagen response lower than that of control platelets, which is most probably due to a depressed sensitivity towards the aggregating effect of TxA_2.

The production of TxA_2 (measured as HHT) and HETE (the lipoxygenase product of AA) by platelets activated with collagen is higher, the larger the collagen dose. The dose–response curves are significantly influenced by the type of dietary fat. The same holds for the HETE/HHT ratio which, at higher activation levels, is very high in animals fed cod-liver oil. This finding together with some other results reported in Chapter 7, section 7.1.2 led us to assume that timnodonic acid (TA) is liberated from platelet phospholipids only after a strong stimulus. Moreover, indications were obtained for at least two different TA-pools, one of which was more easily released from platelet phospholipids than the other(s). Finally, there is strong evidence that endogenous TA does not inhibit the conversion of AA by the cyclooxygenase system.

9. EFFECT OF DIETARY LINOLEIC ACID ON PLATELET FUNCTION IN MAN

9.1. INTRODUCTION

The studies reported in Chapters 4, 5 and 6 show that replacing dietary saturated fatty acids by polyunsaturated fatty acids contributes to the prevention of arterial thrombosis in rats. Although these experimental results have been confirmed by many other investigators using a great variety of animal models (for reviews, see refs. 390 and 687), it is not justified to extrapolate these animal data to the human situation. Animal data only provide a guideline for human studies and therefore it is particularly worthwhile to investigate whether replacement of saturated fats by linoleic acid-rich oils also has an antithrombotic and antiatherosclerotic effect in human subjects. Epidemiological studies would suggest this to be likely because the intake of saturated fat is the environmental factor most closely associated with coronary heart disease [363, 743, 781, 782]. The value of epidemiological studies is rather limited, however, because they only detect associations and do not prove any cause-effect relationships. For this purpose, prospective clinical trials have been performed, which all indicate a favourable effect on atherosclerotic complications of a diet low in saturated fats and enriched with linoleic acid [175, 487, 552]. To find out whether this effect is associated with changes in platelet thrombotic functions, as was shown to be the case in rats (Chapter 5), we investigated the influence of a linoleic acid enriched diet on platelet aggregability in man [388].

9.2. METHODS

9.2.1. *Experimental groups and diets*

The aggregation study was performed at the end of the 'Helsinki primary prevention trial', conducted by Turpeinen and coworkers in two mental hospitals in the Helsinki region [552]. In one hospital the normal Finnish diet was given, which is rich in saturated fats and contains only 4% of digestible energy (en%) as linoleic acid. In the other hospital, the diet was modified: milk was replaced with soyabean oil-filled skim milk while butter and ordinary margarines were replaced with so-called 'soft' margarines, resulting in a dietary linoleic acid content of 16 en% (Table 9.1.).
After six years, the diets were reversed, the total experimental period being twelve

Table 9.1. Approximate daily dietary intake and dietary lipid composition for both groups

Parameter	Unit	Hospital N (control)	Hospital K (experimental)
Tatal energy	10^6J	11.5	11.7
Total fats	g	97	138
Total fat energy	%	31	44
Cholesterol	mg	556	275
Saturated fatty acids	g	48	31
Polyunsaturated fatty acids	g	14	58
Energy from linoleic acid	%	3.8	16.4

years. It then appeared in men, not in women, that the high linoleic acid diet was associated with a 50% reduction in the incidence of coronary heart disease [552, 817, 820]. At the end of the second 6-year period, male subjects were selected at random from patients of both hospitals, the only reasons for exclusion being medication with aspirin-like drugs and expected difficulties in obtaining a clean venepuncture. Although 88 men on the control diet (hospital N) and 69 men on the high linoleic acid diet (hospital K) were included in the study, data from a slightly smaller number of subjects are reported because of some technical difficulties. Both groups did not differ as to average age, body weight and cigarette smoking habits (Fig. 9.3, data obtained from hospital records). All patients participating had been in hospital for at least four years. Platelet aggregation was measured with a newly developed device, the Filtragometer ® which is described in the next section.

9.2.2. *The Filtragometer* ®, *a device to measure platelet aggregation in flowing venous blood*

From the rat studies it appeared that dietary fats modify platelet aggregation in circulation blood; no effects could be observed, however, when aggregation was measured in PRP (Chapter 5, section 3). A very distinct influence of the dietary fat type was seen on the frequency and degree of spontaneous aggregation in circulating arterial blood. These parameters were higher on saturated fat feeding as compared with the administration of a diet rich in polyunsaturated fatty acids (Chapter 5, section 3.3.). These results were obtained using the 'filter-loop technique' [385]. However, this technique is difficult to apply in humans because its use requires arterial punction which often leads to spasm and consequently to a low blood flow. Moreover it has a high incidence of thrombotic complications [503]. Therefore, we developed a venous modification of the technique for which a new device, the filtragometer, was constructed.

The filtragometer (Fig. 9.1.) has been described in detail before [392]. Briefly, it consists of a motor-driven syringe, with which blood from a forearm vein is drawn through a filter, similar to that used in the 'filter-loop technique'. Pressures are measured at both sides of the filter and subtracted electronically to obtain the pressure difference across the filter (ΔP). Since blood is drawn at a constant velocity (2ml.min^{-1}), the ΔP-value is determined by the resistance of the filter and, therefore is a measure for the amount of aggregates which have been 'collected' on the filter. Apart from this ΔP-value, P_2, which is the pressure between arm and filter, is also monitored in order to check blood supply.

Heparin, infused just behind the puncture needle (5 IU.ml^{-1} final concentration) prevents the blood from clotting. Moreover it may stabilize intravascular aggregates which then obstruct the filter, resulting in a change in the ΔP-value, the time course of which is shown schematically in Fig. 9.2. The start of the measurement is indicated by an upward deflection of the tracing. From this moment on, blood is drawn from the arm and heparin is administered. Due to the internal resistance of the system, the viscosity of the saline causes a small pressure difference, which increases when the more viscous blood replaces the priming saline. A further increase in ΔP indicates that aggregates obstruct the filter, which has been confirmed by scanning electron microscopy. A downward deflection marks the moment when $\Delta P = -5$ mmHg. At this moment heparin in replaced by sodium citrate and after a short period the decrease of ΔP indicates cleaning of the filter as a result of disaggregation. From this ΔP-curve, the following parameters can be calculated.

- the aggregation time, t_A, which is the time (s) necessary to reach a ΔP-value of 5 mm Hg.
- the aggregation velocity, T_S, defined as tg α, where α is the angle between the tangent to the curve at $\Delta P = 5$ mm Hg and the horizontal ($=$ time) axis.
- the maximum aggregation, A_{max}, which is the maximum height of the aggregation curve in mm Hg.
- the disaggregation induction time, t_{DI}, being the time (s) between termination of heparin infusion and start of disaggregation.

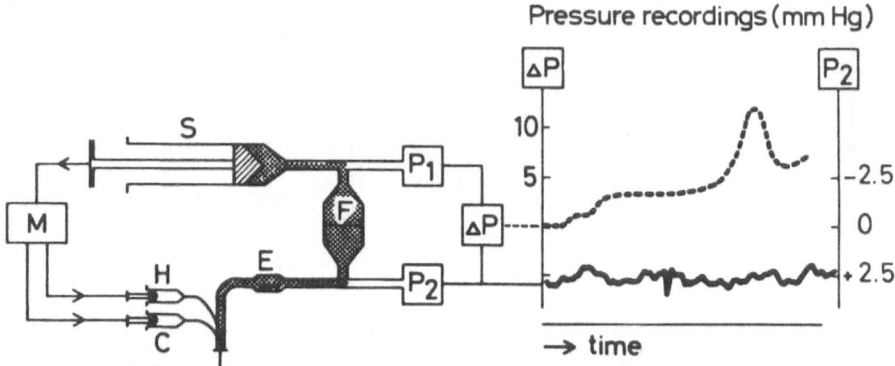

Fig. 9.1 Diagram of filtragometer. M: Motor; S: Syringe; F. Filter; E. Mixing chamber; H. Heparin infusion; C: Citrate infusion. For explanation of P_1, P_2 and ΔP, see text.

For most purposes t_A appeared the most practical aggregation parameter.

Although formation of aggregates within the filtragometer cannot be excluded, there is good evidence that the apparatus measures – at least for the greater part – the platelet aggregates present in the blood before it entered the device (394). Model experiments showed that the filtragometer reacts reproducibly to a standard filter obstruction (399). Reproducibility studies, however, demonstrated that platelet aggregation show large fluctuations. These findings, together with the results of studies concerning the interrelationship between the aggregation criteria t_A and T_S, strongly indicate that, in a given subject, the aggregation tendency of platelets in venous blood may vary from ml to ml [392].

The filtragometer appeared a suitable instrument to demonstrate the anti-aggregating effect of PGE_1 ex vivo and oral aspirin [392]. No significantly different filtragometer response has been observed in patients deficient in coagulation factors VIII, IX, X, and XII, but patients suffering from von Willebrand's disease, Glanzmann's thrombasthenia, Hermanski-Pudlak syndrome and uremia, showed, a diminished filtragometer response (i.e. a longer aggregation time). Male patients suffering from angina pectoris have an increased aggregation tendency and a decreased disaggregation tendency compared with healthy controls. These patients have a significantly higher aggregation tendency than female angina pectoris patients [394]. In acute myocardial infarction, a highly increased filtragometer response has been reported by Fleischman et al. [250] but these findings could not yet be confirmed by others (Hugenholz, P.: personal communication). Patients with a history of myocardial infarction show an increased aggregation tendency and a

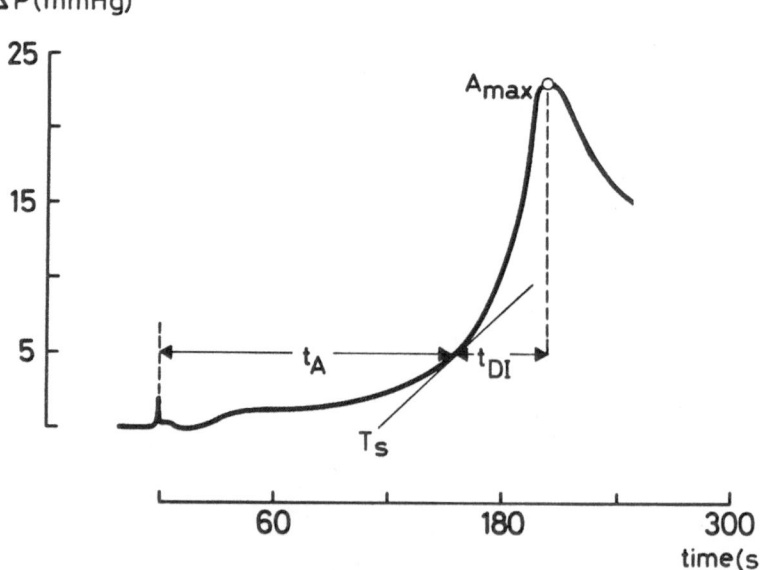

Fig. 9.2. Schematic representation of aggregation curve. T_A: aggregation time; T_S: aggregation velocity/ A_{max}: maximum aggregation; t_{DI}: disaggregation induction time.

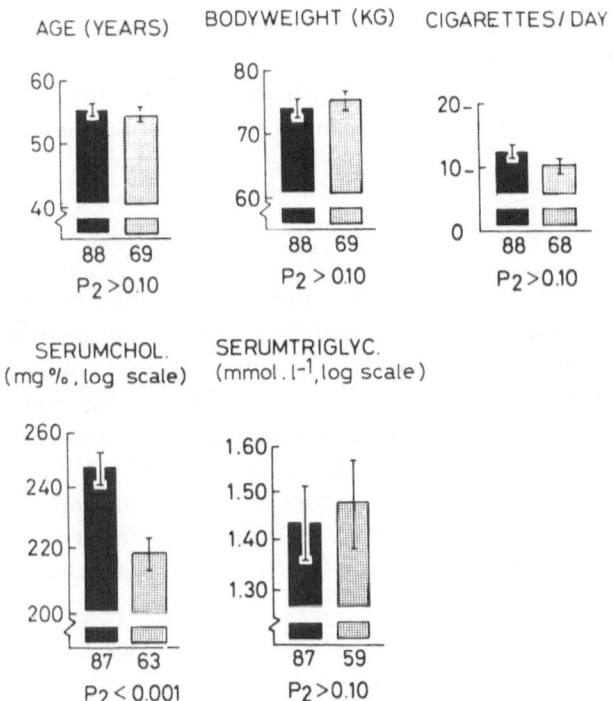

AGE (YEARS)   BODYWEIGHT (KG)   CIGARETTES/DAY

SERUMCHOL.   SERUMTRIGLYC.
(mg %, log scale)   (mmol . l⁻¹, log scale)

Fig. 9.3. Characterization of both experimental groups (mean ± SEM). ■ diet containing 4en% linoleic acid; ▓ diet containing 16 en% linoleic acid. Numbers under bars indicate number of subjects; P_2: degree of significance (Student's two-sample test).

diminished frequency and degree of disaggregation. The filtragometer response has been reported to be significantly enhanced in acute stroke [250], in stress [253] and in diabetes mellitus [254]. Smoking was shown to increase the filtragometer response [59] but we were unable to confirm this finding. Finally, the use of oral contraceptives was associated with a higher filtragometer response [60]. It should be noted that, in most cases discussed so far, the overlap between experimental and control groups is considerable.

9.2.3 *Experimental procedure*

Subjects were studied between 7 a.m. and 11 a.m. after an overnight fast. First, the template bleeding time was measured [551], using an apparatus devised by Praga and coworkers [667]. The subjects were then placed in a recumbent position after which an indwelling catheter was inserted into an antecubital vein while applying minimum stasis. After some blood had drained away, samples were carefully taken for the following measurements:

- platelet and red cell counts, (using a Celloscope ® particle counter)
- serum triglyceride and serum cholesterol contents. These measurements were performed by Finnish colleagues and the results are given in Fig. 9.3.

172

- platelet retention, using 2 ml heparinized whole blood and the rotating bulb technique, as described by Wright [875].

After completion of blood sampling, the indwelling catheter was connected to the filtragometer and platelet aggregation in flowing venous blood was measured as described in section 9.2.2.

9.3. *Results*

Data on platelet retention, bleeding times and platelet- and red-cell counts are given in Fig. 9.4. For none of these criteria, was a pronounced difference observed between the two groups. As shown in Fig. 9.5. platelet aggregation measured with the filtragometer is significantly decreased in the high-linoleic acid group: the aggregation time is longer, aggregation velocity and maximum aggregation are lower and disaggregation occurs more quickly as compared with the control, low-linoleic acid group. Although the difference in filtragometer response between both groups is highly significant, there is a considerable overlap between the groups. Now it might be argued that the difference in platelet aggregation between both groups is not

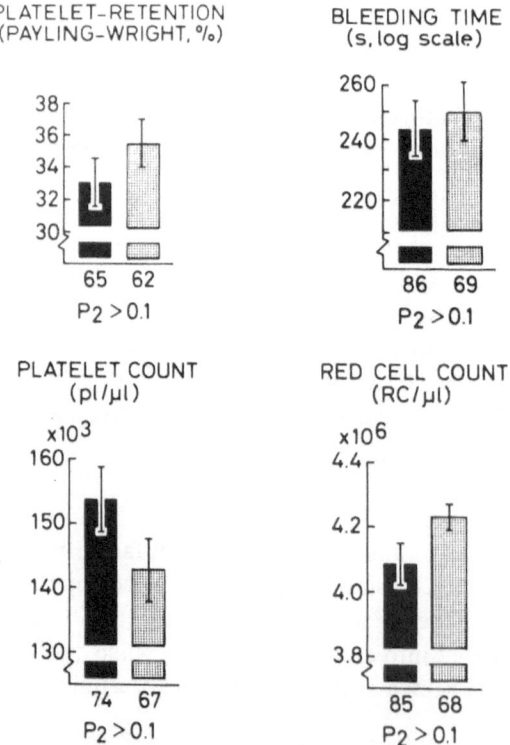

Fig. 9.4. Effect of dietary linoleic acid content on several haematological parameters (mean ± SEM). ■ 4 en% linoleic acid; ▨ 16 en% linoleic acid. Numbers under bars refer to number of subjects; P_2: degree of significance (Student's two-sample test).

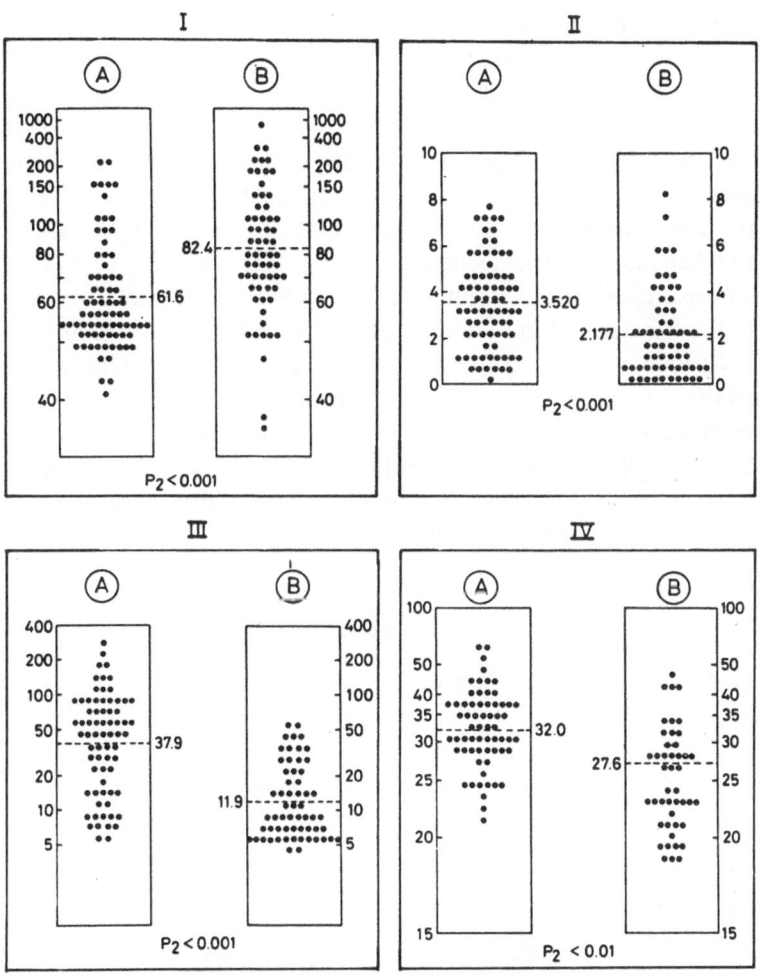

Fig. 9.5. Effect of dietary linoleic acid content on platelet aggregation in male subjects.
A: 4 en% linoleic acid; B: 16 en% linoleic acid.
I: Aggregation time (s, reciprocal scale).
II: Aggregation velocity (T$_s$, see Fig. 9.2).
III:Maximum aggregation (mmHg, log scale).
IV:Disaggregation induction time (s, reciprocal scale).
P$_2$: Degree of significance (Student's two-sample test); dashed lines are group means.

attributable to the diets but to other environmental differences between the hospitals. To be sure on this point, platelet aggregation was measured again one year later, which was three months after diet-normalization in hospital K. However, several patients participating in the first study, were discharged so that they could not be measured again. As a result, only 38 patients from each hospital were measured twice.

The results shown in Fig. 9.6., demonstrate that the difference in aggregation observed between patients of the two hospitals during the first measurement, was greatly reduced three months after the dietary switch in hospital K, although it had not yet disappeared completely. In connection with a technical modification to the filtragometer, which was still in an experimental stage at that time, platelet aggregation *values* during the second measurement were considerably lower as compared to those during the first measurement. Since in hospital N (the control hospital), no dietary switch had taken place, platelet aggregation values in this hospital were taken as 100% for both measurements. The results obtained in hospital K were expressed as a percentage of those measured in hospital N, thereby correcting for the modification to the filtragometer. When computed in this way, the dietary switch in hospital K caused the aggregation time to become shorter (from 156 to 133%), the aggregation velocity to increase from 58 to 70% and maximum aggregation to increase from 43 to 86% of those measured in the control hospital. These results demonstrate that the dietary linoleic acid content has, indeed, a decreasing effect on platelet aggregation as measured with the filtragometer.

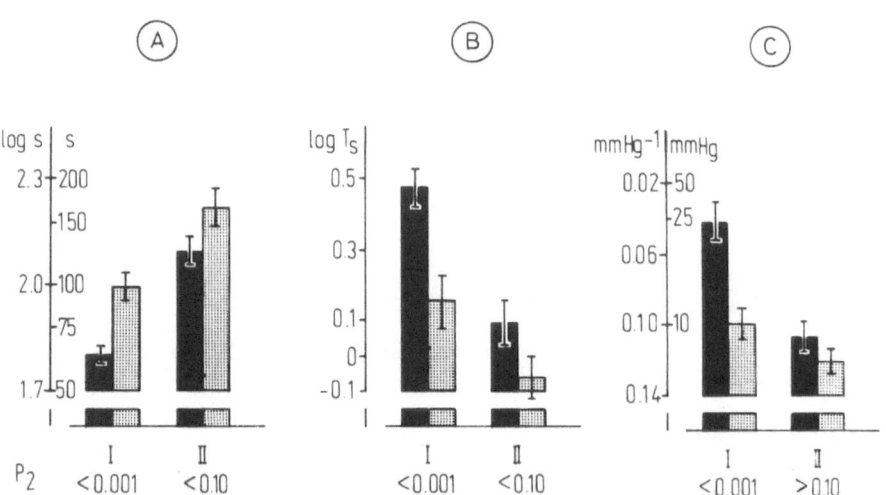

Fig. 9.6. Platelet aggregation (Filtragometer, mean ± SEM), measured twice in the same subjects (n = 38)

■ Hospital N, dietary linoleic acid content 4 en%;

▓ Hospital K, dietary linoleic acid content 16 en%;

I: Results of first measurement performed after a dietary period of four to six years.

II: Results of second measurement carried out one year later and three months after lowering the linoleic content of the diet in hospital K towards that in hospital N.

A: Aggregation time (s, log scale); B: Aggregation velocity (T_s, log scale); C: Maximum aggregation (mmHg, reciprocal scale).

P_2: Degree of significance (Student's two-sample test).

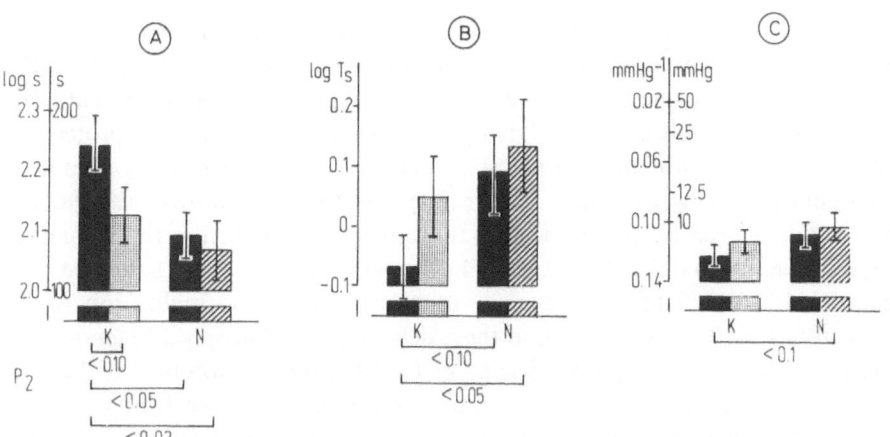

Fig. 9.7. Platelet aggregation (Filtragometer) three months after diet normalization in the experimental hospital (no change of diet in control hospital).
■ subjects participating in original trial (n = 35 − 42);
▓ subjects not participating in original trial eating the experimental diet for less than nine months before diet normalisation (n = 34 − 37);
▨ subjects not participating in original trial, eating the control diet all the time (n = 31 − 37).
A: Aggregation time (s); B: Aggregation velocity (T_s);
C: Maximum aggregation (mmHg); P_2; Degree of significance.
K: Experimental hospital, three months after diet normalisation.
N: Control hospital

9.4. DISCUSSION

Turpeinen et al. [552, 817, 820] demonstrated that administration of the high linoleic acid diet was associated with a significantly reduced incidence in coronary heart disease (CHD) in men, measured by the appearence of certain ECG-patterns and by the occurrence of coronary deaths. Since myocardial infarction largely results from occlusive coronary thrombosis, in which platelet aggregation in involved [13, 321–324, 647, 753, see also Chapter 1, section 1], it is conceivable that the lower platelet aggregation observed in the present study, contributed to this reduced CHD indicence.

The dietary groups showed no difference in platelet retention, but it should be emphasised that there was a considerable time lapse between blood sampling and retention measurements (approximately 30 min). During this period, unstable aggregation-modulating substances possibly present in blood, may have become inactivated.

The slow response of platelet aggregation to the decrease in dietary linoleate is rather surprising because Fleischman and co-workers, who confirmed the anti-aggregating effect of linoleic acid in humans, had shown that this effect is readily reversible when returning to a low-linoleic acid diet [251, 252]. However, their high-linoleic acid feeding period lasting only two to three weeks whereas the subjects participating in our studies had been on the high-linoleic acid diet for at least five years before their linoleic acid intake was reduced. This could indicate that long-term feeding of a high-linoleic acid diet provides a long-term thromboprotection. Supporting evidence for this concept was obtained from aggregation values measured in subjects who were admitted to the hospitals in between both measurements. Those who had been hospitalised more than three months before the second investigation were included in this study. The new arrivals of hospital K had been on the high linoleic acid diet for less than nine months before diet normalization. As can be seen from Fig. 9.7, aggregation in these new arrivals of hospital K tends to be higher than that in the original participants (shorter aggregation time and higher aggregation velocity). Moreover, the aggregation in the new arrivals of hospital K does not differ from that in both groups in hospital N. This is in contrast to the aggregation in the initial participants of hospital K, which is significantly lower than that in both groups in hospital N. From this finding it seems justified to conclude that the anti-aggregating effect of a diet rich in linoleic acid (LA) persists longer, the longer the diet is eaten.

To be absolutely sure that the agreed dietary switch had indeed been carried through, the dietary composition was estimated after the switch by checking the lists of purchases of both hospitals. Unfortunately, this inspection showed that diet normalization in hospital K had occurred only partly: the soyabean oil-filled skim milk had been skipped, but the use of soft margarine instead of butter had been continued. This resulted in a dietary linoleic-acid content of 8 en% (8-LA), which is still twice as high as that in the control group [816]. This finding means that eating an 8-LA diet for three to twelve months does not result in a lower platelet aggre-

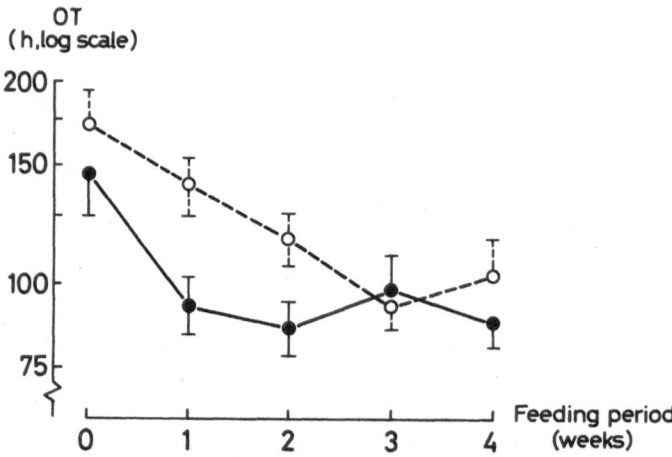

Fig. 9.8. Effect of pre-experimental SO-feeding (50 en%; ●———● one week, ○---○ four weeks) on the course of the prothrombotic effect of HCO (45 en% + 5 en% SO) in rats. Results (OT ± SEM) refer to arterial thrombosis tendencies as measured with the aorta loop (see Chapter 4, section 3).

gation versus a 4-LA diet. Consequently, the anti-aggregating effect of dietary linoleic acid can only been demonstrated at a rather high linoleate intake. This is not in agreement with results obtained by Fleischman and co-workers [251, 252] who noted an aggregation-inhibiting effect already within four days when increasing the dietary linoleic acid content by amounts as low as 0.5–4 en%. The cause of this discrepance is not yet clear. Since they used a filtragometer giving results comparable to ours (unpublished results), a methodological reason seems unlikely.

9.5. THE LONG-TERM THROMBOPROTECTIVE EFFECT OF DIETARY LINOLEIC ACID

As demonstrated in the previous section, subjects who had been on the high linoleic acid diet for almost five years, still showed a diminished aggregation tendency against the control group three months after they had switched to the 8-LA diet, although the latter diet did not appear to have an anti-aggregating effect. As discussed before, a possible explanation may be that long-term feeding of a high LA-diet provides a long-term protection after discontinuation. We tested this possibility in rats in an experiment which is reported in the next section.

9.5.1. *Modulation of the prothrombotic effect of a saturated fat diet in rats by prefeeding an antithrombotic diet*

Two groups of 60 young adult male Wistar rats were fed a diet containing 50 en% sunflowerseed oil (SO). After one or four weeks, arterial thrombosis tendency was measured in 12 rats of each group. In the diet of the remaining animals, 45 en% of the antithrombotic SO was replaced by prothrombotic hydrogenated coconut oil (HCO). One two, three and four weeks later, arterial thrombosis tendency was measured in 12 rats of each group. If the suggestion emerging from the experiments described in the previous section is correct in that the antiplatelet effect of dietary linoleic acid may last longer if the feeding period is extended, the prothrombotic effect of hydrogenated coconut oil should become manifest later, if the animals had been prefed a linoleic acid-rich diet for a longer time. This indeed appeared to be so (fig. 9.8): the course of the thrombosis-promoting effect of dietary HCO greatly depends on the pre-experimental SO-feeding period. This prothrombotic effect was maximal within one week if the animals had been prefed the antithrombotic SO for one week only. After a four-week pre-experimental SO-period, it takes three to four weeks for the expression of the prothrombotic effect of HCO to become maximal, although the initial arterial thrombosis tendencies did not differ significantly. Therefore, it can be concluded that, at least in rats, the thromboprotective role of dietary SO lasts longer, the longer the feeding period. This is in agreement with the suggestion obtained from the human experiment described in the previous section.

9.5.2. *The possible role of adipose tissue linoleate in long-term thromboprotection. A hypothesis*

Results reported in the previous sections show that the maximum dietary fat effects on arterial thrombosis tendency and platelet aggregation take much more time to become perceptible than the mean platelet life-span, which is approximately 10 and 3 days for man and rat, respectively. Consequently, the long-term thromboprotective effect of dietary linoleate we observed cannot have been caused by a direct effect on the platelets but must be the result of some slowly changing factor in the platelet's environment. Upon prolonged feeding, the linoleic acid content of the diet is known to be reflected by that of the adipose tissue. The Helsinki study showed that the LA-content of adipose tissue in the 16- and 4-LA groups was 26.9 ± 3.06 (n = 31) and 10.2 ± 1.93 (n = 35), respectively [819]. The turnover of adipose tissue triglycerides is rather slow as compared with plasma triglycerides (174,249). Consequently, the adipose tissue LA-content might be expected to decrease only slowly when lowering the dietary LA-concentration. Since adipose tissue is the main source of plasma long-chain free fatty acids (Chapter 2), the composition of the latter will largely be determined by that of the adipose tissue.

In stress situations (prolonged fasting, myocardial infarction, fright, etc), a hormone-mediated rapid mobilization of adipose tissue fatty acids occurs, resulting in a rise of the plasma FFA-levels to such an extent that the FFA-binding capacity of plasma proteins is sometimes exceeded. It has been shown very convincingly that this situation causes hyperaggregability of blood platelets [152, 327, 370]. Moreover, it has been shown that these platelet reactions depend on the type of FFA: long-chain saturated fatty acids are much more active in this respect than linoleic acid [371, 671], whereas dihomo-γ-linolenic acid significantly lowers platelet aggregation [677] (see also section 7). Moreover, it has been shown that the quantity and quality of the plasma free fatty acids can affect the ability of the endothelial cells to act as a non-thrombogenic surface [624, 778a]. The adipose tissue fatty acid composition may therefore be expected to affect the (anti) thrombotic functions of blood platelets and vascular endothelium through its effect on the plasma free fatty acid composition [622].

In this respect, the epidemiological findings by Logan and co-workers are of interest. They compared blood and adipose tissue lipid profiles of people from Stockholm and Edinburg and noted that the higher mortality from coronary artery disease in Edinburg is associated with a lower blood lipid- and adipose tissue linoleic acid content, whereas serum total and LDL cholesterol contents appeared to be similar [497]. A thromboregulatory function of plasma FFA is also likely, considering the observation that FFA are able to perturb lipid domains in biological membranes, thereby influencing membrane receptor-mobility and -efficiency [447]. These considerations suggest a possible thromboregulation through modulation of plasma-free fatty acid content and composition, which should be further investigated.

9.6. POSSIBLE MECHANISMS BY WHICH LINOLEIC ACID LOWERS PLATELET
AGGREGABILITY AND ARTERIAL THROMBOSIS TENDENCY

Although feeding LA-rich sunflowerseed oil to rats causes various prothrombotic changes in vitro; e.g. an increase in collagen sensitivity (Chapter 8, section 3.1.) and an enhancement of platelet TxA_2 formation (Chapter 8, section 5.), it lowers platelet aggregation in circulating arterial blood and reduces arterial thrombus formation in vivo. The diminishing effect of dietary linoleate on various thrombotic platelet functions has been confirmed by many investigators [251, 252, 425, 633, 634, 686, 689], but little is known about the mechanisms underlying this effect. An increased dietary LA-concentration causes the platelet LA-content to increase as well [613, 618, 620, 660, 686] (see also Chapter 8). Since endogenous LA may become released upon platelet activation [186] and because it competitively inhibits conversion of arachidonic acid by the cyclo-oxygenase enzyme system [291, 477, 644], an increase in platelet LA may result in a lower endoperoxide and TxA_2 formation upon platelet activation and thus diminish the propagation of platelet aggregation. Another way in which LA may inhibit platelet TxA_2 formation is by inhibiting platelet phospholipase A_2, as demonstrated by Vallee and co-workers [823]. However, our experiments with rats demonstrated that feeding LA-enriched diets did not diminish but stimulated platelet TxA_2-formation. This observation does not necessarily apply to man as well, although it may be recalled that, as far as platelet-AA metabolism is concerned, there is a striking similarity between rat and man (cf. the effect of fish oil, Chapter 7).

Recently, Beitz and coworkers [38] demonstrated that LA-rich cholesterolesters promote the conversion of PGH_2 into PGI_2 by pig aorta microsomes. Since a LA-rich diet does increase the LA-content of cholesterolesters, this finding could be extrapolated to suggest that a LA-rich diet increases vascular prostacyclin production and thereby lowers arterial thrombosis tendency. Although this idea is in line with findings by ten Hoor and co-workers [802] it is not supported by results obtained by us (Chapters 6 and 8) and others [177, 284, 835a].

The enhanced AA metabolism upon feeding an LA-enriched diet, as described in Chapter 8, does not seem to be restricted to platelets. Thus it has been shown that replacement of dietary saturated fatty acids by LA results in an increased prostaglandin (PG) production of stimulated rat adipocytes [491] and in a higher PG-synthesizing potential of rat whole lung [546]. Not all PGs of the same series change to a same extent [809], suggesting that, apart from the precursor level, other factors may play a role as well. One of these factors may be the dietary fat content. In this respect the work of Schoene and coworkers is relevant. They reported that an increase of the ratio between dietary polyunsaturated and saturated fatty acids (P/S ratio) from 0.3 to 1.0 had no effect on the TxB_2-production of platelets pre-labelled with radioactive AA and triggered with thrombin. However, upon lowering the total dietary fat content from 43 to 25 en% the same decrease in P/S ratio caused an almost 50% drop in TxB_2 formation. These results are difficult to interpret, however, since only the metabolism of newly incorporated AA was measured which does not necessarily reflect prostanoid formation from truely endogenous precursors [730].

A stimulating effect of dietary LA on the turnover of total body prostanoids is also indicated by findings that the urinary excretion of PG-metabolites increases proportionally to the LA-intake in rat [629] and man [3, 4, 880]. In infants, however, treatment with Intralipid ® (an LA-rich fat emulsion) causes the urinary excretion of prostaglandin E metabolites (PGE-M) to decrease to a level, comparable to that, found in EFA-deficient infants. When these latter were treated with Intralipid, PGE-M increased to control levels [269] indicating that the relationship between LA intake and prostanoid turnover is not rectilinear. This appears to be true for rats: the urinary prostanoid excretion increases with dietary linoleate levels between 0.2 and 21 en% and decreases slightly at higher LA concentrations [786].

Summarising these literature data it can be stated that, because of its complexity, the relationship between dietary LA intake and total body prostanoid turnover has not yet been elucidated completely. Although there is no unanimity [269, 731], most work indicates an increasing effect of dietary LA on total body prostanoid production, which is not related to changes in tissue fatty acid composition only [204].

The stimulating effect of dietary LA on the peroxidation of arachidonic acid may give rise to an increased formation of PGE_2 and PGD_2, the latter being a very active aggregation inhibitor [638, 766] whereas the former has only weak aggregation-stimulating properties [458, 747]. However, in rats, PGD_2 is inactive as a platelet antiaggregant [852]. Therefore, this explanation for the antiplatelet effect of dietary LA is also rather unlikely, or at least incomplete.

Recently, Lagarde and coworkers [475] reported that platelet FFA are efficiently used in the formation of platelet prostaglandins, although their levels are very low. They also demonstrated that a small enhancement of the dihomo-γ-linolenic acid level (D-LA) caused a much more increased formation of PGE_1 (an active aggregation inhibitor) than a similar enhancement of the arachidonic acid (AA) level did with respect to stimulation of PGE_2 production. Dietary D-LA has been shown to decrease platelet aggregation in animals and man [449, 752, 858, 859] although negative results have been published as well [637]. Since D-LA is an intermediate in the conversion of LA into AA (Chapter 2), an enhanced LA-intake might be expected to increase D-LA synthesis, possibly leading to a higher platelet D-LA level. This was not observed in our experiments with rats (Chapter 8) but since the $\Delta 5$-desaturase, which mediates the conversion of D-LA into AA (see Chapter 2), seems much more active in rats than in man [856], we simply may not expect to observe it. Moreover, as indicated above, we did not investigate the composition of platelet FFA which may be very important in this respect. Therefore, it seems worthwhile to investigate the role of PGE_1 from platelets or other sources in the dietary LA-induced inhibition of platelet aggregation and thrombus formation. Colard and coworkers [148] have recently shown that incorporation of linoleic acid into the membrane phospholipids of rat liver parenchymal cells resulted in a significant increase of the basal, fluoride- of glucagon-stimulated adenylate cyclase activities, in contrast to oleic acid, which had no effect, and arachidonic acid, which caused a decrease at high concentrations. Since a cAMP-increase is associated with a decreased platelet aggregability, (Chapter 3, section 7.) a similar effect of linoleate on platelet membrane adenylate cyclase could possibly explain the antiplatelet effect of linoleic acid.

Finally, the inhibiting effect of dietary LA on platelet aggregation may be an expression of the same LA-effect as that responsible for reduced cell-to-substrate adhesion, demonstrated in cultured BHK-cells which could not be reversed upon indomethacin addition and is, therefore, a prostaglandin-independent phenomenon [381].

9.7. SUMMARY

Filtragometer measurements showed that a diet with 16 en% linoleic acid given to human subjects for over four years produced a significant, 50% reduction in platelet aggregability as compared with a diet containing 4 en% linoleic acid. To attain the anti-platelet effect of dietary linoleic acid, ingestion of a rather high dose is required because 8 en% given for over three months, did not modify platelet aggregability. Indications that the thromboprotective effect of dietary linoleate lasts longer, the longer the feeding period, were confirmed in an experiment with rats. It is hypothesized that the long-term effect of dietary linoleate is mediated by linoleic acid, which is taken up in adipose tissue during the feeding period and slowly released into the plasma after withdrawal of the diet. Platelet TxA_2-formation is most probably not involved in the mechanism(s) underlying the anti-aggregating effect of dietary linoleate. An enhanced formation of PGE_1 by platelets and/or other tissues seems plausible and is not incompatible with our results.

10. SUMMARY AND CONCLUDING REMARKS

Extensive animal experiments, human epidemiological studies and clinical trials all indicate that the type of dietary fat affects the genesis, course and complications of the atherosclerotic process. Since arterial thrombosis is implicated in atherosclerosis, both as an initiating and a complicating factor, the effect of dietary fatty acid composition on arterial thrombogenesis and its underlying processes in animals and man has been investigated extensively. In this volume these investigations are summarised and used as a frame of reference for a discussion of own findings obtained by some newly developed techniques.

In rats, diets rich in saturated fatty acids are thrombogenic, oils rich in mono-unsaturated fatty acids such as olive oil and rapeseed oil seem to behave neutrally and are antithrombotic only when replacing saturated fats. Oils rich in poly-unsaturated fatty acids such as sunflowerseed oil, maize oil, and certain fish oils have a distinct antithrombotic effect.

Except for certain fish oils, changes in blood coagulation are not likely to play a major role in the dietary fat effect on arterial thrombogenesis. However, further research in this field is required. The same holds for fibrinolysis, especially since new techniques are becoming available. It is to be hoped that their use will clarify the rather inconsistent and confusing results appearing from older literature as to the effect of the dietary fat type on fibrinolysis in relation to arterial thrombus formation and lysis.

In rat as well as in man a positive relationship was demonstrated between dietary fat induced changes in arterial thrombosis tendency and blood platelet aggregability. This strongly indicates that changes in platelet thrombotic functions mediate the effects of dietary fat on arterial thrombogenesis.

Since prostanoids, Tromboxane A_2 (TxA_2) and prostacyclin (PGI_2) in particular, are very important modulators of platelet function, the dietary fat effect on pro-stanoid metabolism has also been investigated. These studies showed that in rats the antithrombotic effect of oils rich in polyunsaturated fatty acids of the (n–3) family (linseed oil, certain fish oils) is explained by their decreasing influence on the production of prothrombotic TxA_2 by activated blood platelets. The simultaneously occurring decrease in the vascular production of antithrombotic prostacyclin appeared insufficient to destroy this effect, suggesting that TxA_2 is more important for thromboregulation than PGI_2.

The decreasing effect on the production of platelet thromboxane A_2 and vascular prostacyclin by dietary (n–3) fatty acids is caused by their inhibiting influence on the conversion of linoleic acid into the prostanoid precursor, arachidonic acid. The long-term use of oils rich in (n–3) fatty acids will lead to a systemic depression of tissue arachidonic acid (AA) levels and, consequently, of the production of AA-derived eicosanoids several of which are important physiological modulators. The lower formation of the 2-series prostanoids is not compensated for by the production of prostaglandin-like substances of the 3-family. The ultimate effect of a continuous, generalized depression of prostanoid and AA-derived leukotriene formation is not yet known and should be investigated further before a general use of these oils can be recommended.

Due to species differences in the activities of enzymes involved in the metabolism of α-linolenic acid, the possible antithrombotic effect of linseed oil in man is expected to be less pronounced than that of certain fish oils. The use of these latter oils, which are expected to be antithrombotic, provided they contain only small amounts of saturated fatty acids, is likely to be hampered not only for reasons of taste and technology, but also because of certain pathological conditions thought to be associated with a large intake of long chain poly-unsaturated fatty acids of the (n –3) family.

Linoleic acid, which is abundant in sunflower-, safflower- and maize oil, produces a distinct antithrombotic effect without lowering the formation of platelet and vessel-wall prostanoids. The mechanism of this effect is not yet clear. A detailed study of the platelet lipid profile and fatty acid composition did not indicate the involvement of platelet membrane fluidity. However, more appropiate techniques are required to obtain a definitive answer to this question. The involvement of prostaglandins from sources other than platelets and vascular tissue, which may be a factor in the explanation of the antithrombotic effect of dietary linoleic acid, is not incompatible with our results and deserves further investigation.

Replacing dietary saturated fats with linoleic acid-rich products, considerably reduces platelet aggregation in male human subjects. It is likely that this lower platelet aggregability contributed to the 50% decrease in mortality from coronary heart disease, which was associated with the high-linoleic acid diet. Indications obtained showed that the anti-platelet effect of dietary linoleate lasts longer, the longer the feeding period. It is assumed that this long-term effect of dietary linoleate is mediated by linoleic acid, which is taken up by adipose tissue during the feeding period and slowly released into the plasma after withdrawal from the diet.

After the onset of a myocardial infarct, about 50% of the patients die within a few hours, leaving too little time for successful intervention and/or secondary prevention. This implies that primary prevention of coronary disease is of major importance. Fewer calories, more physical exercise, no smoking and a more relaxed attitude are thought to be important factors in this respect. Moreover, a change in dietary composition may lower the risk of coronary thrombosis. Based on the results of the experimental studies in animals and man described and discussed in this volume, a decreased intake of saturated fatty acids together with an increased consumption of poly-unsaturated fatty acids, especially linoleic acid, may lower not only arterial thrombosis tendency, but other atherosclerosis risk factors as well. Dietary linoleic acid has been shown to decrease serum cholesterol, especially in low-density lipoproteins, lower borderline hypertension and normalise biochemical abnormalities in obesity and maturity-onset diabetes. Moreover, animal studies clearly indicated that a linoleic acid-rich diet improves cardiac perfusion and work capacity [827]. Finally, a high linoleate diet was shown to stop the progression of micro- and macroangiopathy in diabetic patients [403]. After a careful screening of all pertinent data and sources Heyden [363] concluded that any alleged major adverse effect of dietary linoleate can be dismissed.

REFERENCES

1. Aaes-Jørgensen, E.: Essential fatty acids. Physiol. Rev. 41: 1–51 (1961).
2. Ackman, R.G., Eaton, C.A. and Dyerberg, J.: Marine docosenoic acid isomer distribution in the plasma of Greenland Eskimos. Am. J. Clin. Nutr. 33: 1814–1817 (1980).
3. Adam, O., Dill-Wiessner, M., Wolfram, G. and Zöllner, N.: Plätchenaggregation und Prostaglandinumsatz beim Menschen unter definierter Linolsaurezufuhr mit Formeldiäten. Res. Exp. Med. (Berl) 177: 227–235 (1980).
4. Adam, O., Wolfram, G. and Zöllner, N.: Platelet fatty acids and prostaglandin turnover during defined linoleic acid intake with formula diets. Artery 8: 85–89 (1980).
5. Adelson, L. and Hoffman, W.: Sudden death from coronary disease. JAMA 176: 129–135 (1961).
6. Ally, A.I. and Horrobin, D.F.: Thromboxane A_2 in blood vessel walls and its physiological significance: relevance to thrombosis and hypertension. Prost. and Med. 4: 431–438 (1980).
7. Altschul, R.: Endothelium, its development, morphology, function, and pathology. New York, Macmillan Co., 1954, p. 157.
8. Ambrus, J.L., Ambrus, C.M., Gastpar, H., Sapvento, P.J., Weber, F.J. and Thurber, L.E.: Study of platelet aggregation in vitro. I. Effect of bencyclan. J. Med. 7: 439–447 (1976).
9. Andreoli, V.M., Maffei, F., and Tonon, G.C.: Platelet lipid modification induced by fatty acids: experimental studies and correlations with human neuropathology. Haemostasis 2: 118–140 (1973/1974).
10. Annual report from the Chief Medical Officer in Greenland 1963–1967, Cited in: Bang, H.O. and Dyerberg, J.: Plasma lipids and lipoproteins in Greenlandic West coast Eskimos. Acta Med. Scand. 192: 85–94 (1972).
11. Antoniades, H.N. and Scher, C.D.: Radioimmunoassay of a human serum growth factor for Balb/c-3T3 cells: derivation from platelets. Proc. Natl. Acad. Sci. USA 74: 1973–1977 (1977).
12. Antoniades, H.N., Scher, C.D. and Stiles, C.D.: Purification of human platelet-derived growth factor. Proc. Natl. Acad. Sci. USA 76: 1809–1813 (1979).
13. Ardlie, N.G., Kinlough, R.L. and Schwartz, C.J.: In vitro thrombosis and platelet aggregation in myocardial infarction. Br. Med. J. 1: 888–891 (1966).
14. Ardlie, N.G. and Han, P.: Enzymatic basis for platelet aggregation and release: the significance of the 'platelet atmosphere' and the relationship between platelet function and blood coagulation. Br. J. Haematol. 26: 331–356 (1974).
15. Arfors, K.E. and Bergqvist, D.: The red cell in the hemostatic process. Microvasc. Res. 11: 430 (1976).
16. Armitage, P.: Clinical trials in the secondary prevention of myocardial infarction and stroke. Thromb. Haemostas. 43: 90–94 (1980).
17. Aschkenasy, A.: On the pathogenesis of anaemias and leucopenias induced by protein deficiency. Am. J Clin. Nutr. 5: 14–25 (1957).
18. Ashburn, A.D., Weaver, M.M. and Summers, P.A.: Effects of red blood cll injections on diet-induced atrial thrombosis in Swiss mice. Am. J. Anat. 133: 341–348 (1972).
19. Assaf, S.A.: Cyclic AMP-mediated phosphorylation reactions in the regulation of blood platelet aggregation. Int. J. Biochem. J: 535–540 (1976).
20. Axen, U., Lincoln, F.H., Thompson, J.L., Honohan, T. and Nishizawa, E.E.: Chemistry of

prostaglandins in: Scriabine, A., Lefer, A.M. and Kuehl, F.A. Jr. (Eds.): Prostaglandins in cardiovascular and renal function. Spectrum Publications Inc. Jamaica, N.Y. (1980) pp. 3–8.

21. Ball, C.R., Williams, W.L. and Collum, J.M.: Cardiovascular lesions in Swiss mice fed a high fat-low protein diet with and without betaine supplementation. Anat. Rec. 145: 49–59 (1963).

22. Ball, C.R., Clower, B.R., Williams, W.L. and Jackson, M.: Dietary-induced atrial thrombosis in mice. Arch. Path. 80: 391–396 (1965).

23. Ball, C.R.: Hematologic studies in mice fed a thrombogenic diet. Arch. Path. 85: 547–553 (1968).

24. Ball, C.R., Westin, D.C. and Jackson, M.: Anemia induced by thrombogenic diet and remission after normal diet. Arch. Path. 90: 117–124 (1970).

25. Bang, H.O., Dyerberg, J. and Nielsen, A.: Plasma lipids and lipoprotein pattern in Greenlandic West-coast Eskimos. Lancet i: 1143–1146 (1971).

26. Bang, H.O. and Dyerberg, J.: Plasma lipids and lipoproteins in Greenlandic West-coast Eskimos. Acta Med. Scan. 192: 85–94 (1972).

27. Bang, H.O., Dyerberg, J. and Hjørne, N.: The composition of food consumed by Greenland Eskimos. Acta Med. Scand. 200: 69–73 (1976).

28. Bang, H.O. and Dyerberg, J.: The bleeding tendency in Greenland Eskimos. Dan. Med. Bull. 27: 202–205 (1980).

29. Bang, H.O., Dyerberg, J. and Sinclair, H.M.: The composition of the Eskimo food in north western Greenland. Am.J.Clin.Nutr. 33: 2657–2661 (1980).

30. Bang, H.O. and Dyerberg, J.: The lipid metabolism in Greenlanders. Meddr. Grønland, Man & Soc. 2. Copenhagen 1981. 18 pp.

31. Barnard, P.J.: Pulmonary arteriosclerosis and cor pulmonale due to recurrent thromboembolism. Circulation 10: 343–361 (1954).

32. Barndt, R., Blankenhorn, D.H., Crawford, D.W. and Brooks, S.H.: Regression and progression of early femoral atherosclerosis in treated hyperlipoproteinemic patients. Ann. Intern. Med. 86: 139–146 (1977).

33. Baroldi, S., Falzi, G. and Mariani, F.: Sudden coronary death. A postmortem study in 208 selected cases compared to 97 'control' subjects. Am. Heart J. 98: 20–31 (1979).

34. Basista, M.J., Dobranowski, M.J. and Gryglewski, R.J.: Prostacyclin and thromboxane generating systems in rabbits pretreated with aspirin. Pharmacol. Res. Comm. 10: 759–773 (1978).

35. Basnayake, V. and Sinclair, H.M.: The effect of deficiency of essential fatty acids upon the skin. In: Popjak and Le Breton (eds): Biochemical problems of lipids. London, Butterworth (1956) p.p. 476–484.

36. Baumgartner, H.R.: The role of blood flow in platelet adhesion, fibrin deposition and formation of mural thrombi. Microvasc. Res. 5: 167–179 (1973).

37. Beare-Rogers, J.L.: Docosenoic acids in dietary fats. Progr. Chem. Fats 15: 29–56 (1977).

38. Beitz, J., Hoffmann, P. and Förster, W.: Cholesterolesters of rat hearts of linoleic acid fed rats stimulate prostaglandin I_2 (PGI_2) synthetase activity. Post. and Med. 6: 17–21 (1981).

39. Beitz, J., Mest, H.-J. and Förster, W.: Influence of linseed oil diet on the pattern of serum lipids in man. Acta Biol. Med. Germ. 40: K31–K35 (1981).

40. Bell, R.L., Kennerly, D.A., Standford, N. and Majerus, P.W.: Diglyceride lipase: A pathway for arachidonate release from human platelets. Proc. Natl. Acad. Sci. USA 76: 3238–3241 (1979).

41. Benditt, E.P. and Benditt, J.M.: Evidence for a monoclonal origin of human atherosclerotic plaques. Proc. Natl. Acad. Sci. USA 70: 1753–1756 (1973).

42. Benditt, E.P.: Evidence for a monoclonal origin of human atherosclerotic plaques and some implications. Circulation 50: 650–652 (1974).

43. Benson, R.L.: The present status of coronary arterial disease. Arch. Path. 2: 870–916 (1926).

44. Bentzen, A.J., Jacobsen, P.A. and Munck-Petersen, S.: An investigation of the platelet adhesiveness by Hellem's method in elderly patients under longterm psychiatric care, on a controlled diet with an unsaturated fatty acid load. Geront. Clin., Basel 14: 217–234 (1972).

45. Benveniste, J., Henson, P.M. and Cochrane, C.G.: Leucocyte-dependent histamine release from

rabbit platelets. The role of IgE, basophils and a platelet-activating factor. J. Exp. Med. 136: 1356–1377 (1971).

46. Benveniste, J., Le Couedic, J.P. and Kamoun, P.: Aggregation of human platelets by platelet-activating factor. Lancet i: 344–345 (1975).

47. Béréziat, G., Chambaz, J., Trugnan, G., Pépin, D. and Polonovski, J.: Turnover of phospholipid linoleic and arachidonic acids in human platelets from plasma lecithins. J. Lipid. Res. 19: 495–500 (1978).

48. Béréziat, G.: Are phospholipases involved in platelet activation? Agents Actions 9: 390–399 (1979).

49. Béréziat, G.: Comment les modifications des lipides plasmatiques constatées lors de l'athérosclerose peuvent-elles agir sur la physiologie plaquettaire? Sem. Hôp. Paris 55: 753–754 (1979).

50. Bergström, S., Danielsson, H. and Samuelsson, B.: The enzymatic formation of prostaglandin E_2 from arachidonic acid. Biochim. Biophys. Acta 90: 207–210 (1964).

51. Berlin, E., Matusik, E.J. and Young, C.: Effects of dietary fat on the fluidity of platelet membranes. Lipids 15: 604–608 (1980).

52. Bertelé, V., Cerletti, C., Schieppati, A., DiMinno, G. and deGaetano, G.: Inhibition of thromboxane synthetase does not necessarily prevent platelet aggregation. Lancet i: 1057–1058 (1981).

53. Bertelé, V., Roncaglioni, M.C., Donati, M.B. and deGaetano, G.: Heparin counteracts the antiaggregating effect of prostacyclin by potentiating platelet aggregation. Thromb. Res. (Submitted.)

54. Best, L.C., Jones, P.B.B., McGuire, M.B. and Russell, R.G.G.: Thromboxane B_2 production and lipid peroxidation in human blood platelets. Adv. Prost. Thromb. Res. 6: 297–299 (1980).

55. Besterman, E., Myat, G. and Travadi, V.: Diurnal variations of platelet stickiness compared with effects produced by adrenalin. Br. Med. J. 1: 597–600 (1967).

56. Besterman, E.M.M. and Gillet, M.P.T.: Inhibition of platelet aggregation by lysolecithin. Atherosclerosis 14: 323–330 (1971).

57. Besterman, E.M.M. and Gillet, M.P.T.: Influence of lysolecithin on platelet aggregation initiated by 5-hydroxytryptamine. Nature (New Biology) 241: 223–224 (1973).

58. Bevers, E., van Dieijen, G., Rosing, J., Hornstra, G. and Zwaal, R.F.A.: The effect of prostacyclin on the participation of platelets in X-activation and thrombin formation. Thromb. Haemost. 46: 271 (1981).

59. Bierenbaum, M.L., Fleischman, A.I., Stier, A., Somol, H. and Watson, P.: Effect of cigarette smoking upon in vivo platelet function in man. Thromb. Res. 12: 1051–1057 (1978).

60. Bierenbaum, M.L., Fleischman, A.I., Stier, A., Watson, P., Somol, H., Naso, A.M. and Binder, M.: Increased platelet aggregation and decreased high-density lipoprotein cholesterol in woman on oral contraceptives. Am. J. Obstet. Gynecol. 134: 638–641 (1979).

61. Bierman, E.L. and Albers, J.J.: Lipoprotein uptake by cultured human arterial smooth muscle cells. Biochim. Biophys. Acta 388: 198–202 (1975).

62. Billah, M.M., Lapetina, E.G. and Cuatrecasas, P.: Phospholipase A_2 activity specific for phosphatidic acid. A possible mechanism for the production of arachidonic acid in platelets. J. Biol. Chem. 256: 5399–5403 (1981).

63. Billimoria, J.D., Irani, V.J. and MacLagan, N.F.: Blood lipid fractionation and blood clotting in ischaemic heart disease. J. Atheroscler. Res. 5: 102–111 (1965).

64. Bills, T.K., Smith, J.B., Kocsis, J.J. and Silver, M.J.: Metabolism of a potential anti-thrombotic agent (8, 11, 14-eicosatrienoic acid) by human platelets. Fed. Proc. 35: 755 (1976).

64a. Bills, T.K., Smith, J.B. and Silver, M.J.: Platelet uptake, release and oxidation of [^{14}C]arachidonic acid. in: Silver, M.J., Smith, J.B. and Kocsis, J.J. (Eds.): Prostaglandins in hematology. Spectrum Publications Inc. N.Y. 1977, pp. 27–55.

65. Bills, T.K., Smith, J.B. and Silver, M.J.: Metabolism of ^{14}C-arachidonic acid by human platelets. Biochim. Biophys. Acta 424: 303–314 (1976).

188

66. Bills, T.K., Smith, J.B. and Silver, M.J.: Selective release of arachidonic acid from the phospholipids of human platelets in response to thrombin. J. Clin. Invest. 60: 1–6 (1977).

67. Bjøggild, J., Halberg, O. and Jørgenson, F.S.: Sundhedstilstanden i Grønland. Landslaegens årsberetning for årene 1973, 1974, 1975 og 1976, Godthåb, Greenland, 1978, Cited in ref. 30

68. Black, K.L., Culp, B., Madison, D., Randall, O.S. and Lands, W.E.M.: The protective effects of dietary fish oil on focal cerebral infarction. Prost. Med. 3: 257–268 (1979).

69 Blackwell, G.J., Duncombe, W.G., Flower, R.J., Parsons, M.F. and Vane, J.R.: The distribution and metabolism of arachidonic acid in rabbit platelets during aggregation and its modification by drugs. Br. J. Pharmacol. 59: 353–366 (1977).

70. Blackwell, G.J., Flower, R.J., Russell-Smith, N., Salmon, J.A., Thorogood, P.B. and Vane, J.R.: Prostacyclin is produced in whole blood. Br. J. Pharmacol. 64: 436P (1978).

70a. Blair, I.A., Barrow, S.E., Waddell, K.A., Lewis, P.J. and Dollery, C.T.: Prostacyclin is not a circulating hormone in man. Prostaglandins 23: 579–590 (1982).

71. Bligh, E.G. and Dyer, W.J.: A rapid method of total lipid extraction and purification. Can. J. Biochem. Physiol. 37: 911–917 (1959).

72. Bloj, B., Morero, R.D. and Farías, R.N.: Membrane fluidity, Cholesterol and allosteric transitions of membrane boud Mg^{2+}-APTase, $(Na^+ + K^+)$-APTase and acetyl cholinesterase from rat erythrocytes. FEBS Lett. 38: 101–105 (1973).

73. Bloj, B., Morero, R.D., Farias, R:N. and Trucco, R.E.: Membrane lipid fatty acids and regulation of membrane bound enzymes. Biochim. Biophys. Acta 311: 67–69 (1973).

74. Blumgart, H.L., Schlesinger, M.J. and Davis, D.: Studies on the relation of the clinical manifestations of angina pectoris, coronary thrombosis and myocardial infarction to the pathologic findings. Am. Heart J. 19: 1–91 (1940).

75. Böhle, E., Bauke, J., Harmuth, E. and Breddin, K.: Untersuchungen über die Agglutination der Blutplättchen nach Zufuhr verschiedener Nahrungsfette. Klin. Wschr. 43: 555–562 (1965).

76. Bonne, C., Martin, B., Watada, M. and Regnault, F.: The antagonism of prostaglandins I_2, E_1 and D_2 by prostaglandin E_2 in human platelets. Tromb. Res. 21: 13–22 (1981).

77. Borchgrevink, C.F., Berg, K.J., Skaga, E., Skjaeggestad, Ö and Stormorken, H.: Effect of linseed oil on platelet adhesiveness and bleeding time in patients with coronary heart disease. Lancet ii: 980–982 (1965).

78. Borchgrevink, C.F., Berg, K.J., Skaga, E. and Skjaeggestad, Ö.: Absence of prophylactic effect of linolenic acid in patients with coronary heart disease. Lancet ii: 187–189 (1966).

79. Borda, E.S., Lazzari, M.A., Gimeno, M.F. and Gimeno, A.L.: Human platelet rich plasma and human serum protects from inactivation the antiaggregatory capacity of prostacyclin-like material (PGI$_2$) produced by the rat stomach fundus. Prostaglandins 19: 899–905 (1980).

80. Borgeat, P., Hamberg, M., and Samuelsson, B.: Tranformation of arachidonic acid and homo-γ-linolenic acid by rabbit polymorphonuclear leucocytes. Monohydroxy acids from novel lipoxygenases. J. Biol. Chem. 251: 7816–7820 (1976).

81. Borgeat, P. and Samuelsson, B.: Arachidonic acid metabolism in polymorphonuclear leukocytes: Effects of ionophore A 23187. Proc. Natl. Acad. Sci. USA 76: 2148–2152 (1979).

82. Born, G.V.R.: Aggregation of blood platelets by adenosine diphosphate and its reversal. Nature 194: 927–929 (1962).

83. Born, G.V.R. and Cross, M.J.: The aggregation of blood platelets. J. Physiol. (Lond.) 168: 178–195 (1963).

84. Born, G.V.R. and others. In: Wolfe, S (ed.): The artery and the Process of Arteriosclerosis: pathogenesis. Adv. Exp. Med. Biol. 16A: 175–184 (1971). Plenum Press, New York.

85. Born, G.V.R., Bergqvist, D. and Arfors, K.E.: Evidence for inhibition of platelet activation in blood by a drug effect on erythrocytes. Nature 259: 233–235 (1976).

86. Born, G.V.R. and Wehmeier, A.: Inhibition of platelet thrombus formation by chlorpromazine acting to diminish haemolysis. Nature 282: 212–213 (1979).

87. Born, G.V.R., Görög, P. and Kratzer, M.A.A.: Aggregation of platelets in damaged vessels. Phil.

Trans. R. Soc. London [Biol] 294: 241–250 (1981).

88. Böttcher, C.J.F., van Gent, C.M. and Pries, C.: A rapid and sensitive submicro phosphorus determination. Anal. Chim. Acta 24: 203–204 (1961).

89. Bottecchia, D. and Doni, M.G.: Artero-venous differences in blood platelet clumping by ADP. Experientia 29: 211–212 (1973).

90. Bowie, E.J.W., Fuster, V., Fass, D.N. and Owen, C.A.Jr.: The role of Willebrand factor in platelet blood vessel interaction including a discussion of resistance to atherosclerosis in pigs with von Willebrand's disease. Proc. Royal Soc. London [Biol] 294: 267–279 (1981).

91. Branemark, P.I.: Intravascular anatomy of blood cells in man. Basel, S. Karger 1971, p. 81.

92. Braunwald, E., Friedewald, W.T. and Furberg. C.T. (eds): Proceedings of the workshop on platelet-active drugs in the secondary prevention of cardiovascular events. Circulation 62 (Suppl. V): 1–135 (1980).

93. Breddin, K. und Bauke, J.: Thrombocytenagglutination und Gefässkrankheiten. Blut 11: 144–165 (1965).

94. Brenner, R.R. and Peluffo, R.O.: Regulation of unsaturated fatty acid biosynthesis. I. Effect of unsaturated fatty acids of 18 carbons on the microsomal desaturation of linoleic acid into γ-linolenic acid. Biochim. Biophys. Acta 176: 471–479 (1969).

95. Le Breton, G.C., Dinerstein, R.J., Roth, L.J. and Feinberg, H.: Direct evidence for intracellular divalent cation redistribution associated with platelet shape change. Biochem. Biophys. Res. Comm. 71: 362–370 (1976).

96. Le Breton, G.C. and Dinerstein, R.J.: Effect of the calcium antagonist TMB-6 on intracellular calcium redistribution associated with platelet shape change. Tromb. Res. 10: 521–523 (1977).

97. Broekhuyse, R.M.: Quantitative two-dimensional thin layer chromatography of blood phospho-lipids. Clin. Chim. Acta 23: 457–461 (1969).

98. Broekman, M.J., Ward., J.W. and Marcus, A.J.: Phospholipid metabolism in stimulated human platelets. Changes in phosphatidylinositol, phosphatidic acid and lysophospholipids. J. Clin. Invest. 66: 275–283 (1980).

99. Broekman, M.J., Ward, J.W. and Marcus, A.J.: Fatty acid composition of phosphatidylinositol and phosphatidic acid in stimulated platelets: persistence of arachidonyl-stearyl structure. J. Biol. Chem. 256: 8271–8274 (1981).

100. Broersma, R.J., Dickerson, G.D. and Sullivan, M.S.: The determination of platelet aggregation by filtration pressure in circulating dog blood. Thrombos. Diathes. Haemorrh. 29: 201–210 (1973).

101. Brox, J. and Østerud. B.: The effect of prostacyclin (PGI_2) on the procoagulant activity of human platelets. Thromb. Haemost. 46:271 (1981).

102. Brox, J.H., Kille, J.-E., Gunne, S. and Nordøy, A.: The effect of cod liver oil and corn oil on platelets and vessel wall in man. Thromb. Haemostas. 46: 604–611 (1981).

103. Bschor, F. and Deiniger, R.: Einfluss der Hyperlipämie auf die Thrombogenese im Coronarsystem des isolierten Katzenherzens. Klin. Wochenschr. 42: 435–450 (1964).

104. Buchanan, M.R., Blajchman, M.A., Dejana, E., Mustard, J.F., Senyi, A.F. and Hirsch, J.: Shortening of bleeding time in thrombocytopenic rabbits after exposure of jungular vein to high aspirin concentration. Prost. Med. 3: 333–342 (1979).

105. Buchwald, H., Moore, R.B. and Varco, R.L.: The partial ileal bypass operation in treatment of hyperlipemias. Advan. Exp. Med. Biol. 63: 221–230 (1974).

106. Büller, J. and Vles, R.O.: Dietary fats and atherosclerosis in the rabbit. Voeding 27: 223–231 (1966).

107. Bult, H. and Bonta, I.L.: Rat platelets aggregate in the absence of endogenous precursors of prostaglandin endoperoxides. Nature 264: 449–451 (1976).

108. Bunting, S., Gryglewski, R.J., Moncada, S. and Vane, J.R.: Arterial walls generate from prosta-glandin endoperoxides a substance (prostaglandin X) which relaxes strips of mesenteric and coeliac arteries and inhibits platelet aggregation. Prostaglandins 12: 897–913 (1976).

109. Bunting, S., Moncada, S. and Vane, J.R.: Antithrombotic properties of vascular endothelium.

190

Lancet ii: 1075–1076 (1977).

110. Bunting, S., Simmons, P.M. and Moncada, S.: Inhibition of platelet activation by prostacyclin: possible consequences in coagulation and anticoagulation. Thromb. Res. 21: 89–102 (1981).

111. Burch, J.W., Baenziger, N.L., Stanford, N. and Majerus, P.W.: Sensitivity of fatty acid cyclooxygenase from human aorta to acetylation by aspirin. Proc. Natl. Acad. Sci USA 75: 5181–5184 (1978).

112. Burke, J.M. and Ross, R.: Collagen synthesis by monkey arterial smooth muscle cells during proliferation and quiescence in culture. Exp. Cell. Res. 107: 387–395 (1977).

113. Burr, G.O. and Burr, M.M.: Deficiency disease, produced by the rigid exclusion of fat from the diet. J. Biol. Chem. 82: 345–367 (1929).

114. Bushfield, D. and Tomich, E.G.: Acute intravascular haemolysis and platelet behaviour. Nature 218: 696–697 (1968).

115. Capurro, N.L., Lipson, L.C., Bonow, R.O., Goldstein, R.E., Shulman, N.R. and Epstein, S.E.: Relative effects of aspirin on platelet aggregation and prostaglandin-mediated coronary vasodilatation in the dog. Circulation 62: 1221–1227 (1980).

116. Carroll, K.K.: Digestibility of individual fatty acids in the rat. J. Nutr. 64: 399–410 (1958).

117. Carroll, K.K. and Richards, J.F.: Factors affecting digestibility of fatty acids in the rat. J. Nutr. 64: 411–424 (1958).

118. Cazenave, J.P.: Personal communication.

119. Cazenave, J.P., Packham, M.A. and Mustard, J.F.: Adherence of platelets to a collagen-coated surface: development of a quantitative method. J. Lab. Clin. Med. 82: 978–990 (1973).

120. Cazenave, J.P., Reimers, H.J., Kinlough-Rathbone, R.L., Packham, M.A. and Mustard, J.F.: Effects of sodium periodate on platelet functions. Lab. Invest. 34: 471–481 (1976).

121. Cazenave, J.P., Benveniste, J. and Mustard, J.F.: Aggregation of rabbit platelets by platelet-activating factor is independent of the release reaction and the arachidonate pathway and inhibited by membrane-active drugs. Lab. Invest. 41: 275–285 (1979).

122. Cazenave, J.P., Sutter, A., Hemmendinger, S., Wiesel, M.-L., Lanza, F. and Daver, J.: Adrenaline activates human platelets but does not cause primary aggregation if thrombin generation is inhibited by hirudin. Thromb. Haemostas. 46: 95 (1981).

123. Chambaz, J., Béréziat, G., Pépin, D. and Polonovski, J.: Turnover of platelet arachidonic and linoleic acids. Biochimie 61: 127–130 (1979).

124. Chambaz, J., Robert, A., Wolf, C., Béréziat, G. and Polonovski, J.: Different acylation and accumulation in free form of arachidonic acid or its sodium salt in human platelets. Thromb. Res. 15: 743–753 (1979).

125. Chan, A.C., Allen, C.E. and Hegarty, P.V.J.: The effects of vitamin E depletion and repletion on prostaglandin synthesis in semitendinosus muscle of young rabbits. J. Nutr. 110: 66–73 (1980).

126. Chan, A.C., Hegarty, P.V.J. and Allen, C.E.: The effects of vitamin E depletion and repletion on prostaglandin dehydrogenase activity in tissue of young rabbits. J. Nutr. 110: 74–81 (1980).

127. Chandler, A.B.: In vitro thrombotic coagulation of blood. Lab. Invest. 7: 110–115 (1958).

128. Chandler, A.B. Hand, R.A.: Phagocytozed platelets; a source of lipids in human thrombi and atherosclerotic plaques. Science 134: 946–947 (1961).

129. Chandler, A.B.: The anatomy of a thrombus. In: Thrombosis. Sherry, S., Brinkhous, K.M., Genton, E. and Stengle, J.M. (eds), Washington, National Academy of Sciences, 1969, p. 279–299.

130. Chandler, A.B.: Reversal and repair of vascular injury in thrombosis. Thromb. Diath. haemorrh: (suppl. 40) 273–284 (1970).

131. Chandler, A.B.: Thrombosis and the development of atherosclerotic lesions. In: Atherosclerosis: Proceedings of the second international symposium, Jones, R.J. (ed), New York, Springer Verlag, 1970, p. 88–93.

132. Chandler, A.B.: Thrombosis in the development of coronary atherosclerosis. In: Atherosclerosis and Coronary Heart Disease. Likoff, W., Segal, B.L., Insull, W.Jr. and Moyer, J.H. (eds), New York, Grune and Stratton Inc. 1972, p. 28–34.

133. Chandler, A.B.: Mechanisms and frequency of thrombosis in the coronary circulation. Thromb. Res. 4 (Suppl. 1): 3–23 (1974).

134. Chandler, A.B., Chapman, I., Erhardt, L.R., Roberts, W.C., Schwartz, C.J., Sinapius, D., Spain, D.M., Sherry, S., Ness, P.M. and Simon, T.L.: Coronary thrombosis in myocardial infarction. Report of a workshop on the role of coronary thrombosis in the pathogenesis of acute myocardial infarction. Am. J. Cardiol. 34: 823–833 (1974).

135. Chandler, A.B. and Pope, J.T.: Arterial thrombosis in atherogenesis: A survey of the frequency of incorporation of thrombi into atherosclerotic plaques. In: Blood and Arterial Wall in Atherogenesis and Arterial Thrombosis. Hautvast, J.G.A.J., Hermus, R.J.J., van der Haar, F. (eds), Leiden, the Netherlands, E.J. Brill, 1975, p. 110–118.

136. Chapman, I.: Morphogenesis of occluding coronary artery thrombosis. Arch. Path. 80: 256–261 (1965).

137. Chase, H.P. and Dupont, J.: Abnormal levels of prostaglandins and fatty acids in blood of children with cystic fibrosis. Lancet ii: 236–238 (1978).

138. Chignard, M., Le Couedic, J.P., Tence, M., Vargaftig, B.B. and Benveniste, J.: The role of platelet-activating factor in platelet aggregation. Nature 279: 799–800 (1979).

139. Cho, M.J. and Allen, M.A.: Chemical stability of prostacyclin (PGI$_2$) in aqueous solutions. Prostaglandins 15: 943–954 (1978).

140. Christ-Hazelhof, E. and Nugteren, D.H.: Prostacyclin is not a circulating hormone. Prostaglandins 22: 739–746 (1981).

141. Christ, E.J. and Nugteren, D.H.: The biosynthesis and possible function of prostaglandins in adipose tissue. Biochim. Biophys. Acta. 218: 296–307 (1970).

142. Clark, E., Graef, I. and Chasis, H.: Thrombosis of the aorta and coronary arteries with special reference to 'fibrinoid' lesions. Arch. Path. 22: 183–212 (1936).

143. Claus, A.: Gerinnungsphysiologische Schnellmethode zur Bestimmung des Fibrinogens. Acta Haematol. 17: 237–246 (1957).

144. Clower, B.R.: Relation of levels of dietary fat to atrial thrombosis in RF mice. J. Atheroscler. Res. 8: 885–890 (1968).

145. Clower, B.R. and Lockwood, W.R.: Light and electron microscopy in diet-induced atrial thrombosis in Swiss mice. II. Recovery on return to a balanced diet. Am. J. Path. 66: 65–82 (1972).

146. Cohen, P., Derksen, A. and van den Bosch, H.: Pathway of fatty acid metabolism in human platelets. J. Clin Invest. 49: 128–139 (1970).

147. Cohen, P., Broekman, M.J., Verkley, A., Lisman, J.W.W. and Derksen, A.: Quantification of human platelet inositides and the influence of ionic environment on their incorporation of orthophosphate^{32}P. J. Clin. Invest. 50: 762–772 (1971).

148. Colard, O., Kervabon, A. and Roy, C.: Effects on adenylate cyclase activities of unsaturated fatty acid incorporation into rat liver plasma membrane phospholipids. Specific modulation by linoleate. Biochem. Biophys. Res. Comm. 95: 97–102 (1980).

149. Collaborative Group for the study of stroke in young women: Oral contraception and increased risk of cerebral ischemia or thrombosis. N. Engl. J. Med. 288: 871–877 (1973).

150. Collen, D.: On the regulation and control of fibrinolysis. Thrombos. Haemostas. 43: 77–89 (1980).

151. Colman, R.W.: Platelet function in hyperlipidemia. In: Platelet function testing. Day, H.J., Holmsen, H. and Zucker, M.B. (eds.), Washington, DHEW Pub No (NIH) 78–1087, 1978, p. 618–629.

152. Connor, W.E., Hoak, J.C. and Warner, E.D.: Plasma free fatty acids, hypercoagulability and thrombosis. In: Sherry, S., Brinkhous, K.M., Genton, E. and Stengle, J.M. (eds): Thrombosis. Nat. Acad. Sci. Washington D.C. p.p. 355–373 (1969).

153. Constantinides, P.: Plague fissures in human coronary thrombosis. J. Atheroscler. Res. 6: 1–17 (1966).

154. Cooper, B., Schafer, A.I., Puchalsky, D. and Handin, R.I.,: Desensitization of prostaglandin-activated platelet adenylcyclase. Prostaglandins 17: 561–571 (1979).

155. Cooper, R.A.: Abnormalities of cell-membrane fluidity in the pathogenesis of disease. N Engl. J. Med. 297: 371–377 (1977).

156. Coughlin, S.R., Moskowitz, M.A., Zetter, B.R., Antoniades, H.N. and Levine, L.: Platelet dependent stimulating of prostacyclin synthesis by platelet-derived growth factor. Nature 288: 600–602 (1980).

157. Craig, I.H., Bell, F.P., Goldsmith, C.H. and Schwarz, C.J.: Thrombosis and atherosclerosis: the organization of pulmonary thromboemboli in the pig. Macroscopic observations, protein, DNA and major lipids. Atherosclerosis 18: 277–300 (1973).

158. Craig, I.H., Bell, F.P. and Schwarz, C.J.: Thrombosis and atherosclerosis: the organization of pulmonary thromboemboli in the pig. Individual phospholipids, fatty acid composition of lec-ithin, sphingomyelin, esterified cholesterol and ^{3}H-cholesterol specific activity. Exp. Mol. Pathol. 18: 290–304 (1973).

159. Crawford, M.A., Casperd, N.M. and Sinclair, A.J.: The long chain metabolites of linoleic and linolenic acids in liver and brain in herbivores and carnivores. Comp. Biochem. Physiol. 54B: 395–401 (1976).

160. Crawford, M.A., Hassam, A.G. and Rivers, J.P.W.: Essential fatty acid requirements in infancy Am. J. Clin. Nutr. 31: 2181–2185 (1978).

161. Crawford, T. and Levene, C.I.: Incorporation of fibrin in the aortic intima. J. Path. Bact. 64: 523–528 (1952).

162. Crawford, T.: The healing of puncture wounds in arteries. J. Path. Bact. 72: 547–552 (1956).

163. Crawford, T.: Thrombotic occlusion and the plaque. In: Evolution of the Atherosclerotic Plaque, Jones, R.J. (ed). Chicago, Univ. Chicago Press, 1963, p. 279–290.

164. Cullen, C.F. and Swank, R.L.: Intravascular aggregation and adhesiveness of the blood elements associated with alimentary lipemia and injections of large molecular substances. Effect on blood-brain barrier. Circulation 9: 335–346 (1954).

165. Culp, B.R., Titus, B.G. and Lands, W.E.M.: Inhibition of prostaglandin biosynthesis by eicosap-entaenoic acid. Prost. Med. 3: 269–278 (1979).

166. Culp, B.R., Lands, W.E.M., Lucchesi, B.R., Pitt, B. and Romson, J.: The effect of dietary supplementation of fish oil on experimental myocardial infarction. Prostaglandins 20: 1021–1031 (1980).

167. Czervionke, R.L., Smith, J.B., Fry, G.L., Hoak, J.C. and Haycraft, D.L.: Inhibition of pro-stacyclin by treatment of endothelium with aspirin. Correlation with platelet adherence. J. Clin. Invest. 63: 1089–1092 (1979).

168. Danielsson, H.: Present status of research on catabolism and excretion of cholesterol. In: Paoletti, R. and Kritchevsky, D. (eds): Adv. Lip. Res. I. New York, Academic Press, 1963, p.p. 335–385.

169. Danse, L.H.J.C., Stolwijk, J. and Verschuren, P.M.: Fish oil-induced yellow fat disease in rats. IV. Functional studies in the reticuloendothelial system. Vet. Pathol. 16: 593–603 (1979).

170. Davies, M.J., Woolf, N. and Brandley, J.P.W.: Endothelialisation of experimentally produced mural thrombi in the pig aorta. J. Path. 97: 589–594 (1969).

171. Davies, M.J., Woolf, N. and Robertson, W.B.: Pathology of acute myocardial infarction with particular reference to occlusive coronary thrombi. Brit. Heart J. 38: 659–664 (1976).

172. Davis, T.M.E., Mitchell, M.D. and Turner, R.C.: Prostacyclin and thromboxane metabolites in diabetes. Lancet ii: 789–790 (1979).

173. Day, A.J. and Gould-Hurst, P.R.S.: Esterification of ^{14}C-labelled cholesterol by reticuloendo-thelial cells. Quart. J. Exp. Physiol. 46: 376–382 (1961).

174. Dayton, S.: Composition of lipids in human serum and adipose tissue during prolonged feeding of a diet high in unsaturated fat. J. Lipid Res. 7: 103–111 (1966).

175. Dayton, S., Pearce, M.L., Hashimoto, S. and Dixon, W.J.: A controlled clinical trial of a diet high in unsaturated fat in preventing complications of atherosclerosis. Circulation 40 (Suppl. II): 1–63 (1969).

176. De Deckere, E.A.M., Nugteren, D.H. and ten Hoor, F.: Prostacyclin is the major prostaglandin

released from the isolated perfused rabbit and rat heart. Nature 268: 160–163 (1977).

177. De Deckere, E.A.M., Nugteren, D.H. and ten Hoor, F.: Influence of type of dietary fat on the prostaglandin release from isolated rabbit and rat hearts and from rat aortas. Prostaglandins 17: 947–955 (1979).

178. Deiniger, R.: Einfluss von Fettinfusionen auf Leistung und Sauerstoffverbrauch des isoliert durchströmten Herzens. Arch. Exp. Path. Pharmakol. 245: 414–426 (1963).

179. Dejana, E.: 'Aspirinated' platelets are hemostatic in thrombocytopenic rats with 'nonaspirinated' vessel walls. Evidence from an exchange transfusion model. Blood 56: 959–962 (1980).

180. Delaini, F., Reyers, I., de Bellis Vitti, G., Poggi, A. and Donati, M.B.: Studies on a new model of thrombotic tendency in the rat. In: Breddin, K., Gross, D. and Rotter, W. (eds.): Thrombosemodelle am Tier. Schattauer Verlag, Stuttgart, 1981, pp. 147–155.

181. Dembinska-Kiec, A., Gryglewska, T., Zmuda, A. and Gryglewski, R.J.: The generation of prostacyclin by arteries and by the coronary vascular bed is reduced in experimental atherosclerosis in rabbit. Prostaglandins 14: 1025–1034 (1977).

182. Demel, R.A. and de Kruyff, B.: The function of sterols in membranes. Biochim. Biophys. Acta 457: 109–132 (1976).

183. Demopoulos, C.A., Pinckard, R.N. and Hanahan, D.J.: Platelet-activating factor. Evidence for 1-0-alkyl-2-acetyl-sn-glyceryl-3-phosphoryl-choline as the active component (a new class of lipid mediators). J. Biol. Chem. 254: 9355–9358 (1979).

184. Derksen, A. and Cohen, P.: Extensive incorporation of [2-^{14}C] Mevalonic acid into cholesterol-precursors by human platelets in vitro. J. Biol. Chem. 248: 7396–7403 (1973).

185. Derksen, A.: Failure of rhesus platelets and arterial tissue to convert preformed (^{14}C) lanosterol to (^{14}C) cholesterol in vivo. In: Derksen, A.: Studies on Lipid Metabolism in Human Platelets. Thesis, Fox Run Press, Topsfield, Mass. USA, (1975) p.p. 45–53.

186. Derksen, A. and Cohen, P.: Patterns of fatty acid release from endogenous substrates by human platelet homogenates and membranes. J. Biol. Chem. 250: 9342–9347 (1975).

187. DeWood, M.A., Spores, J., Notske, R., Mouser, L.T., Burroughs, R., Golden, M.S. and Lang, H.T.: Prevalence of total coronary occlusion during the early hours of transmural myocardial infarction. N Engl. J. Med. 303: 897–902 (1980).

188. Deykin, D. and Desser, R.K.: The corporation of acetate and palmitate into lipids by human platelets. J. Clin. Invest. 47: 1590–1602 (1968).

189. Deykin, D.: Altered lipid metabolism in human platelets after primary aggregation. J. Clin. Invest. 52: 483–492 (1973).

190. Deykin, D. and Snyder, D.: Effect of epinephrine on platelet lipid metabolism. J. Lab. Clin. Med. 82: 554–559 (1973).

191. Dhall, D.P. and Matheson, N.A.: Platelet aggregate filtration pressure. A method of measuring platelet aggregation in whole blood. Cardiovasc. Res. 3: 155–160 (1969).

192. Diczfalusy, U., Falardeau, P. and Hammarström, S.: Conversion of prostaglandin endoperoxides to C_{17}-hydroxy acids catalyzed by human platelet thromboxane synthetase. FEBS Letts. 84: 271–274 (1977).

193. Diczfalusy, U. and Hammarström, S.: A structural requirement for the conversion of prostaglandin endoperoxides to thromboxanes. FEBS Letts. 105: 291–295 (1979).

194. Didisheim, P.: Animal models useful in the study of thrombosis and antithrombotic agents; in Spaet: Progress in Hemostasis and Thrombosis, vol. 1, Grune & Stratton, New York, 1972), p.p. 165–197.

195. Dormandy, T.L.: Free radical oxidation and anti-oxidants. Lancet i: 647–650 (1978).

196. Dorp, D.A. van, Beerthuis, R.K., Nugteren, D.H. and Vonkeman, H.: The biosynthesis of prostaglandins. Biochim. Biophys. Acta 90: 204–207 (1964).

197. Dorp, D.A. van: Recent developments in the biosynthesis and the analysis of prostaglandins. Ann. N.Y. Acad. Sci. 180: 181–199 (1971).

198. Dorp, D.A. van, van Evert, W.C. and van der Wolf, L.: 20-Methyl prostacyclin. A powerful

'unnatural' platelet aggregation inhibitor. Prostaglandins 16: 953–955 (1978).

199. Douglas, A.S.: Anticoagulant therapy in coronary artery disease. In: Sherry, S. et al. (eds): Thrombosis. Nat. Acad. Sci., Washington D.C., p.p. 690–704 (1969).

200. Downie, H.G., Murphy, E.A., Rowsell, H.C. and Mustard, J.F.: Extracorporeal circulation: a device for the quantitative study of thrombus formation in flowing blood. Circulat. Res. 12: 441–448 (1963).

201. Dubber, A.H.C., Rifkin, B., Gale, M., McNicol, G.P. and Douglas, A.S.: The effect of fat feeding on fibrinolysis, 'Stypven' time and platelet aggregation. J. Atheroscler. Res. 7: 225–235 (1967).

202. Duguid, J.B.: Thrombosis as a factor in the pathogenesis of coronary atherosclerosis. J. Pathol. Bacteriol. 58: 207–212 (1946).

203. Duguid, J.B.: Thrombosis as a factor in the pathogenesis of aortic atherosclerosis. J. Path. Bacteriol. 60: 57–61 (1948).

204. Dupont, J., Mathias, M.M. and Connally, P.T.: Effects of dietary essential fatty acid concentration upon prostanoid synthesis in rats. J. Nutr. 110: 1695–1702 (1980).

205. Dusting, G.J., Moncada, S. and Vane, J.R.: Disappearance of prostacyclin in the circulation of the dog. Br. J. Pharmacol. 62: 414–415P (1977).

206. Dusting, G.J., Moncada, S. and Vane, J.R.: Recirculation of prostacyclin (PGI_2) in the dog. Br. J. Pharmacol. 64: 315–320 (1978).

207. Dutilh, C.E., Haddeman, E., Jouvenaz, G.H., ten Hoor, F. and Nugteren, D.H.: Study of the two pathways for arachidonate oxygenation in blood platelets. Lipids 14: 241–246 (1979).

208. Dutilh, C.E., Haddeman, E., Don, J.A. and ten Hoor, F.: The role of arachidonate lipoxygenase and fatty acids during irreversible blood platelet aggregation in vitro. Prost. and Med. 6: 111–126 (1981).

209. Dutton, H.J.: Hydrogenation of fats in: Holman, R.T. (Ed.): Progress in the Chemistry of Fats and Other Lipids. Vol. 9 (Polyunsaturated acids.). Pergamon Press, Oxford, 1971, pp. 349–375.

210. Dyerberg, J.: Personal communication.

211. Dyerberg, J., Bang, H.O. and Hjørne, N.: Fatty acid composition of the plasma lipids in Greenland Eskimos. Am. J. Clin. Nutr. 28: 958–966 (1975).

212. Dyerberg, J., Bang, H.O. and Hjørne, N: Plasma cholesterol concentration in Caucasian Danes and Greenland West-coast Eskimos. Dan. Med. Bull 24: 52–55 (1977).

213. Dyerberg, J. and Bang, H.O.: Dietary fat and thrombosis. Lancet i: 152 (1978).

214. Dyerberg, J., Bang, H.O., Stoffersen, E., Moncada, S. and Vane, J.R.: Eicosapentaenoic acid and prevention of thrombosis and atherosclerosis? Lancet ii: 117–119 (1978).

215. Dyerberg, J. and Bang, H.O.: Haemostatic function and platelet polyunsaturated fatty acids in Eskimos. Lancet ii: 433–435 (1979).

216. Dyerberg, J., Bang, H.O. and Aagaard, O.: α-Linolenic acid and eicosapentaenoic acid. Lancet i: 199 (1980).

217. Dyerberg, J.: Platelet-vessel wall interaction: influence of diet. Phil. Trans. R. Soc. Lond. B. 294: 373–381 (1980).

218. Dyerberg, J.: Effect on hemostasis by feeding eicosapentaenoic acid. in: Nutritional Factors: Modulating Effects on Metabolic Processes. Beers, R.F.Jr. and Bassett, E.G. (eds). Raven Press, New York, 1981, pp. 511–521.

219. Dyerberg, J., Jørgensen, K.A. and Arnfred, T.: Human umbilical blood vessel converts all cis-5, 8, 11, 14, 17 eicosapentaenoic acid to prostaglandin I_3. Prostaglandins 22: 857–862 (1981).

220. Stoffersen, E. Jørgensen, K.A. and Dyerberg, J.: Antithrombin III and dietary intake of polyunsaturated fatty acids. Scand. J. Clin. Lab. Invest. 42: 83–86 (1982).

221. Eastham, R.D.: Clinical Haematology, Wright, Bristol (1966).

222. Editorial: Oral contraceptives and health. Lancet i: 1147–1148 (1974).

223. Egan, R.W., Paxton, J. and Kuehl, F.A. Jr.: Mechanism for irreversible self-deactivation of prostaglandin synthetase. J. Biol. Chem. 251: 7329–7335 (1976).

224. Eika, C.: The platelet aggregating effect of eight commercial heparins. Scand. J. Haematol. 9:

480–482 (1972).

225. Einheber, A., Wren, R.E., Carter, D. and Rose, L.R.: A simple collar device for the protection of skin grafts in mice. Lab. An. Care 17: 345–348 (1967).

226. Eldor, A. and Weksler, B.B.: Heparin and dextran sulphate antagonize PGI_2 inhibition of platelet aggregation. Thromb. Res. 16: 617–628 (1979).

227. Elemer, G. and Gabbiani, G.: Modifications of aortic intima during hypertension. Role of angiotensin and mineralocorticoids. In: Carlson, L.A., Paoletti, R., Sirtori, C. and Weber, G. (eds): International Conference on Atherosclerosis. Raven Press, New York, 1978, p.p. 553–560.

228. El-Maraghi, N. and Genton, E.: The relevance of platelet and fibrin thromboembolism of the coronary microcirculation, with special reference to sudden cardiac death. Circulation 62: 936–944 (1980).

229. Emmons, P.R., Hampton, R.J., Harrison, M.J.G., Honour, A.J. and Mitchell, J.R.A.: Effect of prostaglandin E_1 on platelet behaviour in vitro and in vivo. Brit. Med. J. 2: 468–472 (1967).

230. Engelberg, H.: Studies with the Chandler Rotating Loop. Evidence that thrombin generation is responsible for the formation of the artificial in vitro thrombi. Thromb. Diath. haemorrh. 22: 344–350 (1969).

231. Erhardt, L.R., Lundman, T. and Mellstedt, H.: Incorporation of ^{125}I-labelled fibrinogen into coronary arterial thrombi in acute myocardial infarction in man. Lancet i: 387–390 (1973).

232. Erhardt, L.R., Unge, G. and Boman, G.: Formation of coronary arterial thrombi in relation to onset of necrosis in acute myocardial infarction in man. Am. Heart J. 91: 592–598 (1976).

233. Etienne, J., Grüber, A. and Polonovski, J.: L'activité phospholipasidique des plaquettes de rat. Biochimie 61: 433–435 (1979).

234. Evans, G. and Irvine, W.T.: Long-term arterial graft patency in relation to platelet adhesiveness, biochemical factors and anticoagulant therapy. Lancet ii: 353–355 (1966).

235. Evans, G., Mustard, J.F.: Platelet-surface reaction and thrombosis. Surgery 64: 273–280 (1978).

236. Evert, W.C. van, Nugteren, D.H. and van Dorp, D.A.: Inhibition of prostaglandin biosynthesis by c-5, c-8, c-11-eicosatrienoic acid. Prostaglandins 15: 267–272 (1978).

237. Fantl, P. and Ward, H.A.: The thromboplastic component of intact blood is present in masked form. Austr. J. Exp. Biol. Med. Sci. 36: 499–504 (1958).

238. Farías, R.N., Bloj, B., Morero, R.D., Siñeriz, F. and Trucco, R.E.: Regulation of allosteric membrane-bound enzymes through changes in membrane lipid composition. Biochim. Biophys. Acta 415: 231–251 (1975).

239. Fass, D.N., Downing, M.R., Meyers, P., Bowie, E.J.W. and Witte, L.D.: Cell growth stimulation by normal and von Willebrand porcine platelets and endothelial cells. Blood 52 (Suppl. I): 181 (1978).

240. Fearnley, G.R.: Fibrinolysis. Edward Arnold (Publishers) Ltd. London, 1965.

241. Ferguson, J.C., MacKay, N. and McNicol, G.P.: Effect of feeding fat on fibrinolysis. 'Stypven' time and platelet aggregation in Africans, Asians and Europeans. J. Clin. Path. 23: 580–585(1970).

242. Ferguson, J.C., Mackay, N. and McNicol, G.P.: Effect of feeding fat on fibrinolysis, 'Stypven' time and platelet aggregation in elderly Africans. J. Clin. Path. 25: 574–576 (1972).

243. Ferreira, S.H. and Vane, J.R.: Prostaglandins: their disappearance from and release into the circulation. Nature 216: 868–873 (1967).

244. Ferreira, S.H., Moncada, S. and Vance, J.R.: Indomethacin and aspirin abolish prostaglandin release from the spleen. Nature (New biology) 231: 237–239 (1971).

245. Ferretti, A., Schoene, N.W. and Flanagan, V.P.: Identification and quantification of prostaglandin E_3 in renal medullary tissue of three strains of rats fed fish oil. Lipids 16: 800–804 (1981).

246. Fine, K.M., Dupont, J. and Mathias, M.M.: Rat platelet prostaglandin, cyclic AMP and lipid response to variations in dietary fat. J. Nutr. 111: 699–709 (1981).

247. Fischer, S.: Simple and atherogenic thrombosis in the coronary vessels. J. Atheroscler. Res. 4: 230–238 (1964).

247a. FitzGerald, G.A., Brash,A.R., Falardeau, P. and Oates, J.A.: Estimated rate of prostacyclin secretion into the circulation in normal man. J. Clin. Invest. 68: 1272–1276 (1981).

248. Fitzpatrick, F.A., Wijnalda, M.A. and Kaiser, D.G.: Oximes for high performance liquid and electron capture gas chromatography of prostaglandins and thromboxanes. Anal. chem. 49: 1032–1035 (1977).

249. Fleischman, A.I., Hayton, A. and Bierenbaum, M.L.: Objective biochemical determination of dietary adherence in the young coronary male. Am. J. Clin. Nutr. 20: 333–337 (1967).

250. Fleischman, A.I., Bierenbaum, M.L., Justice, D., Stier, A. and Sullivan, A.S.: In vivo platelet function in acute myocardial infarction, acute cerebrovascular accidents and following surgery. Thrombos. Res. 6: 205–207 (1975).

251. Fleischman, A.I., Bierenbaum, M.L., Justice, D., Stier, A., Sullivan, A. and Fleischman, M.: Titrating dietary linoleate to in vivo platelet function in man. Am. J. Clin. Nutr. 28: 601–605 (1975).

252. Fleischman, A.I., Justice, D., Bierenbaum, M.L., Stier, A. and Sullivan, A.: Beneficial effect of increased dietary linoleate upon in vivo platelet function in man. J. Nutr. 105: 1286–1290 (1975).

253. Fleischman, A.I., Bierenbaum, M.L. and Stier, A.: Effect of stress due to anticipated minor surgery upon in vivo platelet aggregation in humans. J. Human Stress, 2: 33–37 (1976).

254. Fleischman, A.I., Bierenbaum, M.L., Stier, A., Somol, H. and Watson, P.B.: In vivo platelet function in diabetes mellitus. Thrombos. Res. 9: 467–471 (1976).

255. Fogelman, A.M., Schechter, I., Seager, J., Hokom, M., Child, J.S. and Edwards, P.A.: Platelet production of pathological LDL. In: Atherosclerosis V, Gotto, A.M. Jr., Smith, L.C., and Allen, B. (eds), New York, Springer-Verlag, 1980, pp. 787–790.

256. Folco, G., Granström, E. and Kindahl, H.: Albumin stabilizes thromboxane A_2. FEBS Letts. 82: 321–324 (1977).

257. Folts, J.D., Crowell, E.B. Jr. and Rowe, G.G.: Platelet aggregation in partially obstructed vessels and its elimination with aspirin. Circulation 54: 365–370 (1976).

258. Fong, J.S.C.: Alpha-tocopherol: its inhibition of human platelet aggregation. Experientia 32: 639–641 (1976).

259. French, J.E.: The fine structure of experimental thrombi. In: Sherry, S., Brinkhous, K.M., Genton, E. and Stengle, J.M. (eds): Thrombosis. National Acad. Sci. Washington, 1969, pp. 300–320.

260. Freuchen, P.: Om Sundhedstilstanden blandt Polareskimoerne. Ugeskr. Laeg 77: 1089–1108 (1915) cited in ref. 28.

261. Friedberg, C.K. and Horn, H: Acute myocardial infarction not due to coronary artery occlusion. JAMA 112: 1675–1679 (1939).

262. Friedman, L.I., Lien, H., Grabowski, E.F., Leonard, E.F. and McCord, C.W.: Inconsequentiality of surface properties of initial platelet adhesion. Trans. Am. Soc. Artif. Int. Org. 16: 63–76 (1970).

263. Friedman, M. and Byers, S.O.: Experimental thrombo-atherosclerosis. J. Clin. Invest. 40: 1139–1152 (1961).

264. Friedman, M., Manwaring, J.H., Roseman, R.H., Donlon, G., Ortega, P. and Grube, S.M.: Instantaneous and sudden deaths. Clinical and pathological differentiation in coronary artery disease. JAMA 225: 1319–1328 (1973).

265. Friedman, R.J., Moore, S., Singal, D.P. and Gent, M.: Regression of injury-induced atheromatous lesions in rabbits. Arch. Path. Lab. Med. 100: 189–195 (1976).

266. Friedman, R.J., Stemerman, M.B., Wenz, B., Moore, S., Gauldie, J., Gent, M., Tiell, M.L. and Spaet, T.H.: The effect of thromboytopenia on experimental arteriosclerotic lesion formation in rabbits. Smooth muscle cell proliferation and re-endothelialization. J. Clin. Invest. 60: 1191–1201 (1977).

267. Friedman, Z., Seyberth, H., Lamberth, E.L. and Oates, J.: Decreased prostaglandin E turnover in infants with essential fatty acid deficiency. Pediat. Res. 12: 711–714 (1978).

268. Friedman, Z. and Frölich, J.C.: Essential fatty acids and the major urinary metabolites of the E prostaglandins in thriving neonates and in infants receiving parenteral fat emulsions. Pediat. Res.

13: 932–936 (1979).

269. Friedman, Z. and Oates, J.: Effects of dietary variation in linoleic acid content on platelet aggregation and the major urinary metabolites of the E prostaglandins (PGE-M) in infants. In: Hegyeli, R.J. (ed) Prostaglandins and Cardiovascular Disease. Raven Press, New York, 1981, pp. 69–80.

270. Frink, R.J., Trowbridge, J.O. and Rooney, P.A. Jr.: Nonobstructive coronary thrombosis in sudden cardiac death. Am. J. Cardiol. 42: 48–51 (1978).

271. Frost, H.: Zur Pathogenese obliterierender Arterienprozesse bei Hypercholesterinämie. Thromb. Diath. Haemorrh. 22: 351–359 (1969).

272. Fry, D.L.: Acute vascular endothelial changes associated with increased blood velocity gradients. Circ. Res. 22: 165–197 (1968).

273. Fukami, H.M., Holsen, H. and Bauer, J.: Thrombin-induced oxygen consumption, malondialdehyde formation and serotonin-secretion in human platelets. Biochim. Biophys. Acta 428: 253–256 (1976).

274. Fulton, W.F.M.: Coronary thrombosis in myocardial infarction. In: Acute and Long-term Medical Management of Myocardial Ischemia. Hjalmarson, A. and Wilhelmsen, L. (eds). Mölndal, Sweden, Lindgren and Soner AB, 1978, p. 59–69.

275. Fulton, W.F.M.: Coronary thrombotic occlusion in myocardial infarction and thrombus in the pathogenesis of atherosclerosis. In: Carlson, L.A., Paoletti, R., Sirtori, C.R. and Weber, G. (eds): International conference on atherosclerosis. Raven Press, New York, 1978, pp. 75–89.

276. Fuster, V. and Bowie, E.J.W.: The von Willebrand pig as a model for atherosclerosis research. Thromb. Haemostas. 39: 322–327 (1978).

277. Fuster, V., Bowie, E.J.W., Lewis, J.C., Fass, D.N., Owen, C.A. Jr. and Brown, A.L. Jr.: Resistance to arteriosclerosis in pigs with von Willebrand's disease. J. Clin. Invest. 61: 722–730 (1978).

278. Fuster, V., Bowie, E.J.W. and Fass, D.N.: Atherosclerosis in homozygous and heterozygous von Willebrand pigs fed a high cholesterol diet. Circulation 60 (Suppl. II): 272 (1979) (Abstract no. 1062).

279. Fuster, V., Bowie, E.J.W., Fass, D.N. and Owen, C.A. Jr.: Long-term prospective study on spontaneous atherosclerosis in normal and von Willebrand pigs. Circulation 60 (Suppl. II): 271 (1979) (Abstract no. 1061).

280. de Gaetano, G., Livio, M., Donati, M.B. and Remuzzi, G.: Platelet and vascular prostaglandins in uraemia, thrombotic microangiopathy and pre-eclampsia. Phil. Trans. Roy. Soc. Lond. [Biol] 294: 339–342 (1981).

281. Galli, C., Petroni, A., Socini, A., Agradi, E., Colombo, C. Folco, G.C. and Tremoli, E.: Platelet-vessel wall interactions: effects of platelets and plasma on the antiaggregatory activity and 6 keto-$PGF_{1\alpha}$ production in isolated perfused aortas. Prostaglandins 22: 703–713 (1981).

282. Galli, C., Spagnuolo, C., Bosisio, E., Tosi, L., Folco, C. and Galli, G.: Dietary essential fatty acids, polyunsaturated fatty acids and prostaglandins in the central nervous system. Adv. Prost. Thromb. Res. 4: 181–189 (1978).

283. Galli, C., Agradi, E., Petroni, A. and Tremoli, E.: Dietary essential fatty acids, tissue fatty acids and prostaglandin synthesis. Progr. Fd. Nutr. Sci. 4: 1–7 (1980).

284. Galli, C., Agradi, E., Petroni, A. and Tremoli, E.: Differential effects of dietary fatty acids on the accumulation of arachidonic acid and its metabolic conversion through the cyclooxygenase and lipoxygenase in platelets and vascular tissue. Lipids 16: 165–172 (1981).

285. Geer, J.C., McGill, H.C. Jr. and Strong, J.P.: The fine structure of human atherosclerotic lesions. Am. J Path. 38: 263–287 (1961).

286. Geer, J.C. and Haust, M.D.: Smooth muscle cells in atherogenesis. Basel, S. Karger, 1972.

287. Geill, T. and Dybkaer, R.: The effect of linolenic acid orally on platelet adhesiveness and fibrinogen concentration. Scand. J. Clin. Lab. Invest. 23: 256–258 (1969).

288. Geiringer, E.: Intimal vascularization and atherosclerosis. J. Path. Bact. 63: 201–211 (1951).

289. Gent, C.M. van, Luten, J.B., Bronsgeest-Schoute, H.C. and Ruiter, A.: Effect, on serum lipid

levels of ω-3 fatty acids, of ingesting fish-oil concentrate. Lancet, ii: 1249–1250 (1979).

290. Genton, E.: A perspective on platelet-suppressant drug treatment in coronary artery and cerebrovascular disease. Circulation 62 (Suppl. V): 111–121 (1980).

291. Gerrard, J.M., White, J.G. and Krivitt, W.: Labile aggregation-stimulating substance, free fatty acids and platelet aggregation. J. Lab. Clin. Med. 87: 73–82 (1976).

292. Gerrard, J.M., Peterson, D., Townsend, D. and White, J.G.: Prostaglandins and platelet contraction. Circulation 54 (Suppl. II): 196 (1976).

293. Gerrard, J.M., White, J.G., Rao, G.H.R. and Townsend, D.: Localization of platelet prostaglandin production in the platelet dense tubular system. Am. J. Pathol. 83: 283–398 (1976).

294. Gerrard, J.M. cited by Smith, J.B.: Lipid-membrane interaction of platelets and coagulation with the arterial wall. Adv. Exptl. Med. Biol. 104: 343–348 (1977).

295. Gerrard, J.M., Townsend, D., Staddard, S., Witkop, C.J. Jr. and White, J.G.: The influence of prostaglandin G_2 on platelet ultrastructure and platelet secretion. Am. J. Pathol. 86: 99–116 (1977).

296. Gerrard, J.M., Kindom, S.E., Peterson, D.A., Peller, J., Krantz, K.E. and White, J.G.: Lysophosphatidic acids. Influence on platelet aggregation and intracellular calcium flux. Am. J. Pathol. 96: 423–438 (1979).

297. Glynn, M.F., Murphy, E.A. and Mustard, J.F.: Effect of clofibrate on platelet economy in man. Lancet ii: 447–448 (1967).

298. Goetzl, E.J., Woods, J.M. and Gorman, R.R.: Stimulation of human eosinophil and neutrophil polymorphonuclear leucocyte chemotaxis and random migration by 12-L-hydroxy-5,8,10,14-eicosatetraenoic acid. J. Clin. Invest. 59: 179–183 (1977).

299. Goodfellow, C.F., Paton, R.C., Moncada, S., Salmon, J.A., Davies, J.A. and McNicol, G.P.: Prostaglandins and uterine bleeding. Thromb. Haemostas. 46: 274 (1981).

299a. Goodnight, S.H., Harris, W.S. and Connor, W.E.: The effects of dietary ω-3 fatty acids on platelet composition and function in man: a prospective, controlled study. Blood 58: 880–885 (1981).

300. Gorman, R.R., Bunting, S. and Miller, O.V.: Modulation of human platelet adenyl cyclase by prostacyclin. Prostaglandins 13: 377–388 (1977).

301. Gorman, R.R. Fitzpatric, F.A. and Miller, O.V.: Reciprocal regulation of human platelet cAMP levels by Thromboxane A_2 and prostacyclin. Adv. Cycl. Nucl. Res. 9: 597–609 (1978).

302. Gorman, R.R.: Modulation of human platelet function by prostacyclin and thromboxane A_2. Fed. Proc. 38: 83–88 (1979).

303. Gorman, R.R., Wierenga, W. and Miller, O.V.: Independence of the cyclic AMP-lowering activity thromboxane A_2 from the platelet release reaction. Biochim. Biophys. Acta 572: 95–104 (1979).

304. Gorman, R.R. and Hopkins, N.K.: Agonist-specific desensitization of PGI_2-stimulated cyclic AMP accumulation by PGE_1 in human foreskin fibroblasts. Prostaglandins 19: 2–16 (1980).

305. Gospodarowicz, D.: Purification of a fibroblast growth factor from bovine pituitary. J. Biol. Chem. 250: 2515–2520 (1975).

306. Gospodarowicz, D. and Moran, J.S.: Mitogenic effect of fibroblast growth factor on early passage cultures of human and murine fibroblasts. J. Cell Biol. 66: 451–457 (1975).

307. Gottenbos, J.J. and Thomasson, H.J.: Aorta atheromatosis in rabbits on feeding cholesterol or fats. Coll. Int. Centr. Nat. Rech. Sci. 99: 221–239 (1961).

308. Gould, S.E.: Pathology of the heart and blood vessels. Thomas, Springfield, Ill., 1968.

309. Griggs, T.R., Reddick, R.L., Sultzer, D. and Brinkhous, K.M.: Susceptibility to atherosclerosis in aortas and coronary arteries of swine with von Willebrand's disease. Am. J. Path. 102: 137–145 (1981).

310. Gromnatskii, N.I.: Viscous metamorphosis of platelets and functional changes in the blood clotting system under influence of alimentary lipemia. Bull. Exp. Biol. Med. USSR 71: 518–519 (1971).

311. Gross, R. and Schneider, W.: Energy metabolism in: Johnson, S.A. (ed.) The Circulating Platelet. Academic Press, New York & London, 1971, p.p. 123–188.

312. Gröttum, K.A.: Influence of aggregating agents on electrophoretic mobility of blood platelets from healthy individuals and from patients with cardiovascular diseases. Lancet i: 1406–1408 (1968).

313. Gryglewski, R.J., Bunting, S., Moncada, S., Flower, R.J. and Vane, J.R.: Arterial walls are protected against deposition of platelet thrombi by a substance (PGX) which they make from prostaglandin edoperoxides. Prostaglandins 12: 685–713 (1976).

314. Gryglewski, R.J., Korbut, R. and Ocetkiewicz, A.C.: Generation of prostacyclin by lungs in vivo and its release into the arterial circulation. Nature 273: 765–767 (1978).

315. Gryglewski, R.J., Salmon, J.A., Ubatuba, F.B., Weatherly, B.C., Moncada, S. and Vane, J.R.: Effect of all cis 5, 8, 11, 14, 17 eicosapentaenoic acid and PGH_3 on platelet aggregation. Prostaglandins 18: 453–478 (1979).

316. Gryglewski, R.J., Slpawinski, J. and Korbut, R.: Endogenous mechanisms that regulate prostacyclin release. Adv. Prost. Thromb. Res. 7: 777–785 (1980).

317. Gudbjarnason, S.: Prostaglandins and polyunsaturated fatty acids in heart muscle. J. Mol. Cell. Cardiol. 7: 443–449 (1975).

318. Gudbjarnason, S. and Hallgrimsson, J.: The role of myocardial membrane lipids in the development of cardiac necrosis. Acta Med. Scand. (Suppl. 587): 17–27 (1976).

319. Gudbjarnason, S.: Pathophysiology of long-chain polyenoic fatty acids in heart muscle. Nutr. Metabol. 24 (Suppl. 1): 142–146 (1980).

320. Gunning, A.J., Pickering, G.W., Robb-Smith, A.H.T. and Russell, R.R.: Mural thrombosis of the internal carotid artery and subsequent embolism. Q J. Med. 33: 155–195 (1964).

321. Haerem, J.W.: Sudden coronary death: the occurrence of platelet aggregates in the epicardial arteries of man. Atherosclerosis 14: 417–432 (1971).

322. Haerem, J.W.: Platelet aggregates in intramyocardial vessels of patients dying suddenly and unexpectedly of coronary artery disease. Atherosclerosis 15: 199–213 (1972).

323. Haerem, J.W.: Mural platelet microthrombi and major acute lesions of main epicardial arteries in sudden coronary death. Atherosclerosis 19: 529–541 (1974).

324. Haerem, J.W.: Platelet aggregates and mural microthrombi in the early stages of acute, fatal coronary disease. Thrombos. Res. 5: 243–249 (1974).

325. Haerem, J.W.: Sudden, unexpected coronary death. Acta Path. Microbiol. Scand., Sect. A. (Suppl. 265): 1–47 (1978).

326. Haertly, G.S. (1936) cited in Gitler, C.: Plasticity of biological membranes. Ann. Rev. Biophys. Bioeng. 1: 51–92 (1972).

327. Haft, J.I. and Fani, K.: Intravascular platelet aggregation in the heart, induced by stress. Circulation 47: 353–358 (1973).

327a. Hal ushka, P.V., Rogers, R.C., Loadholt, C.B. and Colwell, J.A.: Increased platelet thromboxane synthesis in diabetes mellitus. J. Lab. Clin. Med. 97: 87–96 (1981).

328. Hamazaki, T., Hirai, A., Terano, T., Sajiki, J., Kondo, S., Fujita, T., Tamura, Y. and Kumagai, A.: Effects of orally administered ethyl ester of eicosapentaenoic acid (EPA; C20:5ω3) on PGI_2-like substance production by rat aorta. Prostaglandins 23: 557–568 (1982).

329. Hamazaki, T., Hirai, A., Terano, T., Tamura, Y., Kumagai, A. and Sajiki, J.: Oral administration of eicosapentaenoic acid (EPA) stimulates production of prostacyclin by rat aorta. Thromb. Haemostas. 46: 179 (1981).

330. Hamberg, M. and Samuelsson, B.: Detection and isolation of an endoperoxide intermediate in prostaglandin biosynthesis. Proc. Natl. Acad. Sci. USA 70: 899–903 (1973).

331. Hamberg, M. and Samuelsson, B.: Prostaglandin endoperoxides. Novel transformations of arachidonic acid in human platelets. Proc. Natl. Acad. Sci. USA 71: 3400–3404 (1974).

332. Hamberg, M., Svensson, J. and Samuelsson, B.: Prostaglandin endoperoxides. A new concept concerning the mode of action and release of prostaglandins. Proc. Natl. Acad. Sci. USA 71: 3824–3828 (1974).

333. Hamberg, M., Svensson, J. and Samuelsson, B.: Thromboxanes, a new group of biologically active

compounds derived from prostaglandin endoperoxides. Proc. Natl. Acad. Sci. USA 72: 2994–2998 (1975).

334. Hamberg, M.: Transformations of 5, 8, 11, 14, 17-eicosapentaenoic acid in human platelets. Biochim. Biophys. Acta 618: 389–398 (1980).

335. Hammarström, S. and Falardeau, P.: Resolution of prostaglandin endoperoxide synthase and thromboxane synthase of human platelets. Proc. Natl. Acad. Sci. USA 74: 3691–3695 (1977).

336. Hammarström, S. and Diczfalusy, U.: Biosynthesis of Thromboxanes. Adv. Prost. Thromb. Res. 6: 267–274 (1980).

337. Hampton, J.R. and Mitchell, J.R.A.: A transferable factor causing abnormal platelet behaviour in vasular disease. Lancet ii: 764–768 (1966).

338. Hand, R.A. and Chandler, A.B.: Atherosclerotic metamorphosis of autologous pulmonary thromboemboli in the rabbit. Am. J. Pathol. 40: 469–486 (1962).

339. Hansen, P.F.T., Geill, T., and Lund, E.: Dietary fats and thrombosis. Lancet ii: 1193–1194 (1962).

340. Hansen, A.E., Stewart, R.A., Hughes, G. and Söderhjelm, L.: Relation of linoleic acid to infant feeding: a review. Acta Paediat. 51 (Suppl. 137) 1962.

341. Hardisty, R.M. and Hutton, R.A.: Platelet aggregation and the availability of platelet factor 3. Br. J. Haematol. 12: 764–776 (1966).

342. Harker, L.A., Slichter, S.J., Scott, C.R.: Homocysteinemia: vascular injury and arterial thrombosis. N Engl. J. Med. 291: 537–543 (1974).

343. Harker, L.A., Ross, R., Slichter, S.J. and Scott, C.R.: Homocystine-induced arteriosclerosis. The role of endothelial cell injury and platelet response in its genesis. J. Clin. Invest. 58: 731–741 (1976).

344. Harland, W.A. and Holburn, A.M.: Coronary thrombosis and myocardial infarction. Lancet ii: 1158–1159 (1966).

344a. Harris, W.S., Connor, W.E. and Goodnight, S.H. Jr.: Dietary fish oils, plasma lipids and platelets in man. Progr. Lip. Res. 20: 75–79 (1981).

345. Hársfalvi, J., Muszbek, L., Stadler, I. and Fésüs, L.: Inhibition of platelet factor 3 availability by prostacyclin. Prostaglandins 20: 935–945 (1980).

346. Haslam, R.J. and McClenaghan, M.D.: An assay for activators of platelet adenylate cyclase present in rabbit blood: Evidence that prostacyclin (PGI$_2$) is not a circulating hormone. Thromb. Haemostas. 42: 117 (1979).

346a. Haslam, R.J. and McClenaghan, M.D.: Measurement of circulating prostacyclin. Nature 292: 364–366 (1981).

347. Haust, M.D., Movat, H.Z. and More, R.H.: The role of fibrin thrombi in the genesis of the common white plaque in arteriosclerosis. Circulation 14: 483 (1956).

348. Haust, M.D., More, R.H., Movat, H.Z.: The mechanism of fibrosis in arteriosclerosis. Am. J. Path. 35: 265–273 (1959).

349. Haust, M.D., More, R.H. and Movat, H.Z.: The role of smooth muscle cells in the fibrogenesis of arteriosclerosis. Am. J Path. 37: 377–389 (1960).

350. Haust, M.D.: The morphogenesis and fate of potential and early atherosclerotic lesions in man. Hum. Path. 2: 1–29 (1971).

351. Hawkey, C.W. and Symons, C.: Variation in ADP-induced platelet aggregation in vitro in primates as a result of differences in plasma ADP inhibitor levels. Thrombos. Diathes. haemorrh. 19: 29–35 (1968).

352. Hayashida, T. and Portman, O.W.: Swelling of liver mitochondria from rats fed diets deficient in essential fatty acids. Proc. Soc. Exptl. Biol. Med. 103: 656–659 (1960).

353. Heard, B.E.: An experimental study of thickening of pulmonary arteries of rabbits produced by organization of fibrin. J. Path. Bact. 64: 13–19 (1952).

354. Hellem, A.J.: The adhesiveness of human blood platelets in vitro. Scand. J. Clin. Invest. 12 (Suppl. 51) (1960).

355. Hellem, A.J., Ödegaard, A.E. and Skålhegg, B.A.: Investigations on adenosine diphosphate (ADP) induced platelat adhesiveness in vitro. Thromb. Diath. Haemorrh. 10: 61–70 (1963).

356. Hemker, H.C.: Unpublished results.
357. Hemker, H.C., Muller, A.D. and Gonggrijp, R.: The estimation of activated human blood coagulation factor VII. J. Mol. Med. 1: 127–134 (1976).
358. Henry, R.L.: Methods for inducing experimental thrombosis. An annotated bibliography. Angiology, Baltimore 13: 554–557 (1962).
359. Henry, R.L.: Effect of pyridinolcarbamate on specific components of hemostasis in Crutz's model. In: Shimamoto, T. and Numano, F. (eds): Atherogenesis. Excerpta Medica, Amsterdam, 1969, pp. 75–81.
360. Hensby, C.N., Barnes, P.J., Dollery, C.T. and Dargie, H.: Production of 6-oxo-PGF$_{1\alpha}$ by human lung in vivo. Lancet ii: 1162–1163 (1979).
361. Hensen, A. and Loeliger, E.A.: Antithrombin III: Its metabolism and its function in blood coagulation. Thromb. Diathes. Haemorrh. 9 (Suppl. 1): 1–84 (1963).
362. Henson, P.M. and Pinckard, R.N.: Platelet-activating factor (PAF). A possible direct mediator of anaphylaxis in the rabbit and a trigger for the vascular deposition of circulating immune complexes. Monogr. Allergy. 12: 13–26 (1977).
363. Heyden, S.: Epidemiological data on dietary fat intake and atherosclerosis with an appendix on possible side-effects. In: Vergroesen, A.J. (ed): The Role of Fats in Human Nutrition. Academic Press London, New York, 1975, pp. 43–113.
364. Heyns, A. du P., van den Berg, D.J., Potgieter, G.M. and Retief, F.P.: The inhibition of platelet aggregation by an aorta intima extract. Thromb. Diathes. haemorrh. 32: 417–431 (1974).
365. Heyns, A. du P., Badenhorst, C.J. and Retief, F.P.: ADP-ase activity of normal and atherosclerotic human aortic intima. Thromb. Haemost. 37: 429–435 (1977).
366. Heyns, A. du P., Badenhorst, C.J. and Retief, F.P.: A stable non-prostaglandin inhibitor of platelet aggregation in human aorta intima extracts. SA Med. J. 55: 908–910 (1979).
367. Hirai, A., Hamazaki, T., Nishikawa, T., Tamura, Y., Kumagai, A. and Sajiki, J.: Eicosapentaenoic acid and platelet function in Japanese. Lancet ii: 1132–1133 (1980).
368. Hirsh, P.D., Hillis, L.D., Campbell, W.B., Firth, B.G. and Willerson, J.T.: Release of prostaglandins and thromboxane into the coronary circulating in patients with ischemic heart disease. N Engl. J. Med. 304: 685–691 (1981).
369. Hissen, W., Fleming, J.S., Bierwagen, M.E. and Pindell, M.H.: Effect of prostaglandin E$_1$ on platelet aggregation in vitro and in hemorrhagic shock. Microvasc. Res. 1: 374–378 (1969).
370. Hoak, J.C., Poole, J.C.F. and Robinson, D.S.: Thrombosis associated with mobilization of fatty acids. Am. J. Pathol. 43: 987–997 (1963).
371. Hoak, J.C., Spector, A.A., Fry, G.L. and Warner, E.D.: Effect of free fatty acids on ADP-induced aggregation. Nature (London) 228: 1330–1332 (1970).
372. Hoak, J.C., Spector, A.A., Fry, G.L. and Barnes, B.C.: Localization of free fatty acids taken up by human platelets. Blood 40: 16–22 (1972).
373. Hohage, R., Hiemeyer, V.: Methodische Untersuchungen zur Plättchen-aggregation bei der Ratte: 1. Verwendbarkeit für rekalzifizierten Zitrat-Heparin-Plasma im Rahmen tierexperimenteller Untersuchungen. Thrombos. Diathes. Haemorrh. 26: 393–398 (1971).
374. Holman, R.T.: The ratio of trienoic: tetraenoic acids in tissue lipids as a measure of essential fatty acid requirement. J. Nutr. 70: 405–409 (1960).
375. Holman, R.T.: Essential fatty acid deficiency. In: Holman, R.T. (ed): Progress in the Chemistry of Fats and Other Lipids. Vol. 9. No. 2, Pergamon Press, London, 1971, pp. 275–348.
376. Holman, R.T.: Essential fatty acid deficiency in humans. In: Galli, C., Jacini, G. and Pecile, A. (eds): Dietary Lipids and Postnatal Development. Raven Press, New York, 1973, pp. 127–143.
377. Holman, R.T.: Effect of dietary *trans* fatty acids upon prostaglandin precursors in: Beers, R.F. Jr. and Bassett, E.G. (eds.): Nutritional Factors: Modulating Effects on Metabolic Processes. Raven Press, New York, 1981, pp. 523–537.
378. Holmsen, H.: Platelet secretion. Current concepts and methodological aspects in: Day, H.J., Holmsen, H. and Zucker, M.B. (eds) Platelet function testing. DHEW Publication No (NIH)

78–1087, US Department of Health, Education and Welfare, 1978, pp. 112–132.

379. Hong, S.L. and Levine, L.: Stimulation of prostaglandin synthesis by bradykinin and thrombin and their mechanisms of action on MC 5–5 fibroblasts. J. Biol. Chem. 251: 5814–5816 (1976).

380. Hong, S.L.: Effect of bradykinin and thrombin on prostacyclin synthesis in endothelial cells from calf and pig aorta and human umbilical cord vein. Thromb. Res. 18: 787–785 (1980).

381. Hoover, R.L., Lynch, R.D., Karnovsky, M.J.: Decrease in adhesion of cells cultured in polyunsaturated fatty acids. Cell 12: 295–300 (1977).

382. Hope W., Martin, T.J., Chesterman, C.N. and Morgan, F.J.: Human β-thromboglobulin inhibits PGI_2 production and binds to specific site in bovine aortic endothelial cells. Nature 282: 210–212 (1979).

383. Horlick, L.: Platelet adhesiveness in normal persons and subjects with atherosclerosis. Effect of high fat meals and anticoagulants on the adhesive index. Am. J. Cardiol. 8: 459–470 (1961).

384. Horn, H., Finkelstein, L.E.: Arteriosclerosis of the coronary arteries and the mechanism of their occlusion. Am Heart J. 19: 655–682 (1940).

385. Hornstra, G.: Method to determine the degree of ADP-induced platelet aggregation in circulating rat blood ('Filter-loop technique'). Br. J. Haematol. 19: 321–329 (1970).

386. Hornstra, G.: Degree and duration of prostaglandin E_1-induced inhibition of platelet aggregation in the rat. Eur. J Pharmacol. 15: 343–349 (1971).

387. Hornstra, G.: The influence of dietary sunflowerseed oil and hardened coconut oil in intra-arterial occlusive thrombosis in rats. Nutr. Metabol. 13: 140–149 (1971).

388. Hornstra, G., Chait, A., Karvonen, M.J., Lewis, B., Turpeinen, O., Vergroesen, A.J.: Influence of dietary fat on platelet function in men. Lancet i: 1155–1157 (1973).

389. Hornstra, G. and Vendelmans-Starrenburg, A.: Induction of experimental arterial occlusive thrombi in rats. Atherosclerosis 17: 369–382 (1973).

390. Hornstra, G.: Dietary fats and arterial thrombosis. Haemostas 2: 21–52 (1973/1974).

391. Hornstra, G. and Haddeman, E.: Prostaglandins, essential fatty acids, platelet function and thrombosis. Thromb. Res. 4 (Suppl. 1): 91–92 (1974).

392. Hornstra, G. and ten Hoor, F.: The filtragometer: a new device for measuring platelet aggregation in venous blood of man. Thromb. Diathes. Haemorrh. 34: 531–544 (1975).

393. Hornstra, G. and Lussenburg, R.N.: Relationship between the type of dietary fatty acid and arterial thrombosis tendency in rats. Atherosclerosis 22: 499–516 (1975).

394. Hornstra, G.: The filtragometer in thrombosis research. In: Day, H.J., Holmsen, H. and Zucker, M.B., eds.: Platelet Function Testing. DHEW Publication (no. NIH) 78–1087. US Department of health, education and welfare, Public Health Service, National Institute of Health, 1978, pp. 416–427.

395. Hornstra, G. and Haddeman, E.: Diet-induced changes in arterial thrombosis not primarily mediated by arachidonate peroxidation. Biblthca Haemat. 45: 9–13 (1978).

396. Hornstra, G., Haddeman, E. and Don, J.A.: Some investigations into the role of prostacyclin in thromboregulation. Thromb. Res. 12: 367–374 (1978).

397. Hornstra, G., Haddeman, E. and Don, J.A.: Blood platelets do not provide endoperoxides for vascular prostacyclin production. Nature 279: 66–68 (1979).

398. Hornstra, G. and Hemker, H.C.: Clot promoting effect of platelet-vessel wall interaction: influence of dietary fats in relation to arterial thrombus formation in rats. Haemostasis 8: 211–226 (1979).

399. Hornstra, G.: New experimental models for the investigation of arterial thrombosis tendency and platelet aggregability. In: Hornstra, G.: Dietary fats and arterial thrombosis. Thesis. Maastricht, the Netherlands, 1980, pp. 92–156.

400. Hornstra, G.: Platelet-vessel wall interaction: role of blood clotting. Phil. Trans. Roy. Soc. Lond. [Biol] 294: 355–371 (1981).

401. Hornstra, G., Christ-Hazelhof, E., Haddeman, E., ten Hoor, F. and Nugteren, D.H.: Fish oil feeding lowers thromboxane and prostacyclin production by rat platelets and aorta and does not

result in the formation of prostaglandin I_3. Prostaglandins 21: 727–738 (1981).

402. Horton, E.W.: Molecular insight into thrombosis: Nature 263: 637 (1976).

403. Houtsmuller. A.J., van Hal-Ferwerda, J., Zahn, K.J. and Henkes, H.E.: Favourable influences of linoleic acid on the progression of diabetic micro-and macro-angiopathy. Nutr. Metabol. 24 (Suppl. 1): 105–118 (1980).

404. Houtsmuller, U.M.T.: Differentiation in the biological activity of polyunsaturated fatty acids. In: Galli, C., Jacini, G. and Pecile, A. (eds): Dietary Lipids and Postnatal Development. Raven Press,New York, 1973, pp. 145–155.

405. Houtsmuller, U.M.T.: Biochemical properties of *trans*-fatty acids. Proc. 13th World Congress ISF, Symp. 3, pp. 79–97, ITERG, Paris (1976).

406. Houtsmuller, U.M.T.: Columbinic acid, a new type of essential fatty acid. Progr. Lipid Res. 20: 889–896 (1981).

407. Hovig, T., Jørgensen, L., Rowsell, H.C. and Mustard, J.F.: The structure of thrombus-like deposits formed in extra corporeal shunts. Am. J. Path. 59: 75–99 (1970).

408. Howard, A.N. and Gresham, G.A.: The dietary induction of thrombosis and myocardial infarction. J. Atheroscler. Res. 4: 40–56 (1964).

409. Howard, A.N., Gresham, G.A. and Lindgren, F.T.: Lipoportein studies on rats fed thrombogenic and atherogenic diets. J. Atheroscler. Res. 8: 739–743 (1968).

410. Howard, C.F.Jr.: The relationship of diet and atherosclerosis in diabetic *Macaca nigra*. Adv. Exp. Med. biol. 60: 13–31 (1975).

411. Hwang, D.H. and Kinsella, J.E.: The effects of trans linoleic acid on the concentration of serum prostaglandin $F_{2\alpha}$ and platelet function. Prost. Med. 1: 121–130 (1978).

412. Hwang, D.H. and Kinsella, J.E.: The effects of trans trans methyl linoleate on the concentration of prostaglandins and their precursors in rat. Prostaglandins 17: 543–559 (1978).

413. Hwang, D.H. and Carrol, A.E.: Decreased formation of prostaglandin derived from arachidonic acid by dietary linolenate in rats. Am. J. Clin. Nutr. 33: 590–597 (1980).

414. Imai, S. and Matsubara, I.: Effects of prostacyclin on platelet aggregation as studied with 'Filter-loop' technique in the flowing blood of the dog. Artery 8: 63–72 (1980).

415. Ingerman, C.M., Smith, J.B., Shapiro, S., Sedar, A. and Silver, M.J.: Hereditary adnormality of platelet aggregation attributable to nucletde storage pool deficiency. Blood 52: 332–344 (1978).

416. Ingerman-Wojenski, C., Silver, M.J., Smith, J.B., Nissenbaum, M. and Sedar, A.W.: Prostacyclin production in rabbit arteries in situ: inhibition by arachidonic acid-indiced endothelial cell damage or by low-dose aspirin. Prostaglandins 21: 655–666 (1981).

417. International anticoagulant review group. Collaborative analysis of longterm anticoagulant administration after acute myocardial infaction. Lancet i: 203–209 (1970).

418. Isakson, P.C., Raz, A., Denny, S.E., Pure, E. and Needleman, P.: A novel prostaglandin is the major product of arachidonic acid metabolism in rabbit heart. Proc. Natl. Acad. Sci. USA 74: 101–105 (1977).

419. Jackson, R.L., Taunton, O.D., Morrisett, J.D. and Gotto, A.M. Jr.: The role of dietary polyunsaturated fat in lowering blood cholesterol in man. Circ. Res. 42: 447–453 (1978).

420. Jaffe, E.A., Minick, C.R., Adelman, B., Becker, C.G., Nachman, R.: Synthesis of basement membrane collagen by cultured human endothelial cells. J. Exp. Med. 144: 209–225 (1976).

421. Jaffe, E.A. and Weksler, B.B.: Recovery of endothelial cell prostacyclin production after inhibition by low dose of aspirin. J. Clin. Invest. 63: 532–535 (1979).

422. Jager, F.C.: Linoleic acid intake and vitamin E requirement. In: Vergroesen A.J. (ed): The role of fats in human nutrition. Acad. Press, London, New York, 1975, p. 381–432.

423. Jager, F.C.: High linoleic acid intake and Vitamin E requirement in rats. Nutr. Dieta 11: 270–279 (1969).

424. Jakobson, K. and Papahadjopoulos, D.: Phase transitions and phase separations in phospholipid membranes induced by changes in temperature, pH and concentraton of bivalent cations. Biochemistry 14: 152–161 (1975).

425. Jakubowski, J.A. and Ardlie, N.G.: Modification of human platelet function by a diet enriched in saturated or polyunsatured fat. Atherosclerosis 31: 335–344 (1978).

426. Jakubowski, J.A. and Ardlie, N.G.: Evidence for the mechanism by which eicosapentaenoic acid inhibits human platelet aggregation and secretion – implications for the prevention of vascular disease. Thromb. Res. 16: 205–217 (1979).

427. Jeffcoat, R.: The biosynthesis of unsaturated fatty acids and its control in mammalian liver. In: Campbell,P.N. (ed): Essays in Biochemistry 15: 1–36 (1980).

428. Johnson, M., Reece, A.H. and Harrison, H.E.: An inbalance in arachidonic acid metabolism in diabetes. Adv. Prost. Thromb. Res. 8: 1283–1286 (1980).

429. Johnson, R.A., Morton, D.R., Kinner, J.H., Gorman, R.R., McGuire, J.C., Sun, F.F., Whittaker, N., Bunting, S. and Salmon, J.: The chemical structure of prostaglandin X (Prostacyclin) Prostaglandins 12: 915–928 (1976).

430. Joist, J.H., Dolezel, G., Lloyd, J.V., Kinlough-Rathbone, R.L. and Mustard, J.F.: Platelet factor-3 availability and the platelet release reaction. J. Lab. Clin. Med. 84: 474–482 (1974).

431. Joist, J.H., Dolezel, G., Lloyd, J.V. and Mustard, J.F.: Phospholipid transfer between plasma and platelets in vitro. Blood 48: 199–211 (1976).

432. Joist, J.H., Dolezel, G., Cucuianu, M.P., Nishizawa, E.E. and Mustard, J.F.: Inhibition and potentiation of platelet function by lysolecithin. Blood 49: 101–112 (1977).

433. Joist, J.H., Baker, R.K. and Schonfeld, G.: Increased in vivo and in vitro platelet function in type II- and type IV-hyperlipoproteinemia. Thromb. Res. 15: 95–108 (1979).

434. Jones, D.,Gresham, G.A., Lloyd, H.G. and Howard, A.N.: Yellow fat in the wild rabbit. Nature 207: 205–206 (1965).

435. Jones, R.L., Kerry, P.J., Poyser, N.L., Walker, I.C. and Wilson, N.H.: The identification of trihydroxyeicosatrienoic acids as products from the incubation of arachidonic acid with washed blood platelets. Prostaglandins 16: 853–589 (1978).

436. Jørgensen, L., Rowsell, H.C., Hovig, T., Glynn, M.F. and Mustard, J.F.: Adenosine diphosphate-induced aggregation and myocardial infarction in swine. Lab. Invest. 17: 616–644 (1967).

437. Jørgensen, L., Rowsell, H.C., Hovig, T. and Mustard, J.F.: Resolution and organization of platelet-rich mural thrombi in carotid arteries of swine. Am. J. Path. 51: 681–719 (1967).

438. Jørgensen, L., Haerem, F., Chandler, A.B. and Borchgrevink, C.F.: The pathology of acute coronary death. Acta Anaesth. Scand. (Suppl. 29): 193–199 (1968).

439. Jørgensen, L., Chandler, A.B. and Borchgrevink, C.F.: Acute lesions of coronary arteries in anticoagulant-treated and in untreated patients. Atherosclerosis 13: 21–44 (1971).

440. Jørgensen, L., Packham, M.A., Rowsell, H.C. and Mustard, J.F.: Deposition of formed elements of blood on the intima and signs of intimal injury in the aorta of rabbit, pig and man. Lab. Invest. 27: 341–350 (1972).

441. Kannagi, R., Koizumi, K., Hata-Tanoue, S. and Masude, T.: Mobilization of arachidonic acid from phosphatidylethanolamine fraction to phosphatidylcholine fraction in platelets. Biochem. Biophys. Res. Comm. 96: 711–718 (1980).

442. Kannel, W.B.: Results of the epidemiologic investigation of ischaemic heart disease: Illustrated by the Framingham study. In: de Haas, Hemker and Snellen (eds.) Ischaemic Heart Disease, University Press, Leiden, 1970, pp. 272–310.

443. Kannel, W.B.: Soms lessons in cardiovascular epidemiology from Framingham. Am. J. Cardiol. 37: 269–282 (1976).

444. Kaplan, K.L., Broekman, M.J., Chernoff, A., Lesznik, G.R. and Drillings, M.: Platelet α-granule proteins: studies on release and subcellular localization. Blood 53: 604–618 (1979).

445. Kaplan, D.R., Chao, F.C., Stiles, C.D., Antoniades, H.N. and Scher, C.D.: Platelet α granules contain a growth factor for fibroblasts. Blood 53: 1043–1052 (1979).

446. Kapp, J.P., Duckert, F. and Hartmann, G.: Platelet adhesiveness and serum lipids during and after Intralipid ®-infusions. Nutr. Metab. 13: 92–99 (1971).

447. Karnovski, M.J.: Lipid domains in biological membranes. Their structural and functional per-

turbation by free fatty acids and the regulation of receptor mobility. Am. J. Pathol. 97: 212–221 (1979).

448. Käser-Glanzmann, R., Jakábová, M., Géorge, J.N. and Lüscher, E.F.: Stimulation of calcium uptake in platelet membrane vesicles by adenosine 3′,5′-cyclic monophosphate and protein kinase. Biochim. Biophys. Acta 466: 429–440 (1977).

449. Kernoff, P.B.A., Willis, A.L., Stone K.J., Davies, J.A. and McNicol, G.P.: Antithrombotic potential of dihomo-gamma-linolenic acid in man. Br. Med. J. 2: 1441–1444 (1977).

450. Kerr, J.W., Pirrie, R., MacAulay, I. and Bronte Stuart, B.: Platelet aggregation by phospholipids and free fatty acids. Lancet i: 1296–1299 (1965).

451. Kim, W.M., Merskey, C., Deming, Q.B., Adel, H.N. and Welinsky, H.: Hyperlipidemia, hyper-coagulability and accelerated thrombosis. Studies in congenitally hyperlipidemic rats and in rats and monkeys with induced hyperlipidemia. Blood 47: 275–285 (1976).

452. Kinlough-Rathbone, R.L., Packham, M.A. and Mustard, J.F.: The effect of prostaglandin E_1 on platelet function in vitro and in vivo. Br. J. Haematol. 19: 559–571 (1970).

453. Kinlough-Rathbone, R.L., Reimers, H.J., Mustard, J.F. and Packham, M.A.: Sodium arachidonate can induce platelet shape change and aggregation which are independent of the release reaction. Science 192: 1011–1012 (1976).

454. Kinsella, J.E., Hwang, D.H., Yu, P., Mai, J. and Shimp, J.: Prostaglandins and their precursors in tissues from rats fed on trnas, trans-linoleate. Biochem. J. 184: 701–704 (1979).

455. Kitada, S., Hays, E.F. and Mead, J.F.: Characterization of a lipid mobilizing factor from tumors. Progr. Lipids Res. 20: 823–826 (1981).

456. Kitchen, E.A., Boot, J.R. and Dawson, W.: Chemotactic activity of Thromboxane B_2, prostaglandins and their metabolites for polymorphonuclear leucocytes. Prostaglandins 16: 239–244 (1978).

457. Kloeze, J.: Influence des graisses alimentaires sur l'adhésivité des plaquettes. In: Extrait des Journées de Diabétologie de l'Hôtel-Dieu, Flammarion, Paris, 1966, pp.227–233.

458. Kloeze, J.: Influence of prostaglandins on platelet adhesiveness and platelet aggregation. In: S. Bergström and B. Samuelsson (eds.): Prostaglandins. Almqvist and Wiksell, Stockholm, 1967 pp. 241–252.

459. Kloeze, J., Houtsmuller, U.M.T. and Vles, R.O.: Influence of dietary fat mixtures on platelet adhesiveness, atherosclerosis and plasma cholesterol content in rabbits. J. Atheroscler. Res. 9: 319–334 (1969).

460. Kloeze, J.: Prostaglandins and platelet aggregation in vivo. I. Influence of PGE_1 and ω-homo-PGE_1 on transient thrombocytopenia and of PGE_1 on the LD_{50} of ADP. Thromb. Diathes. haemorrh. 23: 286–292 (1970). II. Influence of PGE_1 and $PGF_{1\alpha}$ on platelet thrombus formation induced by an electric stimulus in veins of the rat brain surface. Ibid pp. 293–298.

461. Kohler, N. and Lipton, A.: Platelets as a source of fibroblast growth-promoting activity. Exp. Cell Res. 87: 297–301 (1974).

462. Kommerell, B., Barth, P. and Pfleiderer, T.: Coagulation changes with intravenous administration of fat after blocking the RES. Thromb. Diath. haemorrh. 15: 381–389 (1966).

463. Kramár, J. and Levine, V.E.: Influence of fats and fatty acids on the capillaries. J. Nutr. 50: 149–160 (1953).

464. Krebs, H.A. and Henseleit, K.: Untersuchungen über die Harnstoffbilding in Tierkörper. Hoppe-Seiler's Z. Phys. Chem. 210: 33–66 (1932).

465. Kreneman, J. and Wensvoort, P.: Muscular dystrophy and yellow fat disease in Shetland pony foals. Neth. J. Vet. Sci. 1: 42–48 (1968).

466. Kritchevsky, D.: Experimental atherosclerosis in primates and other species. Ann. N. Y. Acad. Sci. 162: 80–88 (1969).

467. Kronmann, N. and Green, A.: Epidemiological studies in the Upernavik district, Greenland. Incidence of some chronic diseases. 1950–1974. Acta Med. Scand. 208: 401–406 (1980).

468. Kulkarni, P.S., Roberts, R. and Needleman, P.: Paradoxical endogenous synthesis of a coronary

dilating substance from arachidonate. Prostaglandins 12: 337–353 (1976).

469. Kunau, W.-H. and Dommes, P.: Degradation of unsaturated fatty acids. Identification of intermediates in the degradation of cis-4-decenoyl-CoA by extracts of beef liver mitochondria. Eur. J. Biochem. 91: 533–544 (1978).

470. Kuo, P.T.: Whereat, A.F., Altman, A.A. and West, J.W.: Effects of fat on coronary circulation in dogs. Circulat. Res. 8: 1157–1163 (1960).

471. Ladbrooke, B.D. and Chapman, D.: Thermal analysis of lipids, proteins and biological membranes. A reveiw and summary of some recent studies. Chem. Phys. Lipids, 3: 304–356 (1969).

472. Lagarde, M., Charib, A. and Dechavanne, M.: A simple radiochemical assay of thromboxane B_2, 12-hydroxyeicosatetraenoic acid (HETE) and 12-hydroxyheptadecatrienoic acid (HHT) synthetized by human platelets. Clin. Chim. Acta 79: 255–259 (1977).

473. Lagarde, M., Velardo, B., Blanc, M. and Dechavanne, M: Fatty acids bound to serum albumin decrease the half-life of thromboxane A_2. Prostaglandins 20: 275–283 (1980).

474. Lagarde, M., Burtin, M., Sprecher, H., Dechavanne, M. and Renaud, S.: Potentiating effect of 5, 8, 11-eicosatrienoic acid (20: 3ω9) on platelet aggregation. Thromb. Haemostas: 46: 208 (1981).

475. Largarde, M., Guichardant, M. and Dechavanne, M.: Human platelet PGE_1 and dihomo gamma linolenic acid. Comparison to PGE_2 and arachidonic acid. Progr. Lip. Res. 20: 439–443 (1981).

476. Lands, W.E.M. and Samuelsson, B.: Phospholipid precursors of prostaglandins. Biochim. Biophys. Acta 164: 426–429 (1968).

477. Lands, W.E.M., LeTellier, P.R., Rome, L.H. and Vanderhoek, J.Y.: Inhibition of prostaglandin biosynthesis in: Samuelsson, B. and Bernhard, S. (eds): Adv. Biosciences 9: 15–28 (1973).

479. Lapetina, E.G., Schmitges, C.J., Chandrabose, K. and Cuatrecasas, P.: Cyclic adenosine 3′, 5′-monophosphate and prostacyclin inhibit membrane phsopholipase activity in platelets. Biochem. Biophys. Res. Comm. 74: 828–835 (1977).

480. Lapetina, E.G. and Cuatrecasas, P.: Stimulation of phosphatidic acid production in platelets precedes the formation of arachidonate and parallels the release of serotonin. Biochim. biophys. Acta 573: 394–402 (1979).

481. Lapetina, E.G., Billah, M.M. and Cuatrecasas, P.: The initial action of thrombin on platelets. Conversion of phosphatidylinositol to phosphatidic acid preceeding the production of arachidonic acid. J. Biol. Chem. 256: 5037–5040 (1981).

482. Latour, J.G., Leger, C. and Renaud, S.: Activation of Hageman factor and initiation of hepatic vein thrombosis in hyperlipemic rats. Am. J. Pathol. 76: 178–193 (1974).

483. Layman, D.L., Epstein, E.H. Jr., Dodson, R.F. and Titus, J.L.: Biosynthesis of type I and III collagens by cultured smooth muscle cells from human aorta. Proc. Natl. Acad. Sci. USA 74: 671–675 (1977).

484. Leary, T.: Experimental atherosclerosis in the rabbit compared with human (coronary) atherosclerosis. Arch. Path. 17: 453–492 (1934).

485. Lee, M.O.: Determination of the surface of the white rat with its application to the expression of metabolic results. Am. J. Physiol. 39: 24–34 (1939).

486. Lees, R.S. and Carvalho, A.C.A.: Hypercholesterolenvla and platelets. In: The thrombotic process in atherogenesis. Chandler, A.B., Eurenius, K., McMillan, G.C., Nelson, C.B., Schwartz, C.J. and Wessler, S. (eds). New York, Plenum Publishing Corp., 1978, pp. 301–308.

487. Leren, P.: The Oslo diet–heart study. Circulation 42: 935–942 (1970).

488. Leung, N.L., Kinlough- Rathbone, R.L. and Mustard, J.F.: Incorporation of $^{32}PO_4$ into phospholipids of blood platelets. Br. J. Haematol. 36: 417–425 (1977).

489. Lieberman, G.E., Lewis, G.P. and Peters. T.J.: A membrane-bound enzyme in rabbit aorta capable of inhibiting adenosine diphosphate-induced platelet aggregation. Lancet ii: 330–332 (1977).

490. Likar, I.N., Likar, L.J., Robison, R.W. and Gouvelis, A.: Microthrombi and intimal thickening in bovine coronary arteries. Arch. Pathol. 87: 146–153 (1969).

491. Lipinski, B.A. and Mathias, M.M.: Prostaglandin production and lipolysis in isolated rat adipocytes as affected by dietary fat. Prostaglandins 16: 957–963 (1978).

492. Lloyd, J.V. and Mustard, J.F.: Changes in ^{32}P-content of phosphatidic acid and the phosphoinositides of rabbit platelets during aggregation induced by collagen or thrombin. Br. J. Haematol. 26: 243–253 (1974).

493. Lloyd, J.V., Nishizawa, E.E., Haldar, J. and Mustard, J.F.: Changes in ^{32}P-labelling of platelet phospholipids in response to ADP. Br. J. Haematol. 23: 571–585 (1972).

494. Lloyd, J.V., Nishizawa, E.E., Joist, H.J. and Mustard, J.F.: Effect of ADP – induced aggregation on^{32}PO$_4^-$ incorporation into phosphatidic acid and the phosphoinositides of rabbit platelets. Br. J. Haematol. 24: 589–604 (1973).

495. Lloyd, J.V., Nishizawa, E.E., and Mustard, J.F.: Effect of ADP-induced shape change on incorporation of ^{32}P into platelet phosphatidic acid and mono-, di- and triphosphatidylinositol. Br. J. Haematol. 25: 77–99 (1973).

496. Lockwood, W.R., Clower, B.R. and Hetherington, F.: Light and electron microscopy of diet-induced aterial thrombosis in TS mice. I. Primary changes in the endocardium. Am. J. Anat. 125: 185–200 (1969).

497. Logan, R.L., Thomson, M., Riemersma, R.A., Oliver, M.F., Olsson, A.G., Rössner, S.. Callmer, E., Walldius, G., Kaijser, L., Carlson, L.A., Lockerbie, L. and Lutz, W.: Risk factors for ischemic heart disease in normal men aged 40. Edinburgh-Stockholm study. Lancet i: 949–955 (1978).

498. Long, E.R.: The development of our knowledge of arteriosclerosis. In: Arteriosclerosis. Cowdry E.V. (ed.). New York, Macmillan, 1933. pp. 19–52.

499. Lossonczy, T.O. von, Ruiter, A., Bronsgeest-Schoute, H.C., van Gent, C.M. and Hermus, R.J.J.: The effect of a fish diet on serum lipids in healthy human subjects. Am. J. Clin. Nutr. 31: 1340–1346 (1978).

500. Lowry, O.H., Rosebrough, N.J., Farr, A.L. and Randall, R.J.: Protein measurement with the folin phenol reagent. J. Biol. Chem. 193: 265–275 (1951).

501. Lucas, C.T., Call II, F.L. and Williams, W.J.: The biosynthesis of phosphatidylinositol in human platelets. J. Clin. Invest. 49: 1949–1955 (1970).

502. Lyman, D.J., Klein, K.G., Brash, J.L. and Fritzinger, B.K.: The interaction of platelets with polymer surfaces. I. Uncharged hydrophobic polymer surfaces. Thrombos. Diathes. haemorrh. 23: 120–128 (1970).

503. Machleder, H.I., Sweeny, J.P. and Barker, W.F.: Pulseless arm after brachial artery catheterization. Lancet i: 407–409 (1972).

504. Machlin, L.J., Filipski, R., Willis, A.L., Kuhn, D.C. and Brin, M.: Influence of vitamin E on platelet aggregation and thrombocythemia in the rat. Proc. Soc. Exp. Biol. Med. 149: 275–277 (1975).

505. MacIntyre, D.E., Pearson, J.D. and Gordon, J.L.: Localization and stimulation of prostacyclin production in vascular cells. Nature 271: 549–551 (1978).

506. MacIntyre, D.E., Salzman, E.W. and Gordon, J.L.: Prostaglandin receptors on human platelets. Structure-activity relationships of stimulatory prostaglandins. Biochem. J. 174: 921–929 (1978).

507. MacIntyre, D.E., Handin, Z.I., Roseneber, R. and Salzman, E.W.: Heparin opposes prostanoid and non-prostanoid platelet inhibitors by direct enhancement of aggregation. Thromb. Res. 22: 167–175 (1981).

508. Maclouf, J., Kindahl, H., Granström, E. and Samuelsson, B.: Interactions of prostaglandin H$_2$ and thromboxane A$_2$ with human serum albumin. Eur. J. Biochem. 109: 561–566 (1980).

509. MacMillan, A.L. and Sinclair, H.M.: The structure and function of essential fatty acids. Proc. Intern. conf. Biochem. Problems of Lipids, London, Butterworth, 1958, p. 208.

510. Madri, J.A., Dreyer, B., Pitlick, F.A., Furthmayr, H.: The collagenous components of the subendothelium. Lab. Invest. 43: 303–315 (1980).

511. Maguire, K.F. and Doran, G.A.: Surface morphology of endocardial thrombus induced by a high fat diet. Am. J. Anat. 135: 153–157 (1972).

208

512. Majerus, P.W., Baenziger, N.L. and Brody, G.N.: Lipid metabolism in human platelets. Ser. Haemat. IV: 59–74 (1971).

513. Majno, G. and Joris, I.: Endothelium 1977: A review. In: The thrombocyte Process in Atherogenesis, Chandler, A.B., Eurenius, K., Macmillian, G.C., Nelson, C.B., Schwartz, C.J. and Wessler, S. (eds). New York, Plenum, 1978, p. 169–225; 481–526.

514. Mallory, F.B.: The infectious lesions of blood vessels. In: The Harvey lectures, Philadelphia, J.B. Lippincott, Co., 1912–1913, p. 150–166.

515. Malmsten, C., Hamberg, M., Svensson, J. and Samuelsson, B.: Physiological roles of an endoperoxide in human platelets: Hemostatic defect due to platelet cyclo-oxygenase deficiency. Proc. Natl. Acad. Sci. USA 72: 1446–1450 (1975).

516. Malmsten, C., Granström, E. and Samuelsson, B.: Cyclic AMP inhibits synthesis of prostaglandin endoperoxide (PGG_2) in human platelets. Biochem. Biophys. Res. comm. 68: 569–576 (1976).

517. Malmros, H.: Dietary prevention of atherosclerosis. Lancet ii: 479–484 (1969).

518. Mann, J.I. and Inman, W.H.W.: Oral contraceptives and death from myocardial infarction. Br. Med. J. 2: 245–248 (1975).

519. Mann, J.I., Thorogood, M., Waters, W.E. and Powell, C.: Oral contraceptives and myocardial infarction in young women: a further report. Br. Med. J. 3: 631–632 (1975).

520. Mann, J.I., Inman, W.H.W. and Thorogood, M.: Oral contraceptive use in older women and fatal myocardial infarction. Br. Med. J. 2: 445–447 (1976).

521. Marcus, A.J., Ullman, H.L. and Safier, L.B.: Lipid composition of subsellular particles of human blood platelets. J. Lipid Res. 10: 108–114 (1969).

522. Marcus, A.J.: The role of lipids in platelet function: with particular reference to the arachidonic acid pathway. J. Lipid Res. 19: 793–826 (1978).

523. Marcus, A.J., Weksler, B., Jaffe, E., Safier, L., Ullman, H., Broekman, M., Dorso, C. and Brown, S.: Arachidonic acid metabolism in platelets and endothelial cells. Progr. Lipid Res. 20: 431–434 (1981).

524. Margolis, L.B., Tikhonov, A.N. and Vasilieva, E.Y.: Platelet adhesion to fluid and solid phospholipid membranes. Cell 19: 189–195 (1980).

525. Masotti, G., Poggesi, L., Galanti, G., Abbate, R. and Neri Serneri, G.G.: Differential inhibition of prostacyclin production and platelet aggregation by aspirin. Lancet ii: 1213–1216 (1979).

526. Mathias, M.M. and Dupont, J.: The relationship of dietary fats to prostaglandin biosynthesis. Lipids 14: 247–252 (1979).

527. Mathues, J.K., Wolff, C.E., Cevallos, W.H. and Holmes, W.L.: Platelet adhesiveness and thrombosis in rabbits on an atherogenic diet. Med. Exp. 18: 121–128 (1968).

528. Mauco, G., Chap, H., Simon, M.F. and Douste-Blazy, L.: Phosphatidic and lysophosphatidic acid production in phopholipase C and thrombin-treated platelets. Possible involvement of a platelet lipase. Biochimie 60: 653–661 (1978).

529. Mauco, G., Chap, H. and Douste-Blazy, L.: Characterization and properties of a phosphatidylinositol phosphodiesterase (phospholipase C) from platelet cytosol. FEBS Letts. 100: 367–370 (1979).

530. McDonald, L. and Edgill, M.: Dietary restriction and coagulability of the blood in ischaemic heart disease. Lancet ii: 996–998 (1958).

531. McGregor, L. and Renaud, S.: Effect of dietary linoleic acid deficiency on platelet aggregation and phospholipid fatty acids of rats. Thromb. Res. 12: 921–927 (1978).

532. McGregor, L., Morazain, R. and Renaud, S.: A comparison of the effects of dietary short and long chain saturated fatty acids on platelet functions, platelet phospholipids and blood coagulation in rats. Lab. Invest. 43: 438–442 (1980).

533. McGregor, L., Morazain, R. and Renaud, S.: Platelet functions and fatty acid composition of platelet phospholipids in spontaneously hypertensive rats fed saturated or polyunsaturated fats. Atherosclerosis 38: 129–136 (1981).

534. McKean, M.L., Smith, J.B. and Silver, M.J.: Regulation of the fatty acid composition of platelet phospholipids. Thromb. Haemostas. 46: 321 (1981).

534a. McKean, M.L., Smith, J.B. and Silver, M.J.: Phospholipid biosynthesis in human platelets. 1. Formation of phosphatidylcholine from 1-acyl lysophosphatidylcholine by AcylCoA: 1-Acyl-*sn*-glycero-3-phosphocholine acyltransferase. J. Biol. Chem. (In press).

534b. McKean, M.L., Smith, J.B. and Silver, M.J.: Formation of lysophosphatidylcholine by human platelets in response to thrombin. Support for the phospholipase A_2 pathway for the liberation of arachidonic acid. J. Biol. Chem. 256: 1522–1524 (1981).

535. McMillan, G.C.: The onset of plaque formation in arteriosclerosis. Acta Cardiol. (Suppl. 11) 43–62 (1965).

536. McPherson, V.J., Zucker, M.B., Friedberg, N.M. and Rifkin, P.L.: Platelet retention in glass bead columns: further evidence for the importance of ADP. Blood 44: 411–425 (1974).

537. Mead, J.F.: The metabolism of the polyunsaturated fatty acids. In: Holman, R.T. (ed): Progress in the chemistry of Fats and Other Lipids. Oxford, Pergamon, 9: 161–189 (1971).

538. Mead, J.F. and Fulco, A.J.: The Unsaturated and Polyunsaturated Fatty Acids in Health and Disease. 1976. Charles C. Thomas, Springfield, Ill., USA.

539. Meade, T.W., Chakrabarti, R., Haines, A.P., North, W.R.S., Stirling, Y., Thompson, S.G. and Brozović, M.: Haemostatic function and cadiovascular death: early result of a prospective study. Lancet i: 1050–1054 (1980).

540. Meade, T.W. and Thompson, S.G.: Anticoagulants after myocardial infarction. Lancet i: 717 (1981).

541. Meer, J. van der, Stoepman-van Dalen, E.A. and Jansen, J.M.S.: Antithrombin III deficiency in a Dutch family. J. Clin. Pathol. 26: 532–538 (1973).

542. Meeuwissen, O.J.A. Th.: The influence of fatty meals on fibrinolysis. Thesis, Utrecht 1966.

543. Merskey, C., and Marcus A.J.: Lipids, blood coagulation and fibrinolysis. Ann. Rev. Med. 14: 323–338 (1963).

544. Merskey, C. and Wolh, H.: Changes in blood coagulation and fibrinolysis in rats fed atherogenic diets. Thromb. Diath. haemorrh. 10: 295–303 (1964).

545. Mestel, F., Oetliker, O., Beck, E., Felix, R., Imback, P. and Wagner, H.P.: Severe bleeding associated with defective thromboxane synthetase. Lancet i: 157 (1980).

546. Meydani, S.N., Mathias, M.M. and Schatte, C.L.: Dietary fat type and ambient oxygen tension influence pulmonary prostaglandin synthetic potential. Prost. Med. 1: 241–249 (1978).

547. Meyers, K.M., Seachord, C.L., Holmsen, H., Smith, J.B. and Prieur, D.J.: A dominant role of thromboxane formation in secondary aggregation of platelets. Nature 282: 331–333 (1979).

548. Michal, F. and Born, G.V.R.: Effect of the rapid shape change of platelets on the transmission and scattering of light through plasma. Nature 231: 220–222 (1971).

549. Michal, F.: Measurement of platelet aggregation and shape change. Adv. Exptl. Med and Biol. 34: 257–262 (1972).

550. Michell, R.H.: Inositol phospholipids and cell surface receptor function. Biochim. Biophys. Acta 415: 81–147 (1975).

551. Mielke, C.H., Ramos, J.C. and Britten, A.F.H.: Aspirin as an antiplatelet agent: template bleeding time as a monitor of therapy. Am. J. Clin. Pathol. 59: 236–242 (1973).

552. Miettinen, M., Turpeinen, O., Karvonen, M.J., Elosuo, R. and Paavilainen, E.: Effect of cholesterol-lowering diet on mortality from coronary heart disease and other causes. A twelve-year clinical trial in men and women. Lancet ii: 835–838 (1972).

553. Millar, J.H.D., Zilka, K.J., Langman, M.J.S., Wright, H.P., Smith, A.D., Belin, J. and Thompson, R.H.S.: Double blind trial of linoleate supplementation of the diet in multiple sclerosis. Br. Med. J. 1: 765–768 (1973).

554. Miller, O.V., Johnson, R.A. and Gorman, R.R.: Inhibition of PGE_1-stimulated cAMP accumulation in human platelets by thromboxane A_2. Prostaglandins 13: 599–609 (1977).

555. Miller, O.V. and Gorman, R.R.: Evidence for distinct prostaglandin I_2 and D_2 receptors in human platelets. J. Pharmacol. Exp. Ther. 210: 134–140 (1979).

556. Miller, O.V., Aiken, J.W., Shebuski, R.J. and Gorman, R.R.: 6-keto-prostaglandin E_1 is not

equipotent to prostacyclin (PGI$_2$) as an antiaggregatory agent. Prostaglandins 20: 391–400 (1980).

557. Miller, R.D., Burchell, H.B. and Edwards, J.E.: Myocardial infarction with and without acute coronary occlucion. Arch. Int. Med. 88: 597–604 (1951).

558. Mills, D.C.B. and Smith, J.B.: The influence on platelet aggregation of drugs that affect the accumulation of adenosine 3′:5′-cyclic monophospate in platelets. Biochem. J. 121: 185–196 (1971).

559. Mills, D.C.B. and MacFarlane, D.E.: Stimulation of human platelet adenylate cyclase by prostaglandin D$_2$. Thromb. Res. 5: 401–421 (1974).

560. Ministery of Greenland: Grønland 1978. Copenhagen, Danmark 1979.

561. Minkes, M., Stanford, N., Chi, M.M.-Y., Roth, G, Raz, A., Needleman, P. and Majerus, P.: Cyclic adenosine 3′, 5′-monophosphate inhibits the availability of arachidonate to prostaglandin synthetase in human platelet suspensions. J. Clin. Invest. 59: 449–454 (1977).

562. Miyamoto, T., Ogino, N., Yamamoto, S. and Hayaishi, O.: Purification of prostaglandin endoperoxide synthetase from bovine vesicular gland microsomes. J. Biol. Chem. 251: 2629–2636 (1976).

563. Moncada, S., Gryglewski, R.J., Bunting, S. and Vane, J.R.: A lipid peroxide inhibits the enzyme in blood vessel microsomes that generates from prostaglandin endoperoxides the substance (prostaglandin X) which prevents platelet aggregation. Prostaglandins 12: 715–737 (1976).

564. Moncada, S., Gryglewski, R., Bunting, S. and Vane, J.R.: An enzyme isolated from arteries transforms prostaglandin endoperoxides to an unstable substance that inhibits platelet aggregation. Nature 263: 663–665 (1976).

565. Moncada, S., Korbut, R., Buntin, S. and Vane, J.R.: Prostacyclin is a circulating hormone. Nature 273: 767–768 (1978).

566. Moncada, S. and Vane, J.R.: Unstable metabolites of arachidonic acid and their role in haemostasis and thrombosis. Br. Med. Bull. 34: 129–135 (1978).

567. Moolten, S.E. and Vroman, L.: The adhesiveness of blood platelets in thromboembolism and hemorrhagic disorders. I. Measurement of platelet ahesiveness by the glass wool filter. Am. J. Clin. Path. 19: 701–709 (1949).

568. Moolten, S.E., Jennings, P.B. and Solden, A.: Dietary fat and platelet adhesiveness in arteriosclerosis and diabetes. Am. J. Cardiol. 11: 290–300 (1963).

569. Moore, S. and Mersereau, W.A.: Microembolic renal ischemia, hypertension and nephrosclerosis. Arch. Path. 85: 623–630 (1968).

570. Moore, S.: Thrombosis and atherosclerosis. Thromb. Diathes. Haemorrh. (Suppl. 60): 205–212 (1974).

571. Moore, S., Friedman, R.J., Singal, D.P., Gauldie, J. and Blajchman, M.: Inhibition of injury-induced thrombo-atherosclerotic lesions by antiplatelet serum in rabbits. Thromb. Diathes. haemorrh. 35: 70–81 (1976).

572. Moore, S. Belbeck, L.W., Evans, G. and Pineau, S.: Effects of complete or partial occlusion of a coronary artery. Lab. Invest. 44: 151–157 (1981).

573. More, R.H., Movat, H.Z., Haust, M.D.: Role of mural fibrin thrombi of the aorta in the genesis of arteriosclerotic plaques. Report of two cases. Arch. Path. 63: 612–620 (1957).

574. Moretti, R.L. and Abraham, S.: Stimulation of microsomal prostaglandin synthesis by a blood plasma constituent which augments autoregulation and maintenance of vascular tone in isolated rabbit hearts. Circ. Res. 42: 317–323 (1978).

575. Morgan, A.D.: The Pathogenesis of Coronary Occlusion. Oxford, Blackwell Scientific Pub. 1956, p. 171.

576. Morgenstern, E., Pfleiderer, T., Zebisch, P. und Weber, E.: Über die Wirkung von Lipidemulsionen auf Blutplätchen. II. Licht- und elektronenmikroskopische Studien. Thromb. Diath. haemorrh. 22: 525–543 (1969).

577. Morrison, W.R. and Smith, L.M.: Preparation of fatty acid methyl esters and dimethylacetals from lipids with boron fluoride-methanol. J. Lipid Res. 5: 600–608 (1964).

578. Moschos, C.B., Lahiri, K., Lyons, M., Weisse, A.B., Oldewurtel, H.A., Regan, T.J.: Relation of microcirculatory thrombosis to thrombus in the proximal coronary artery. Effect of aspirin, dipyridamole and thrombolysis. Am. Heart J. 86: 61–68 (1973).

579. Movat, H.Z., Haust, M.D. and More, R.H.: The morphologic elements in the early lesions of arteriosclerosis. Am. J. Path. 35: 93–101 (1959).

580. Muirhead, C.R.: The filter-loop technique as a method for measuring platelet aggregation in the flowing blood of the rat; the inhibitory activity of 5-oxo-1-cyclopentene-1-heptanoic acid (AY-16,804) on platelet aggregation. Thrombos. Diathes. Haemorrh. 30: 138–147 (1973).

580a. Muller, A.D.: Personal communication.

581. Murphy, E.A., Rowsell, H.C., Downie, H.G., Robinson, G.A. and Mustard, J.F.: Encrustation and atherosclerosis: the analogy between early in vivo lesions and deposits which occur in extra corporeal circulation. J. Can. Med. Ass. 87: 259–274 (1962).

582. Murphy, R.C., Mathews, R. and Pickett, W.: Leukotrienes and thromboxanes: metabolites of essential fatty acids with significant untoward pharmacological properties. in: Beers, R.F.Jr. and Bassett, E.G. (Eds.): Nutritional factors: Modulating Effects on Metabolic Processes. Raven Press, New York, 1981, pp. 495–509.

583. Mustard, J.F.: Effects of intravenous phospholipid containing phosphatidyl serine on blood clotting with particular reference to the Russell's viper venom time. Nature 196: 1063–1065 (1962).

584. Mustard, J.F. and Murphy, E.A.: Effect of different dietary fats on blood coagulation, platelet economy and blood lipids. Br. med. J. i: 1651–1655 (1962).

585. Mustard, J.F. and Murphy, E.N.: Effect of smoking on blood coagulation and platelet survival in man. Br. Med. J. 1: 846–849 (1963).

586. Mustard, J.F., Rowsell, H.C., Murphy, E.A. and Downie, H.G.: Diet and thrombus formation: quantitative studies using an extra corporeal circulation in pigs. J. Clin. Invest. 42: 1783–1789 (1963).

587. Mustard, J.F., Glynn, M.F., Nishizawa, E.E. and Packham, M.A.: Platelet surface interactions: relationship to thrombosis and hemostasis. Fed. Proc. 26: 106–114 (1967).

588. Mustard, J.F. and Packham, M.A.: Factors influencing platelet function: adhesion, release and aggregation. Pharmacol. Rev. 22: 97–187 (1970).

589. Mustard, J.F. and Packham, M.A.: The reaction of the blood to injury. In: Inflammation, Immunity and Hypersensitivity, Movat H.Z. (ed) Hagerstown, Maryland, Harper & Row, 1979, pp. 557–664.

590. Myatt, L. and Elder, M.G.: Inhibition of platelet aggregation by a placental substance with prostacyclin-like activity. Nature 268: 159–160 (1977).

591. Naeye, R.L.: Thrombotic state after a hemorrhagic diathesis a possible complication of therapy with epsilon-amino caproic acid. Blood 19: 694–701 (1962).

592. Nathaniel, E.J.H. and Chandler, A.B.: Electron microsopic study of adenosine diphosphate-induced platelet thrombi in the rat. J. Ultrastruc. Res. 22: 348–359 (1968).

593. Nathaniel, E.J., Nathaniel, D.R., Nordøy, A and Chandler, A.B.: Electron microscopic observations of platelets in rats fed on different fat diets. J. Ultrastruc. Res. 38: 360–370 (1972).

594. Needleman, P., Minkes, M. and Raz, A.: Thromboxanes: selective biosynthesis and distinct biological properties. Science 193: 163–165 (1976).

595. Needleman, P., Kulkarni, P.S. and Raz, A.: Coronary tone modulation: Formation and actions of prostaglandin endoperoxides and thromboxanes. Science 195: 409–412 (1977).

596. Needleman, P., Wyche, A., Bronson, S.D., Eakins, K. Ferrendelli, J.A. and Minkes, M.: Thromboxane synthetase inhibitors as pharmacological tools: differential biochemical and biological effects of platelet suspensions. Prostaglandins 14: 897–907 (1977).

597. Needleman, P., Bronson, S.D., Wyche, A., Sivakoff, M. and Nicolaou, K.C.: Cardiac and renal prostaglandin I_2. Biosynthesis and biological effects in isolated perfused rabbit tissues. J. Clin. Invest. 61: 839–849 (1978).

598. Needleman, P., Raz, A., Minkes, M.S., Ferrendelli, J.A. and Sprecher, H.: Triene prostaglandins:

prostacyclin and thromboxane biosynthesis and unique biological properties. Proc. Natl. Acad. Sci. USA 76: 944–948 (1979).

599. Needleman, P., Wyche, A. and Raz, A.: Platelet and blood vessel arachidonate metabolism and interactions. J. Clin. Invest. 63: 345–349 (1979).

600. Nelson, A.M.: Diet therapy in coronary disease. Effect on mortality of high-protein, high-seafood, fat-controlled diet. Geriatrics 27: 103–116 (1972).

601. Nemerson, Y. and Pitlick, F.A.: The tissue factor pathway of blood coagulation in: Spaet, T.H. (ed): Progress in Haemostasis and Thrombosis. 1. Grune & Stratton, New York, 1972, pp. 1–37.

602. Newman, H.A.I. and Zilversmit, D.B.: Quantitative aspects of cholesterol flux in rabbit atheromatous lesions. J. Biol. Chem. 237: 2078–2084 (1962).

603. Nidy, E.G. and Johnson, R.A.: Synthesis of prostaglandin PGI$_3$. Tetrahedron Lett. 27: 2375–2378 (1978).

604. Niewiarowski, S., Bankowski, E. and Rogowicka, I.: Studies on the absorption and activation of the Hageman Factor (Factor XII) by collagen and elastin. Thromb. Diathes. haemorrh. 14: 387–444 (1965).

605. Nijkamp, F.P., Moncada, S., White, H.L. and Vane, J.R.: Diversion of prostaglandin endoperoxide metabolism by selective inhibition of thromboxane A$_2$ synthesis in lung, spleen or platelets. Eur. J Pharmacol. 44: 179–186 (1977).

606. Nishikawa, M., Tanaka, T. and Hidaka, H.: Ca^{2+}-calmodulin-dependent phosphorylation and platelet secretion. Nature 287: 863–865 (1980).

607. Nishizawa, E.E., Hovig, T., Lotz, F., Rowsell, H.C. and Mustard, J.F.: Effect of a natural phosphatidyl serine fraction on blood coagulation, platelet aggregation and haemostasis. Brit. J. Haematol. 16: 487–499 (1969).

607a. Nishizawa, E.A. and Mustard, J.F.: The effect of synthetic phosphatidyl serines on platelet aggregation, blood coagulation and haemostasis. Brit. J. Haematol. 20: 45–54 (1971).

608. Nørby, J.G. Effects of giving a fat free diet for up to 10 weeks on the male weanling rat. Br. J. Nutr. 19: 209–224 (1965).

609. Nordøy, A. and Chandler, A.B.: Platelet thrombosis induced by adenosine diphosphate in the rat. Scand. J. Haemat. 1: 16–25 (1964).

610. Nordøy, A. and Chandler, A.B.: The influence of dietary fats on the adenosine diphosphate induced platelet thrombosis in the rat. Scand. J. Haemat. 1; 202–211 (1964).

611. Nordøy, A.: The influence of saturated fats, cholesterol, corn oil and linseed oil on experimental venous thrombosis in rats. Thromb. Diath. haemorrh. 13: 244–256 (1965).

612. Nordøy, A.: The influence of saturated fat, cholesterol, corn oil and linseed oil on the ADP-induced platelet adhesiveness in the rat. Thromb. Diathes. haemorrh. 13: 543–549 (1965).

613. Nordøy, A., Hamlin, J.T., Chandler, A.B. and Newland, H.: The influence of dietary fats on plasma and platelet lipids and ADP-induced platelet thrombosis in the rat. Scand. J. Haemat. 5: 458–473 (1968).

614. Nordøy, A. and Lund, S.: Platelet factor 3 activity, platelet phospholipids and their fatty acid and aldehyde pattern in normal male subjects. Scand. J. Clin. Lab. Invest. 22: 328–338 (1968).

615. Nordøy, A., Rødset, J.M.: Platelet phospholipids and their function in patients with ischemic heart disease. Acta Med. Scand. 188: 133–137 (1970).

616. Nordøy, A., Rødset, J.M.: Platelet phospholipids and their function in patients with juvenile diabetes and maturity onset diabetes. Diabetes 19: 698–702 (1970).

617. Nordøy, A., Rødset, J.M.: Platelet function and platelet phospholipids in patients with hyperbetalipoproteinemia. Acta med. Scand. 189: 385–389 (1971).

618. Nordøy, A. and Rødset, J.M.: The influence of dietary fats on platelets in man. Acta Med. Scand. 190: 27–34 (1971).

619. Nordøy, A., Bjørge, J.M. and Strøm, E.: Comparison of the main lipids in platelets and plasma in man. Acta Med. Scand. 193: 59–64 (1973).

620. Nordøy, A., Strøm, E. and Gjesdal, K.: The effect of alimentary hyperlipaemia and primary

hypertriglyceridaemia on platelets in man. Scand. J. Haemat. 12: 329–340 (1974).

621. Nordøy, A., Svensson, B., Wiebe, D. and Hoak, J.C.: Lipoproteins and the inhibitory effect of human endothelial cells on platelet function. Circ. Res. 43: 527–534 (1978).

622. Nordøy, A.: Albumin bound fatty acids, platelets and endothelial cells in thrombogenesis. Haemostasis 8: 193–202 (1979).

623. Nordøy, A. and Svensson, B.: The simultaneous effect of albumin bound fatty acids on platelets and endothelial cells. Thromb. Res. 15: 215–226 (1979).

624. Nordøy, A., Svensson, B. and Hoak, J.C.: The effects of albumin bound fatty acids on the platelet inhibitory function of human endothelial cells. Eur. J. Clin. Invest. 9: 5–10 (1979).

625. Nugteren, D.H.: Inhibition of prostaglandin biosynthesis by 8-*cis*, 12-*trans*, 14-*cis*-eicosatrienoic acid and 5-*cis*, 8-*cis*, 12-*trans*, 14-*cis*-eicosatetraenoic acid. Biochim. Biophys. Acta 210: 171–176 (1970).

626. Nugteren, D.H. and Hazelhof, E.: Isolation and properties of intermediates in prostaglandin biosynthesis. Biochim. Biophys. Acta 326: 448–461 (1973).

627. Nugteren, D.H.: Arachidonate lipoxygenase in blood platelets. Biochim. Biophys. Acta 380: 299–307 (1975).

628. Nugteren, D.H., Jouvenaz, G.H. and Dutilh, C.E.: Determination of prostaglandins and other products of arachidonate oxygenation in perfusates and during platelet aggregation. Acta. Biol. Med. Germ 37: 701–706 (1978).

629. Nugteren, D.H., van Evert, W.C., Soeting, W.J. and Spuy, J.H.: The effect of different amounts of linoleic acid in the diet on the excretion of urinary prostaglandin metabolites in the rat. Adv. Prostagl. Thrombox. Res. 8: 1793–1796 (1980).

630. O'Brien, J.R.: Platelet aggregation. II. Some results from a new method of study. J. Clin. Path. 15: 452–455 (1962).

631. O'Brien, J.R. and Heywood, J.B.: A comparison of platelet stickiness tests during an Atromid-S trial. Thrombos. Diathes. Haemorrh. 16: 768–777 (1966).

632. O'Brien, J.R.: Effects of salicylates on human platelets. Lancet i: 799–783 (1968).

633. O'Brien, J.R., Etherington, M.D. and Jamieson, S.: Acute platelet changes after large meals of saturated and unsaturated fats. Lancet i: 878–880 (1976).

634. O'Brien, J.R., Etherington, M.D., Jamieson, S., Vergroesen, A.J. and Ten Hoor, F.: Effect of a diet of polyunsaturated fats on some platelet function tests. Lancet ii: 995–997 (1976).

635. O'Donnell, M.C., Henson, P.M. and Fiedel, B.A.: Activation of human platelets by platelet-activating factor (PAF) derived from sensitized rabbit basophils. Immunology 35: 953–958 (1979).

636. O'Donnell, T.F.Jr., Carvalho, A.C.A., Colman, R.W. and Clowes, G.H.A.: Platelet function abnormalities in a family with recurrent arterial thrombosis. Surgery 83: 144–150 (1978).

637. Oelz, O., Seyberth, H.W., Knapp, H.R., Sweetman, B.J. and Oates, J.A.: Effects of feeding ethyl-dihomo-γ-linolenate on prostaglandin biosynthesis and platelet aggregation in the rabbit. Biochim. Biophys. Acta 431: 268–277 (1976).

638. Oelz, O., Oelz, R., Knapp, H.R., Sweetman, B.J. and Oates, J.A.: Biosynthesis of prostaglandin D_2. I. Formation of prostaglandin D_2 by human platelets. Prostaglandins 13: 225–234 (1977).

639. Okuma, M., Steiner, M. and Baldini, M. Studies on lipid peroxides in platelets. I. Method of assay and effect of storage. J. Lab. Clin. Med. 75: 283–296 (1970).

640. Ouderaa, F.J. van der, Buytenhek, M., Nugteren, D.H. and van Dorp, D.A.: Purification and characterization of prostaglandin endoperoxide synthethase from sheep vesicular glands. Biochim. Biophys. Acta 487: 315–331 (1977).

641. Owren, P.A. and Aas, K.: The control of dicumarol therapy and the quantitative determination of prothrombin and proconvertin. Scand. J. Clin. Invest. 3: 201–208 (1951).

642. Owren, P.A., Hellem, A.J. and Ödegaard, A.: Linolenic acid for the prevention of thrombosis and myocardial infarction. Lancet ii: 975–978 (1964).

643. Owren, P.A., Hellem, A.J. and Ödegaard, A.: Linolenic acid and platelet adhesiveness. Lancet ii: 849–850 (1965).

214

644. Pace-Asciak, C and Wolfe, L.S.: Inhibition of prostaglandin synthesis by oleic, linoleic and linolenic acids. Biochim. Biophys. Acta 152: 784–787 (1968).
645. Pace-Asciak, C. and Wolfe, L.S.: A novel prostaglandin derivative formed from arachidonic acid by rat stomach homogenates. Biochemistry 10: 3657–3664 (1971).
646. Pace-Asciak, C.R.: Oxidative biotransformations of arachidonic acid. Prostaglandins 13: 811–817 (1977).
647. Packham, M.A. and Mustard, J.F.: Platelet aggregation: Relevance to thrombotic tendencies. In: Thrombosis, Animal and Clinical Models, Day, H.J., Molony, B.A., Nishisawa, E.E. and Rynbrandt, R.H. (eds). New York, Plenum, 1978, pp. 51–69.
648. Pareti, F.I., Mannucci, P.M., d'Angelo, A., Smith, J.B., Sautebin, L. and Galli, G.: Congenital deficiency of thromboxane and prostacyclin. Lancet i: 898–901 (1980).
649. Pearl, F. and Friedman, M.: Experimental coronary thromboatherosclerosis in the dog. Arch. Path. 77: 370–377 (1964).
650. Pearson, T.A., Dillman, J., Solez, K. and Heptinstall, R.H.: Clonal markers in the study of the origin and growth of human atherosclerotic lesions. Circ. Res. 43: 10–18 (1978).
651. Pearson, T.A., Wang, A., Solez, K. and Heptinstall, R.W.: Clonal characteristics of fibrous plaques and fatty streaks of human aortas. Am. J. Pathol. 81: 379–388 (1975).
652. Pearson, T.A., Solez, K., Dillman, J. and Heptinstall, R.H.: Monoclonal characteristics of organizing arterial thrombi: significance in the origin and growth of human atherosclerotic plaques. Lancet i: 7–11 (1979).
653. Petersen, G.L.: Review of the folin phenol protein quantitation method of Lowry, Rosebrough, Farr and Randall. Anal. Biochem. 100: 201–220 (1979).
654. Pfleiderer, T., Kommerell, B. und Barth, P.: Uber die Wirking einer Fettemulsion auf menschliche Thrombocyten in vitro. Verh. Dtsch. Ges. Inn. Med. 71: 741–744 (1965).
655. Pfleiderer, T., Morgenstern, E. and Weber, E.: Über die Wirkung von Lipidemulsionen auf Blutplättchen. 1. Zunahme der Plättchenaggregation unter dem Einfluss verschiedener Lipidemulsionen in vitro. Thromb. Diath. haemorrh. 22: 513–524 (1969).
656. Philp, R.B. and Payling Wright, H.: Effect of adenosine on platelet adhesiveness in fasting and lipaemic bloods. Lancet ii: 208–209 (1965).
657. Pinckard, R.N., Farr, R.S. and Hanahan, D.J.: Physicochemical and functional identity of rabbit platelet-activating factor (PAF) released in vivo during IgE anaphylaxis with PAF, released in vitro from IgE sensitized basophils. J. Immunol. 123: 1847–1857 (1979).
658. Piper, P.J. and Vane, J.R.: Release of additional factors in anaphylaxis and its antagonism by anti-inflammatory drugs. Nature 223: 29–35 (1969).
659. Pitas, R.E., Nelson, G.J., Jaffe, R.M. and Mahley, R.W.: $\triangle$ 15,18-Tetracosadienoic acid content of sphingolipids from platelets and erythrocytes of animals fed diets high in saturated or polyunsaturated fats. Lipids 13: 551–556 (1978).
660. Pitas, R.E., Nelson, G.J., Jaffe, R.M. and Mahley, R.W.: Effects of diets high in saturated fat and cholesterol on the lipid composition of canine platelets. Lipids 14: 469–477 (1979).
661. Piver, D.D. Cagen, L.M. and Chesney, C.McI.: Stability of prostaglandin I_2 in human blood. Prostaglandins 21: 165–175 (1981).
662. Poggi, A., Kornblihtt, L., Delaini, F., Colombo, T., Mussoni, L., Reyers, I. and Donati, M.B.: Delayed hypercoagulability after a single dose of adriamycin to normal rats. Thromb. Res. 16: 639–650 (1979).
663. Poole, A.R., Howell, J.I. and Lucy, J.A.: Lysolecithin and cellfusion. Nature 227: 810–814 (1970).
664. Poole, J.C.F.: Effect of diet and lipemia on coagulation and thrombosis. Fed. Proc. 21: 20–24 (1962).
665. Pope, J.T., Chandler, A.B., Asokan, S.K. and Pollard, D.: Metamorphosis of experimental coronary thrombi into arteriosclerotic plaques. Circulation 50 (Suppl. III): 295 (1974) (Abstract).
666. Porter, N.A., Wolf, R.A., Pagels, W.R. and Marnett, L.J.: A test for the intermediacy of 11-hydroperoxyeicosa-5, 8, 12, 14-tetraenoic acid (11-HPETE) in prostaglandin biosynthesis. Bio-

chem. Biophys. Res. Commun. 92: 349–355 (1980).

667. Praga, C., Valentini, L., Maiorano, M. and Cortellaro, M.: A new antomatic device for the standardized Ivy bleeding time. Adv. Exp. Med. Biol. 34: 271–279(1972).

668. Prathap, K.: The natural history of platelet-rich mural thrombi in systemic arteries of hyper-cholesterolemic monkeys: light and electron microscope observations. J. Pathol. 110: 203–212 (1973).

669. Prescott, S.M. and Majerus, P.W.: The fatty acid composition of phosphatidylinositol from thrombin-stimulated human platelets. J. Biol. Chem. 256: 579–582 (1981).

670. Preston, F.E., Whipps, S., Jackson, C.A., French, A.J., Wyld, P.J. and Stoddard, C.J.: Inhibition of prostacyclin and platelet thromboxane A_2 after low dose aspirin. N Engl. J. Med. 304: 76–79 (1981).

671. Prost-Dvojakovic, R.J. and Samama, M.: Clot promoting and platelet-aggregating effects of fatty acids. Haemostasis 2: 73–84 (1973/1974).

672. Proudlock, J.W., Day, A.J., Tume, R.K.: Cholesterol-esterifying enzymes of foam cells isolated from atherosclerotic rabbit intima. Atherosclerosis 18: 451–457 (1973).

673. Raymond, S.L. and Dodds, W.J.: Characterization of the Fawn-Hooded rat as a model for hemostatic studies. Thromb. Diath. haemorrh. 33: 361–369 (1975).

674. Raz, A., Isakson, P.C., Minkes, M.S. and Needleman, P.: Characterization of a novel metabolic pathway of arachidonate in coronary arteries which generates a potent endogenous coronary vasodilator. J. Biol. Chem. 252: 1123–1126 (1977).

675. Raz, A., Aharoni, D. and Kenig-Wakshal, R.: Biosynthesis of Thromboxane B_2 and 12-L-hydroxy-5, 8, 10-heptadecatrienoic acid in human platelets. Evidence for a common enzymatic pathway. Eur. J. Biochem. 86: 447–454 (1978).

676. Reches, A., Eldor, A. and Salomon, Y.: Heparin inhibits PGE_1-sensitive adenylate cyclase and antagonizes PGE_1 antiaggregating effect in human platelets. J. Lab. Clin. Med. 93: 638–644 (1979).

677. Refsum, N., Lowery, C. and Nordøy, A: The effects of albumin-bound unsaturated fatty acids on platelets. Haemostasis 10: 3–13 (1981).

678. Reman, F.C., Demel, R.A., de Gier, J., van Deenen, L.L.M., Eibl, H. and Westphal, O.: Studies on the lysis of red cell and bimolecular lipid leaflets by synthetic lysolecithin, lecithins and structural analogs. Chem. Phys. Lipids 3: 221–224 (1969).

679. Remuzzi, G., Cavenaghi, A.E., Mecca, G., Donati, M.B. and de Gaetano, G.: Prostacyclin (PGI_2) and bleeding time in uremic patients. Thromb. Res. 11: 919–920 (1977).

680. Remuzzi, G., Livio, M., Cavenaghi, A.E., Marchesi, D., Mecca, G., Donati, M.B. and Gaetano, G. de: Unbalanced prostaglandin synthesis and plasma factors in uraemic bleeding. A hypothesis. Thromb. Res. 13: 531–536 (1978).

681. Renaud, S., Allard, C. and Latour, J.G.: Influence of the type of dietary saturated fatty acid on lipemia, coagulation and the production of thrombosis in the rat. J. Nutr. 90: 433–440 (1966).

682. Renaud, S.: Thrombogenicity and atherogenicity of dietary fatty acids in rat. J. Atheroscler. Res. 8: 625–636 (1968).

683. Renaud, S.: The recalcification plasma clotting time. A valuable general clotting test in man and rats. Can. J. Physiol. Pharmacol. 47: 689–693 (1969).

684. Renaud, S. and Godu, J.: Induction of large thrombi in hyperlipemic rats by epinephrine and endotoxin. Lab. Invest. 21: 512–518 (1969).

685. Renaud, S., Kinlough, R.L., Mustard, J.F.: Relationship between platelet aggregation and the thrombotic tendency in rats fed hyperlipemic diets. Lab. Invest. 22: 339–343 (1970).

686. Renaud, S., Kuba, K., Goulet, C., Lemire, Y. and Allard, C.: Relationship between fatty acid composition of platelets and platelet aggregation in rat and man. Relation to thrombosis. Cir. Res. 26: 553–564 (1970).

687. Renaud, S. and Gautheron, P.: Dietary fats and experimental (cardiac and venous) thrombosis. Haemostasis 2: 53–72 (1973/1974).

216

688. Renaud, S.: Dietary fats and thrombosis. Biblthca Nutr. Dieta 25: 92–101 (1977).
689. Renaud, S., Morazain, R., McGregor, L. and Baudier, F.: Dietary fats and platelet functions in relation to atherosclerosis and coronary heart disease. Haemostasis 8: 234–251 (1979).
690. Rentrop, P., Blanke, H, Karsch, K.R., Kaiser, H., Köstering, H. and Leitz, K.: Selective intracoronary thrombolysis in acute myocardial infarction and unstable angina pectoris. Circulation 63: 307–317 (1981).
691. Reyers, I., Mussoni, L., Donati, M.B. and de Gaetano, G.: Severe thrombocytopenia delays but does not prevent the occlusion of an arterial prosthesis in rats. Thromb. Haemostas. 46: 558–560 (1981).
692. Riba, A.L., Thakur, M.L., Gottschalk, A. and Zaret, B.L.: Imaging experimental coronary artery thrombosis with indium-III platelets. Circulation 60: 767–775 (1979).
693. Richardson, P.D.: Rheological factors in platelet-vessel wall interactions. Phil. Trans. Roy. Soc. London [Biol] 294: 251–266 (1981).
694. Ridolfi, R.L. and Hutchins, G.M.: The relationship between coronary artery lesions and myocardial infarcts: Ulceration of atherosclerotic plaques precipitating coronary thrombosis. Am. Heart J. 93: 468–486 (1977).
695. Rittenhouse-Simmons, S.: Production of diglyceride from phosphatidylinositol in activated human platelets. J. Clin. Invest. 63: 580– 587 (1979).
696. Robison, G.A., Arnold, A. and Hartman, R.C.: Divergent effects of epinephrine and prostaglandin E_1 on the level of cyclic AMP in human blood platelets. Pharmacol. Res. Comm. 1: 325–332 (1969).
697. Rokitansky, C.A.: Manual of Pathological Anatomy. Swaine, W.E., Sieveking, E., More, C.H. and Day, G.E. (transl.) Vol. 4, Philadelphia, Blanchard & Lea, 1855, p. 198.
698. Romo, M.: Factors related to sudden death in acute ischaemic heart disease. A comunity study in Helsinki. Acta Med Scand. (Suppl. 547): 1–92 (1972).
699. Roncaglioni, M.C., Di Minno, G., Pangrazzi, J., Reyers, I., Mussoni, L. de Gaetano, G. and Donati, M.B.: Plasmatic and vascular factors of the hemostatic system in rats receiving an estrogen-progestogen combination. Contraception 22: 249–257 (1980).
699a. Roncaglioni, M.C., Bertelé, V., de Gaetano, G. and Donati, M.B.: Lack of interaction of heparin with ADP and prostacyclin on rat platelets. Thromb. Res. (Submitted).
700. Ross, R., Glomset, J.A., Kariya, B. and Harker, L.A.: A platelet-dependent serum factor that stimulates the proliferation of arterial smooth muscle cells in vitro. Proc. Nat. Acad. Sci. USA 71: 1207–1210 (1974).
701. Ross, R. and Glomset, J.A.: The pathogenesis of atherosclerosis. N Engl. J Med. 295: 369–377 and 420–425 (1976).
702. Ross, R. and Harker, L.: Hyperlipidemia and atherosclerosis. Science 193: 1094–1100 (1976).
703. Roth, G.J. and Majerus, P.W.: The mechanism of the effect of aspirin on human platelets. I. Acetylation of a particulate fraction protein. J. Clin. Invest. 56: 624–632 (1975).
704. Roth, G.J., Stanford, N. and Majerus, P.W.: Acetylation of prostaglandin synthetase by aspirin. Proc. Natl. Acad. Sci. USA 72: 3073–3076 (1975).
705. Rudland, P.S., Seifert, W. and Godpodarowicz, D.: Growth control in cultured mouse fibroblasts: induction of the pleiotypic and mitogenic responses by a purified growth factor. Proc. Natl. Acad. Sci. USA 71: 2600–2604 (1974).
706. Ruiter, A., Jongbloed, A.W., van Gent, C.M., Danse, L.H.J.C. and Metz, S.H.M.: The influence of dietary mackerel oil on the condition of organs and on blood lipid composition in the young growing pig. Am. J. Clin. Nutr. 31: 2159–2166 (1978).
707. Russell, R.W.R.: Observations on the retinal blood vessels in monocular blindness. Lancet ii: 1422–1428 (1961).
708. Rutherford, R.B. and Ross, R.: Platelet factors stimulate fibroblasts and smooth muscle cells quiescent in plasma serum to proliferate. J. Cell Biol. 69: 196–203 (1976).
709. Rijken, D.C.: Personal communication.

710. Saba, H.I., Saba, S.R., Blackburn, C.A., Hartmann, R.C. and Mason, R.G.: Heparin neutralization: effects upon platelets. Science 205: 499–501 (1979).

711. Saba, S.R. and Mason, R.G.: Studies of an activity from endothelial cells that inhibits platelet aggregation, serotonin release and clot retraction. Thromb. Res. 5: 747–757 (1974).

712. Saeed, S.A., McDonald-Gibson, W.J., Cuthbert, J., Copas, J.L., Schneider, C., Gardiner, P.J., Butt, N.M. and Collier, H.O.J.: Endogenous inhibitor of prostaglandin synthetase. Nature 270: 32–36 (1977).

713. Salmon, J.A.: A radioimmunoassay for 6-keto-prostaglandin $F_{1\alpha}$. Prostaglandins 15: 383–397 (1978).

714. Salmon, J.A., Smith, D.R., Flower, R.J., Moncada, S. and Vane, J.R.: Further studies on the enzymatic conversion of prostaglandin endoperoxides into prostacyclin by porcine aorta microsomes. Biochim. Biophys. Acta 523: 250–262 (1978).

715. Salmon, J.A., Mullane, K.M., Dusting, G.J., Moncada, S. and Vane, J.R.: Elimination of prostacyclin (PGI_2) and 6-oxo-$PGF_{1\alpha}$ in anaesthetized dogs. J. Pharm. Pharmacol. 31: 529–532 (1979).

716. Salzman, E.W. and Levin, L.: Cyclic 3′, 5′-adenosine monophosphate in human blood platelets. J. Clin. Invest. 50: 131–141 (1971).

717. Samuelsson, B., Goldyne, M., Granström, E., Hamberg, M., Hammarström, S., and Malmsten, C.: Prostaglandins and thromboxanes. Ann. Rev. Biochem. 47: 997–1029 (1978).

718. Samuelsson, B., Borgeat, P., Hammarström, S. and Murphy, R.C.: Leukotrienes: A new group of biologically active compounds. Adv. Thromb. Prost. Res. 6. 1–18 (1980).

719. Sanders, T.A.B., Ellis, F.R. and Dickerson, J.W.T.: Polyunsaturated fatty acids and the brain. Lancet i: 751–752 (1977).

720. Sanders, T.A.B. and Nainsmith, D.J.: Conflicting roles of polyunsaturated fatty acids. Lancet i: 654–655 (1980).

721. Sanders, T.A.B., Naismith, D.J., Haines, A.P. and Vickers, M.: Cod-liver oil, platelet fatty acids and bleeding time. Lancet i: 1189 (1980).

722. Sanders, T.A.B., Vickers, M. and Haines, A.P.: Effect on blood lipids and haemostasis of a supplement of cod-liver oil, rich in eicosapentaenoic and docosahexaenoic acids in healthy young men. Clin. Sci. 61: 317–324 (1981).

723. Sanders, T.A.B. and Younger, K.M.: The effect of dietary supplements of $\omega3$ polyunsaturated fatty acids on the fatty acid composition of platelets and plasma choline phosphoglycerides. Br. J. Nutr. 45: 613–616 (1981).

724. Saphir, O., Priest, W.S., Hamburger, W.W. and Katz, L.N.: Coronary arteriosclerosis, coronary thrombosis, and the resulting myocardial changes. An evaluation of their respective clinical pictures including the electrocardiographic records, based on the anatomical findings. Am. Heart J. 10: 567–595; 762–792 (1935).

725. Saynor, R. and Verel, D.: Effect of a marine oil high in eicosapentaenoic acid on blood lipids and coagulation. IRCS Med. Sci. 8: 378–379 (1980).

726. Saynor, R. and Verel, D.: Effect of a fish oil on blood lipids and coagulation. Thromb. Haemost. 46: 65 (1981).

726a. Scherag, R., Kramer, H.J. and Düsing, R.: Dietary administration of eicosapentanoic and linolenic acid increases arterial blood pressure and suppresses vascular prostacyclin synthesis in the rat. Prostaglandins 23: 369–382 (1982).

727. Schafer, A.I., Levine, S., and Handin, R.J.: Regulation of platelet arachidonic acid oxygenation by cyclic AMP. Blood 56: 853–858 (1980).

728. Schick, P.K.: The role of platelet membrane lipids in platelet hemostatic activities. Sem. Hematol. 16: 221–233 (1979).

729. Schoene, N.W. and Iacono, J.M.: The influence of phospholipase A_2 on prostaglandin production in platelets. Adv. Prost. Thromb. Res. 2: 763–766 (1976).

730. Schoene, N.W., Judd, J.T., Marshall, M.W., Reeves, V. and Carvalho, A.: Effects of diets varying

in fat and P/S ratio on arachidonic acid metabolism in human platelets. Adv. Prost. Thromb. Res. 8: 1787–1789 (1980).

731. Schoene, N.W., Reeves, V.B. and Ferretti, A.: Effect of dietary linoleic acid on the biosynthesis of PGE_2 and $PGF_{2\alpha}$ in kidney medullae in spontaneously hypertensive rats. Adv. Prost. Thromb. Res. 8: 1791–1792 (1980).

732. Schoene, N.W., Ferretti, A. and Fiore, D.: Production of prostaglandins in homogenates of medullae and cortices of spontaneously hypertensive rats fed menhaden oil. Lipids 16: 866–869 (1981).

733. Schrör, K., Köhler, P., Müller, M., Peskar, B. and Rösen, P.: Prostacyclin – thromboxane interactions in the platelet perfused in vitro heart. Am. J. Physiol. 241: H18–H25 (1981).

734. Schwartz, C.J. and Gerrity, R.G.: Anatomical pathology of sudden unexpected cardiac death. Circulation 51 and 52 (Suppl. III): 18–26 (1975).

735. Scott, P.J., Hurley, P.J.: Incorporation of radioiodinated serum albumin and low-density lipoprotein into human thrombi in vivo. J. Path. 97: 603–609 (1969).

736. Seiler, D. and Hasselbach, W.: Essential fatty acids deficiency and the activity of the sarcoplasmic calcium pump. Eur. J. Biochem. 21: 385–387 (1971).

737. Sekhar, L.N., Wasserman, J.F., van der Bel-Kahn, J. and Olinger, C.P.: Ultrasonic B-scan echoarteriographic imaging of experimentally induced thrombi in dogs. Neurosurgery 4: 301–307 (1979).

738. Serhan, C., Anderson, P., Goodman, E., Dunham, P. and Weissmann, G.: Phosphatidate and oxidized fatty acids are calcium ionophores. Studies empolying arsenazo III in liposomes. J. Biol. Chem. 256: 2736–2741 (1981).

739. Seyberth, H.W., Oelz, O., Kennedy, T., Sweetman, B.J., Danon, A., Fröhlich, J.C., Heimberg, M. and Oates, J.A.: Increased arachidonate in lipids after administration to man: effects on prostaglandin biosynthesis. Clin. J. Pharm. Ther. 18: 521–529 (1976).

740. Shattil, S.J., Anaya-Galindo, R., Bennett, J., Colman, R.W. and Cooper, R.A.: Platelet hypersensitivity induced by cholesterol incorporation. J. Clin. Invest. 55: 636–643 (1975).

741. Shattil, S.J. and Cooper, R.A.: Membrane microviscosity and human platelet function. Biochem. 15: 4832–4837 (1976).

742. Shattil, S.J., Bennet, J.S., Colman, R.W. and Cooper, R.A.: Abnormalities of cholesterol-phospholipid composition in platelets and low-density lipoproteins of human hyperbetalipoproteinemia. J. Lab. Clin. Med. 89: 341–353 (1977).

743. Shekelle, R.B., MacMillan Shryock, Paul, O., Lepper, M., Stamler, J., Liu, S. and Raynor, W.J.: Diet, serumcholesterol, and death from coronary heart disease. The Western Electric Study. N Engl. J. Med. 304: 65–70 (1981).

744. Shimamoto, T.: Contraction of endothelial cells as a key mechanism in atherogenesis and treatment of atherosclerosis with endothelial cell relaxants. In: Schettler, G. and Weizel, A.: Atherosclerosis. III. Springer Verlag, Berlin, 1974, pp. 64–82.

745. Shimamoto, T.: Drugs and foods on contraction of endothelial cells as a key mechanism in atherogenesis and treatment of atherosclerosis with endothelial cell relaxants (cyclic AMP phosphodiesterase inhibitors). Adv. Exp. Med. Biol. 60: 77–105 (1975).

746. Shinitzky, M. and Inbar, M.: Microviscosity parameters and protein mobility in biological membranes. Biochim. Biophys. Acta 433: 133–149 (1976).

747. Shio, H. and Ramwell, P.: Effect of prostaglandin E_2 and aspirin on the secondary aggregation of human platelets. Nature (New Biology) 236: 45–46 (1972).

748. Siegle, A.M., Smith, J.B. and Silver, M.J.: Specific binding sites for prostaglandin D_2 on human platelets. Biochem. Biophys. Res. Comm. 90: 291–296 (1979).

749. Siess, W., Scherer, B., Böhlig, B., Roth, P., Kurzmann, I., and Weber, P.C.: Platelet membrane fatty acids, platelet aggregation and thromboxane formation during a mackerel diet. Lancet i: 441–444 (1980).

750. Silberbauer, K., Schernthaner, G., Sinzinger, H., Piza-Katzer, H. and Winter, W.: Decreased

vascular prostacyclin in juvenile-onset diabetes. N Engl. J. Med. 300: 366–367 (1979).

751. Silwer, J., Cronberg, S. and Nilsson, I.M.: Occurrence of arteriosclerosis in von Willebrand's disease. Acta Med. Scand. 180: 475–484 (1966).

752. Sim, A.K. and McCraw, A.P.: The activity of γ-linolenate and dihomo-γ-linolenate methyl esters in vitro and in vivo on blood platelet function in non-human primates and in man. Thromb. Res. 10: 385–397 (1977).

753. Sinapius, D.: Beziehungen zwischen Koronarthrombosen und Myokardinfarkten. Dtsch. Med. Wochenschr. 97: 443–448 (1972).

754. Sinclair, A.J. and Collins, F.D.: Fatty livers in rats dificient in essential fatty acids. Biochim. Biophys. Acta 498–510 (1968).

755. Sinclair, H.: Advantages and disadvantages of an Eskimo diet. In: Fumigalli, R., Kritchevsky, D. and Paoletti, R. (eds).: Drugs Affecting Lipid Metabolism. Elsevier/North Holland Biomedical Press, 1980, pp. 363–370.

756. Sinclair, H.M.: The importance of fish in the prevention of chronic degenerative disease. In: Noelle H. (ed): Food from the sea. Springer Verlag, Berlin, 1981, pp. 201–210.

757. Singer, S.J. and Nicholson, G.L.: the fluid mosaic model of the structure of cell membranes. Science 175: 720–731 (1972).

758. Sinha, A.K., Shattil, S.J. and Colman, R.W.: Cyclic AMP metabolism in cholesterol-rich platelets. J. Biol. Chem. 252: 3310–3314 (1977).

759. Sixma, J.J. and Nijessen, J.G.: Characteristics of platelet factor 3 release during ADP-induced aggregation. Comparison with 5-hydroxytryptamine release. Thromb. Diath. Haemorrh. 24: 206–213 (1970).

760. Sixty plus reinfarction study research group: A double-blind trial to assess long-term oral anti-coagulant therapy in elderly patients after myocardial infarction. Lancet ii: 989–994 (1980).

761. Smith, D.R., Weatherly, B.C., Salmon, J.A., Ubatuba, F.B., Gryglewski, R.J. and Moncada, S.: Preparation and biomedical properties of PGH_3. Prostaglandins 18: 423–438 (1979).

762. Smith, E.B.: Quantitative and qualitative comparisons of the lipids in platelets, aortic intima and mural thrombi. Cardiovasc. Res. 1: 111–115 (1967).

763. Smith, H.A. and Jones, Th.E.: Veterinary Pathology. Lea and Febiger, Philadelphia, Penn. (1968).

764. Smith, J.B. and Willis, A.L.: Aspirin selectively inhibits prostaglandin production in human platelets. Nature (New Biology) 231: 235–237 (1971).

765. Smith, J.B. and Silver, M.J.: Phospholipase A_1 of human blood platelets. Biochem. J. 131: 615–618 (1973).

766. Smith, J.B., Ingerman, C.M. and Silver, M.J.: Formation of prostaglandin D_2 during endoperoxyde-induced platelet aggregation. Thromb. Res. 9: 413–418 (1976).

767. Smith, J.B., Ingerman, C.M. and Silver, M.J.: Malondialdehyde formation as an indicator of prostaglandin production by human platelets. J. Lab. Clin. Med. 88: 167–172 (1976).

768. Smith, J.B., Ingerman, C.M. and Silver, M.J.: Persistance of thromboxane A_2-like material and platelet-release inducing activity in plasma. J. Clin. Invest. 58: 1119–1122 (1976).

769. Smith, J.B., Ogletree, M.L., Lefer, A.M. and Nicolaou, K.C.: Antibodies which antagonise the effects of prostacyclin. Nature 274: 64–65 (1978).

770. Smith, J.B. and Willis, A.L.: Formation and release of prostaglandins by platelets in response to thrombin. Br. J. Pharmacol. 40: 545P–546P (1979).

771. Smith, J.B., Araki, H. and Lefer, A.M.: Thromboxane A_2, prostacyclin and aspirin: effects on vascular tone and platelet aggregation. Circulation 62 (suppl. V): 19–25 (1980).

772. Smith, S.K., Kelly, R.W., Abel, M.H. and Baird, D.T.: A role for prostacyclin in excessive menstrual bleeding. Lancet i: 522–524 (1981).

773. Smith, W.L., Rollins, T.E. and DeWitt, D.L.: Subcellular localization of prostaglandin forming enzymes using conventional and monoclonal antibodies. Progr. Lip. Res. 20: 103–110 (1980).

774. Sober, H.A. (ed): Handbook of Biochemistry. Selected data for molecular biology. Buffer solutions, page J-234 No. 4. CRC, Cleveland, Ohio (1970).

775. Spain, D.M. and Bradess, V.A.: The relationship of coronary thrombosis to coronary atherosclerosis and ischemic heart disease. (A necropsy study covering a period of 25 years.). Am. J. Med. Sci. 240: 701–710 (1960).

776. Spearman, Ch.: The proof and measurement of association between two things. Am. J. Psychol. 15: 7214–7217 (1906).

777. Spector, A.A.: Transport and ultilization of free fatty acids. Annals N.Y. Acad. Sci. 149: 768–783 (1968).

778. Spector, A.A., Hoak, J.C., Warner, E.D. and Fry, G.L.: Utilization of long-chain free fatty acids by human platelets. J. Clin. Invest. 49: 1489–1496 (1970).

778a. Spector, A.A., Hoak, J.C., Fry, G.L., Stoll, L.L., Tanke, C.T. and Kaduce, T.L.: Essential fatty acid availability and prostacyclin production by cultured human endothelial cells. Progr. Lip. Res. 20: 471–477 (1981).

779. Sprecher, H. and James, A.T.: Biosynthesis of long-chain fatty acids in mammalian systems. In: Emken, E.A. and Dutton, H.J. (eds): Geometrical and positional fatty acid isomers. Americal Oil Chemist's Society (1979) pp. 303–338.

780. Srivastava, K.C.: Effects of dietary fatty acids, prostaglandins and related compounds on the role of platelets in thrombosis. Biochem. exptl. Biol. 16: 317–338 (1980).

781. Stamler, J.: Epidemiology of coronary heart disease. Med. Clin. North. Am. 57: 5–46 (1973).

782. Stamler, J.: Diet-related risk factors for human atherosclerosis: hyperlipidemia, hypertension, hyperglycemia – current status. Adv. Exp. Med. Biol. 60: 125–158 (1975).

783. Stansby, M.E.: Nutritional properties of fish oils. World Rev. Nutr. Diet 11: 46–105 (1969).

783a. Steer, M.L., MacIntyre, D.E., Levine, L. and Salzman, E.W.: Is prostacyclin a physiologically important circulating anti-platelet agent. Nature 283: 194–197 (1980).

784. Stein, P.D. and Sabbah, H.N.: Measured turbulence and its effect on thrombus formation. Circ. Res. 35: 608–614 (1974).

785. Steinberg, D., Vaughan, M., Nestel, P.J., Strand, O. and Bergström, S.: Effects of prostaglandin on hormone-induced mobilization of free fatty acids. J. Clin. Invest. 43: 1533–1540 (1964).

786. Steinberg, L.Y., Mauldin, R.E. and Mathias, M.M.: The effect of dietary lipids on clotting times and rat serum and urine prostaglandin concentrations. Progr. Lip. Res. 20: 485–489 (1981).

787. Steiner, M., Anastasi, J.: Vitamin E, an inhibitor of the platelet release reaction. J. Clin. Invest. 57: 732–737 (1976).

788. Steiner, M.: Inhibition of platelet aggregation by alpha-tocoherol. In: De Duve, C. and Hayashi, O. (eds.): Tocopherol, Oxygen and Biomembranes. Elsevier/North Holland Biomedical Press, Amsterdam, 1978, pp. 143–163.

789. Struyck, C.B., Beerthuis, R.K., Pabon, H.J.J. and van Dorp, D.A.: Specificity of the enzymic conversion of polyunsaturated fatty acids into prostaglandins. Recl. Trav. Chim. Pays-Bas 85: 1233–1250 (1966).

790. Stuart, M.J., Elrad, H., Graeber, J.E., Hakanson, D.O., Sunderij, S.G. and Barvinchak, M.K. Increased synthesis of prostaglandin endoperoxides and platelet hyperfunction in infants of mothers with mothers with diabetes mellitus. J. Lab. Clin. Med. 94: 12–17 (1979).

791. Stuart, M.J., Gerrard, J.M. and White, J.G.: Effect of cholesterol on production of thromboxane B_2 by platelets in vitro. N Engl. J. Med. 302: 6–10 (1980).

792. Sullivan, L.M. and Mathias, M.M.: Eicosanoid production in rat blood as affected by fasting and dietary fat. Prostaglandins, Leukotrienes and Medicin (in press).

793. Sumiyoshi, A., More, R.H. and Weigensberg, B.I.: Aortic fibro-fatty type atherosclerosis from thrombus in normolipidemic rabbits. Atherosclerosis 18: 43–57 (1973).

793a. Sun, F.F., McGuire, J.C. and Metzler, C.M.: The effect of substrate availability on the metabolism of arachidonic acid in human platelets. Progr. Lip. Res. 20: 275–278 (1981).

794. Svensson, J., Hamberg, M. and Samuelsson, B.: On the formation and effects of thromboxane A_2 in human platelets. Acta Physiol. Scand. 98: 285–294 (1976).

795. Svensson, J. and Oki, T.: Inhibition of platelet aggregation by α-tocopherol and its nicotinate and

acetate esters. Int. J. Vit. Nutr. Res. 48: 250–254 (1978).

796. Swank, R.L.: Effects of high fat feedings on viscosity of blood. Science 120: 427–428 (1954).

797. Swank, R.L., Roth, J.G. and Janssen, J.: Screen filtration pressure method and adhesiveness and aggregation of blood cells. J. Appl. Physiol. 19: 340–346 (1964).

798. Symons, C., De Toszeghi, A. and Cook, I.J.Y.: Effect of ethylchlorophenoxy-isobutyrate with or without androsterone on platelet stickiness. Lancet i: 233–243 (1964).

799. Szczeklik, A., Gryglewski, R.J., Musial, J., Grodzinska, L., Serwonska, M. and Marcinkiewicz, E.: Thromboxane generation and platelet aggregation in survivals of myocardial infarction. Thromb. Haemostas. 40: 66–74 (1978).

800. Tan, W.C. and Privett, O.S.: Studies on the synthesis of prostaglandins in the vesicular glands of essential fatty acid deficient and hypophysectomized rats. Biophys. Biochim. Acta 296: 586–592 (1973).

801. Tateson, J.E., Moncada, S. and Vane, J.R.: Effects of prostacyclin (PGX) on cyclic AMP concentrations in human platelets. Prostaglandins 13: 389–399 (1977).

802. Ten Hoor, F., de Deckere, E.A.M., Haddeman, E., Hornstra, G. and Quadt, J.F.A.: Dietary manipulation of prostaglandin and thromboxane synthesis in heart, aorta and blood platelets of the rat. Adv. Prost. Thromb. Res. 8: 1771–1781 (1980).

803. Thomas, W.A. and Hartroft, W.S.: Myocardial infarction in rats fed diets containing high fat, cholesterol, thiouracil and sodium cholate. Circulation 19: 65–72 (1959).

804. Tomasi, V., Meringolo, G., Bartolini, G. and Orlando, M.: Biosynthesis of prostacyclin in rat liver endothelial cells and its control by prostaglandin E_2. Nature 273: 670–671 (1976).

805. Thomasson, H.J.: Les acides gras essentiels. Revue Française des Corps Gras. Numéro Spécial. Paris (1962).

806. Thomasson, H.J.: Dietary fat and atherosclerosis. In: Dols, M.J.L. (ed): The Physiological and Nutritional Role of Fats in Human Nutrition. Westerbaan, The Haque, 1963, pp. 92–103.

807. Thomasson, H.J.: Über die biologische Wirkung von Nahrungsfetten. In: Fette in der Medizin, Pallas Verlag, Lochham, 1965, pp. 19–21.

808. Thorngren, M. and Gustafson, A.: Effects of 11-week increase in dietary eicosapentaenoic acid on bleeding time, lipids and platelet aggregation. Lancet ii: 1190–1192 (1981).

809. To, D., Smith, F.L. and Carpenter, M.P.: Mammary gland prostaglandin synthesis: effect of dietary lipid and propylgallate. Adv. Prost. Thromb. Res. 8: 1807–1812 (1980).

810. Tomich, E.G.: Effects of potential gradient on the electrophoretic mobility of human blood platelets in the presence of ADP or noradrenaline. Biochem. Pharmacol. 21: 3201–3203 (1972).

811. Trugnan, G., Béréziat, G., Manier, M.C. and Polonovski, J.: Phospholipase activities in subcellular fractions of human platelets. Biochim. Biophys. Acta 573: 61–72 (1979).

812. Ts'ao, C.H., Holly, C.M., Serieno, M.A. and Gallozzo, I.S.: Generation of a PGI_2-like activity by deendothelialized rat aorta. Thromb. Haemost. 42: 873–884 (1979).

813. Tschopp, T.B. and Zucker, M.B.: Hereditary defect in platelet function in rats. Blood 40: 217–226 (1972).

814. Turek, J.V., Houtsmuller, U.M.T., Lussenburg, R.N. and den Ottolander, G.J.H.: Effect of low cholesterol, linoleic acid enriched diet on thrombotic tendency and plasma lipoproteins in patients with angina pectoris. Artery 8: 134–139 (1980).

815. Turner, S.R., Tainer, J.A. and Lynn, W.S.: Biogenesis of chemotactic molecules by the arachidonate system of platelets. Nature 257: 680–681 (1975).

816. Turpeinen, O.: Personal communication.

817. Turpeinen, O.: Effect of cholesterol-lowering diet on mortality from coronary heart disease and other causes. Circulation 59: 1–7 (1979).

818. Turpeinen, O.: Diet and coronary events. J. Am. diet. Ass. 52: 209–213 (1968).

819. Turpeinen, O., Miettinen, M., Karvonen, M.J., Roine, P., Pekkarinen, M., Lehtosuo, E.J. and Alivirta, P.: Dietary prevention of coronary heart disease: long-term experiment. Am. J. Clin. Nutr. 21: 255–276 (1968).

222

820. Turpeinen, O., Karvonen, M.J., Pekkarinin, M., Miettinen, M., Elosuo, R. and Paavilainen, E.: Dietary prevention of coronary heart disease: the Finnish mental hospital study. Int. J. Epidemiol. 8: 99–118 (1979).

821. Uzunova, A.D., Ramey, E.R. and Ramwell, P.W.: Effect of testosterone, sex and age on experimentally induced arterial thrombosis. Nature 261: 712–713 (1976).

822. Uzunova, A.D., Ramey, E.R. and Ramwell, P.W.: Gonadal hormones and pathogenesis of occlusive arterial thrombosis. Am. J. Physiol. 234: H454–H459 (1978).

823. Vallee, E., Gougat, J. and Ageron, M.: Inhibition of platelet phospholipase A_2 as a mechanism for the anti-aggregating effect of linoleic acid. Agents Actions 10: 57–62 (1980).

824. Vanderkooy, J., Fischkoff, S., Chance, B. and Cooper, R.A.: Fluorescent probe analysis of the lipid architecture of natural and experimental cholesterol-rich membranes. Biochemistry 13: 1589–1595 (1974).

824a. Vargaftig, B.B., Chignard, M., Benveniste, J., Lefort, J. and Wal, F.: Background and present status of research on platelet-activating factor (PAF-Acether). Ann. N.Y. Acad. Sci. 370: 119–137 (1981).

825. Vane, J.R.: Inhibition of prostaglandin, prostacyclin and thromboxane synthesis. Adv. Prost. Throm. Res. 4: 27–44 (1978).

826. Vane, J.R. and Moncada, S.: the anti-thrombotic effects of prostacyclin. Acta Med. Scand. (Suppl 642): 11–22 (1980).

827. Vergroesen, A.J.: Dietary prevention of atherosclerosis: new aspects. Compreh. Ther. 5: 19–30 (1979).

828. Vincent, J.E. and Zijlstra, F.J.: Formation by phospholipase A_2 of prostaglandins and thromboxane A_2-like activity in the platelets of normal and essential fatty acid deficient rats. Comparison with effect on human and rabbit platelets. Prostaglandins 14: 1043–1053 (1977).

829. Vles, R.O., Büller, J., Gottenbos, J.J. and Thomasson, H.J.: Influence of type of dietary fat on cholesterol-induced atherosclerosis in the rabbit. J. Atheroscl. Res. 4: 170–183 (1964).

830. Vles, R.O.: Nutritional aspects of rapeseed oil. In.: Vergroesen, A.J. (ed): The Role of Fats in Human Nutrition. Academic Press, London, 1975, pp. 433–477.

831. Vles, R.O., Gottenbos, J.J. and van Pijpen, P.L.: Aspects nutritionnels des huiles de soja hydrogénées et de leurs acides gras insaturés isomériques. Biblthca Nutr. Dieta 25: 186–196 (1977).

832. Vles, R.O. and Kloeze, J.: Effects of feeding alternately maize oil and coconut oil on atherosclerosis in rabbits. J. Atheroscler. Res. 7: 59–68 (1967).

833. Vogt, T.M.: Diet-heart era: premature obituary? N Engl. J. Med. 298: 107 (1978).

834. Volpe, J.J. and Vagelos, P.R.: Mechanisms and regulation of biosynthesis of saturated fatty acids. Physiol. Rev. 56: 339–417 (1976).

835. Vonkeman, H. and van Dorp, D.A.: The action of prostaglandin synthethase on 2-arachidonyl-lecithin. Biochim. Biophys. Acta 164: 430–432 (1968).

835a. Voss, R., ten Hoor, F., Haddeman, E. and Don J.A.: Influence of dietary linoleic acid on the prostacyclin production of the isolated pulsatingly perfused rabbit aorta. Prostaglandins Leukotrienes and Medicin 8: 503–516 (1982).

836. Walker, I.C., Jones, R.L. and Wilson, N.H.: The identification of an epoxy-hydroxy acid as a product from the incubation of arachidonic acid with washed blood platelets. Prostaglandins 18: 173–178 (1979).

837. Walsh, P.N.: The role of platelets in the contact phase of blood coagulation. Br. J. Haematol. 22: 237–254 (1972).

838. Walsh, P.N.: The effects of collagen and kaolin on the intrinsic coagulant activity of platelets. Evidence for an alternative pathway in intrinsic coagulation not requiring Factor XII. Br. J. Haematol. 22: 393–405 (1972).

839. Walsh, P.N. and Griffin, J.H.: Contributions of human platelets to the proteolytic activation of blood coagulation factors XII and XI. Blood 57: 108–118 (1981).

840. Weber, E., Pfleiderer, T., Feder, V. and Morgenstern, E.: Über die Wirkung von Lipidemulsionen

auf Blutplättchen. III. Verhalten von ATP, Glykogen und Glucoseverbrauch. Thromb. Diath. Haemorrh. 23: 99–109 (1970).

841. Weber, G.: Regression of arterial lesions: facts and problems. In: Carlson, L.A., Paoletti, R., Sirtori, C. and Weber, G. (eds.): International Conference on Atherosclerosis. Raven Press, New York, 1978, pp. 1–13.

842. Weigensberg, B.I., More, R.H. and Sumiyoshi, A.: Lipid profile in the evolution of experimental atherosclerotic plaques from thrombus. Lab. Invest. 33: 43–50 (1975).

843. Weigensberg, B.I. and More, R.H.: Uptake of labelled cholesterol by organizing thrombus. In: Atherosclerosis: Metabolic, Morphologic and Clinical aspects. Manning, G.W., Haust, M.D. (eds), New York, Plenum Press, 1977, pp 552–557.

844. Weiss, H.J. and Aledort, L.M.: Impaired platelet/connective tissue reaction in man after aspirin ingestion. Lancet ii: 495–497 (1967).

845. Weiss, H.J., Aledort, L.M. and Kochwa, S.: The effects of salicylates on the hemostatic properties of platelets in man. J. Clin. Invest. 47: 2169–2180 (1968).

846. Weiss, H.J.: Platelet physiology and abnormalities of platelet function. N. Engl. J. Med. 293: 531–541 and 580–588 (1975).

847. Weiss, H.J. and Lages, B.A.: Possible congenital defect in platelet thromboxane synthetase. Lancet i: 157 (1980).

848. Wenger, N.K. and Bauer, S.: Coronary embolism. Review of the literature and presentation of fifteen cases. Am. J. Med. 25: 549–557 (1958).

849. Wessler, S.: The role of stasis in thrombosis. In: Sherry, Brinkhous, Genton and Stengle (eds): Thrombosis, Nat. Acad. Sci., Washington, 1969, pp. 461–468.

850. Westwick, J. and Webb, H.: Selective antagonism of prostaglandin (PG)E₁, PGD₂ and prostacyclin (PGI₂) on human and rabbit platelets by di-4-phloretin phosphate (DPP). Thromb. Res. 12: 973–978 (1978).

851. Whitaker, M.O., Wyche, A., Fitzpatrick, F., Sprecher, H. and Needleman, P.: Triene prostaglandins: Prostaglandin D₃ and icosapentaenoic acid as potential antithrombotic substances. Proc. Natl. Acad. Sci. USA 76: 5919–5923 (1979).

852. Whittle, B.J.R., Moncada, S. and Vane, J.R.: Comparison of effects of prostacyclin (PGI₂) prostaglandin E₁ and D₂ on platelet aggregation in different species. Prostaglandins 16: 373–388 (1978).

852a. Whittle, B.J.R. see ref. 865.

853. Wicks, M.S., Ball, C.R. and Williams, W.L.: Relation of types of dietary fat to cardiovascular damage in mice Am. J. Anat. 124: 481–490 (1969).

854. Wijnalda, M.A. and Fitzpatrick, F.A.: Albumins stabilize prostaglandin I₂. Prostaglandins 20: 853–861 (1980).

855. Williams, M.A., Stancliff, R.C., Packer, L. and Keith, A.D.: Relation of unsaturated fatty acid composition of rat liver mitochondria to oscillation period, spin label motion, permeability and oxidative phosphorylation. Biochim. Biophys. Acta 267: 444–456 (1972).

856. Willis, A.L.: Unanswered questions in EFA and PG research. Progr. Lip. Res. 20: 839–850 (1981).

857. Willis, A.L. and Kuhn, D.C.: A new potential mediator of arterial thrombosis whose biosynthesis is inhibited by aspirin. Prostaglandins, 4: 127–130 (1973).

858. Willis, A.L., Comai, K., Kuhn, D.C. and Paulsrud, J.: Dihomo-γ-linolenate suppresses platelet aggregation when administered in vitro or in vivo. Prostaglandins 8: 509–519 (1974).

859. Willis, A.L. and Smith, J.B.: Some perspectives on platelets and prostaglandins. Progr. Lipid Res. 20: 387–406 (1981).

860. Wilner, G.D., Nossel, H.L. and Le Roy, E.C.: Activation of Hagemen factor by collagen. J. Clin. Invest. 47: 2608–2615 (1968).

861. Wissler, R.W. and Vesselinovitch, D.: Comparative pathogenetic patterns in atherosclerosis. Adv. Lipid Res. 6: 181–206 (1968).

862. Wissler, R.W. and Vesselinovitch, D.: The effects of feeding various dietary fats on the develop-

ment and regression of hypercholesterolaemia and atherosclerosis. Adv. Exp. Med. Biol. 60: 65–76 (1975).

863. Wissler, R.W.: Progression and regression of atherosclerotic lesions. In: The thrombotic Process in Atherogenesis. Chandler, A.B., Eurenius, K., McMillan, G.C., Nelson, C.B., Schwartz, C.J. and Wessler, S. (eds), New York, Plenum Press, 1978, p. 77–109).

864. Witte, L.D., Kaplan, K.L., Nossel, H.L., Lages, B.A., Weiss, H.J. and Goodman, D.S.: Studies of the release from human platelets of the growth factor for cultured human arterial smooth muscle cells. Circ. Res. 42: 402–409 (1978).

865. Whittle, B.J.R., Moncada, S. and Vane, J.R.: Biological activities of some metabolites and analogues of prostacyclin. in: F.G. de la Heras and S. Vega (eds): Medical Chemistry Advances. Perganeon Press. Oxford (1981) pp. 141–158.

866. Wong, P.Y.-K., McGiff, J.C., Sun, F.F. and Lee, W.H.: 6-keto-prostaglandin E_1 inhibits the aggregation of human platelets. Eur. J. Pharmacol. 60: 242–248 (1979).

867. Wong, P.Y.-K., Lee, W.H., Chao, P.H-W, Reiss, R.F. and McGiff, J.C.: Metabolism of prostacyclin by 9-hydroxyprostaglandin dehydrogenase in human platelets. J. Biol. Chem. 255: 9021–9024 (1980).

868. Wong, P.Y-K., Malik, K.U., Desiderio, D.M., McGiff, J.C. and Sun, F.F.: Hepatic metabolism of prostacyclin (PGI_2) in the rabbit: formation of a potent novel inhibitor of platelet aggregation. Biochem. Biophys. Res. Comm. 93: 486–494 (1980).

869. Woolf, N.: The distribution of fibrin within the aortic intima. An immunohistochemical study. Am. J. Path. 39: 521–532 (1961).

870. Woolf, N., Pilkington, J.R.E. and Carstairs, K.C.: The occurrence of lipoproteins in thrombi. J. Path. Bact. 91: 383–387 (1966).

871. Woolf, N. and Carstairs, K.C.: Infiltration and thrombosis in atherogenesis. A study using immunofluorescent techniques. Am. J. Path. 51: 373–386 (1967).

872. Woolf, N.: Thrombosis and atherosclerosis. Adv. Exp. Med. Biol. 104: 145–167 (1978).

873. Woolf, N., Bradley, J.W.P., Crawford, T., Carstairs, K.C.: Experimental mural thrombi in the pig aorta. The early natural history. Br. J. Exp. Path. 49: 257–264 (1968).

874. Wörner, P. and Patcheke, H.: Hyperreactivity by an enhancement of the arachidonate pathway of platelets treated with cholesterol-rich phospholipid-dispersions. Thromb. Res. 18: 439–451 (1980).

875. Wright, H.P.: The adhesiveness of blood platelets in normal subjects with varying concentrations of anticoagulants. J. Path. Bact. 53: 255–262 (1941).

876. Wright, I.S.: Comment on anticoagulant therapy in coronary artery disease. In: Sherry, S. et al. (eds.): Thrombosis. Nat. Acad. Sci. Washington DC., 1969, pp. 705–707.

877. Wu, K.K., Chen, Y-C., Fordham, E., Ts'ao, C-H., Rayudy, G. and Matayoshi, D.: Differential effects of two doses of aspirin on platelet-vessel wall interaction in vivo. J. Clin. Invest. 68: 382–387 (1981).

878. Yamazaki, H.: Changes in blood coagulability, platelet count and platelet aggregation induced by endotoxin or exercise, and the prevention of these changes by pyridinolcarbamate. In: Shimamoto, T. and Numano, F. (eds): Atherogenesis. Excerpta Medica Foundation, Amsterdam, 1969, pp. 93–95.

879. Yoshimoto, T., Yamamoto, S., Okuma, M. and Hayaishi, O.: Solubilization and resolution of thromboxane synthesizing system from microsomes of bovine blood platelets. J. Biol. Chem. 252: 5871–5874 (1977).

880. Zöllner, N., Adam, O. and Wolfram, G.: The influence of linoleic acid intake on the excretion of urinary prostaglandin metabolites. Res. Exptl. Med. 175: 149–153 (1979).

881. Zucker, M.B. and Peterson, J.: Effect of acetylsalicylic acid, other nonsteroidal anti-inflammatory agents and dipyridamole on human blood platelets. J. Lab. Clin. Med. 76: 66–75 (1970).

882. Zwaal, R.F.A.: Membrane and lipid involvement in blood coagulation. Biochim. Biophys. Acta 515: 165–207 (1978).

883. Zwaal, R.F.A., Rosing, J., Tans, G., Bevers, E.M. and Hemker, H.C.: Topological and kinetic aspects of phospholipids in blood coagulation. In: K.G. Mann and F.B. Taylor, Jr. (eds): The regulation of coagulation. Elsevier/North Holland, 1980, pp. 95–115.
884. Zyablitskii, V.M.: Changes in adhesiveness and aggregation of platelets after passage of blood through the lungs. Bull. Exp. Biol. Med. USSR 68: 1073–1075 (1969).

INDEX